AF410865

FOUNDATIONS

NEW LIGHT ON
TIBETAN MEDICINE

ༀ། །བོད་ཀྱི་གསོ་རིག་འོད་སྣང་གསར་པ།།

VOLUME I
FOUNDATIONS

DR. PASANG YONTEN ARYA, MENRAMPA

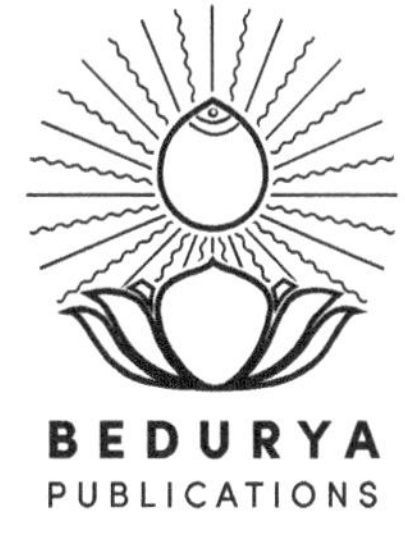

BEDURYA
PUBLICATIONS

Book design: Tiana Morici (abiesco.ch)

Cover illustration: detail from Medical Thangka no. 2
© Dharmapala Thangka Centre, Kathmandu, Nepal (www.thangka.de)

Please refer to the Appendix for other illustration copyright and credit lines.

Disclaimer

This book is not intended as a replacement for medical treatment, nor for consultation with your licensed family physician or specialist. It presents traditional Tibetan medical perspectives on health, disease, diagnosis, and treatment, which may not be recognized or assessed by national health authorities. The author makes no representations or warranties in relation to the information provided here.

ISBN 978-2-9701464-3-8

BEDURYA PUBLICATIONS
www.beduryapublications.org

*Bedurya Publications is a branch of TME - Tibetan Medicine Education Center
Neuchâtel, Switzerland (www.tibetanmedicine-edu.org)*

The author dedicates this book series to all scholars and practitioners, past and present, who contributed to the transmission of Sowa Rigpa. May this work become the cause of healthy developments and thus benefit all sentient beings.

TABLE OF CONTENTS

PART 2 THE THREE HUMORS

CHAPTER 4 MIND AND EMOTIONS   37

CHAPTER 5 INTRODUCTION TO THE THREE HUMORS   49

CHAPTER 6 WIND (_LUNG_)   57

FIGURES

TABLES

EDITOR'S FOREWORD

When I first laid my eyes on TME - Tibetan Medicine Education Center's course materials in January 2012, I was deeply impressed. It felt like a whole new world opened up right before me, like embarking on a life-changing adventure. Greedily reading through the opening chapters and getting a first glimpse of Sowa Rigpa's astounding medical as well as spiritual richness, I was blown away by the rigorous structure of its foundational text—the glorious *Four Tantras* (*Gyüzhi*)—in the overview that followed. These impressions have stayed with me ever since. Literature and enthusiasm alone, however, are not sufficient to effectively navigate this ocean of healing wisdom; we need a skillful guide, an experienced teacher. Listening to Gen. Arya Pasang Yonten's lectures, his generous replies to questions, and later participating in highly rewarding practical workshops and retreats, my heart was convinced time and time again that I had to look no further. It is this deep respect, gratitude, and reverence for Genla's teachings which propelled me since 2016 to help make the extensive materials he accumulated over four decades of study, practice, and instruction into a comprehensive textbook titled *New Light on Tibetan Medicine* (*Bod kyi gso rig 'od snang gsar pa*). Alongside finishing my PhD, setting up my own practice, a postdoctoral research project, and while learning more about *tsalung*, Tibetan medicine, religion, and language, I tried to dedicate as much time and effort as possible to editing his extensive book manuscript. Going through the manuscript chapter by chapter, word by word, it gradually became clear that there was too much material for one—even for two volumes! As I worked my way through the text to improve structure, flow, and layout, Genla had to deal with hundreds of questions and misunderstandings. I cherish our many digital exchanges and especially the days we actually sat next to each other, discussing difficult passages, looking up quotations and references, and sharing many stories on the way. Now, more than five years after the first edits and having set up Bedurya Publications in 2021, we have finally come to the point of publication. Sorry for the long wait! As the editor, it is my hope and wish that the *New Light* volumes bring you the same sense of excitement and discovery that I experienced at the beginning of my journey, acting as a trustworthy reference on your path, and as a direct link to the blessings of the lineage holders of medicine.

Nevertheless, my contribution played only a minor role in how the content of the *New Light* series came together. Already in 2006, Dr. Pasang Yonten was collaborating closely with Sylvie Béguin to prepare the first English-language texts for both the New Yuthok Institute (NYI) in Milan and the future online courses provided by TME, a process which extended up to 2013 and resulted in 11 documents along with a still growing set of audiovisual educational supports. In addition to Sylvie's monumental efforts, these were further checked for language errors by Corine Colette (until she passed away in 2010), and later by Valerie Giese. In parallel, translations to Italian for the NYI students were prepared mainly by Roberto Potocniak, assisted by Carmelo Maiorca and Victorine Cumero. Claudia Bottazzi drew many of the original illustrations, but to standardize the visual appearance of the newly conceived series, these drawings have been recreated, adapted, and/or replaced. Around this time, PADMA also supported the initial development of the book manuscript through a donation, for which TME is grateful.

To get the full picture, though, we need to trace the roots of this book back in time even further. During the 1970s, Pasang Yonten was inspired by the scholarship of his teachers to read and write, and to one day become an author. As lecturer and later college principal at Dharamsala Men-Tsee-Khang (1982–1989), he realized that in order to teach the foundations of humoral theory as expounded in the *Root* and *Explanatory Tantras* in a coherent manner, and to understand the body more fully, supplementary explanations were required. Based on extensive research and personal insights, he penned down a short treatise titled *Ten Sections on the State of the Body* (*Lus gnas skabs bcu pa*, finalized around 1986) in a small notebook, which summarizes the psychological origins of the three humors and their relationships with the elements, organs, channels, and chakras. This, in fact, was the very beginning of the text found in this volume. The *Ten Sections* were later expanded on in another notebook, which ultimately fed into documents that were used when Dr. Pasang started giving short seminars in Germany (in 1992) and later Italy, initially focusing on the medicine trees of the *Root Tantra*. Progressively refining his knowledge and didactical methods by instructing German doctors proficient in biomedical anatomy and physiology, he quickly understood that non-Tibetan students generally do not have the time, interest, or ability to study the *Gyüzhi* verse by verse. Not giving up, he took on the challenge of transmitting the essentials of both theory and practice nonetheless, thus bridging the formidable cultural and geographical gap between the Himalayas and the Alps. From the point when TME's website was launched in December 2005, more and more of his repeatedly updated lecture notes—especially from the newly set up four-year course in Milan—were divided into parts and copy-edited, and several files were freely shared online. These materials were the source of the TME course texts, which were in turn the basis for *New Light*.

Genla long did not have any concrete plans to publish a Sowa Rigpa textbook, but he did write the TME texts in a scholarly way from the outset, adding quotations, references, footnotes, and for instance indicating topics that needed further research. This writing style confirms that the provided explanations were never intended as translations, repetitions of what he received from his teachers, or what can be found in traditional commentaries. Although these are of course indispensable, the emphasis here is placed more on contemporary understanding realized through personal and comparative research, drawing on multiple sources, and confirmed by experience. In this way, Pasang Yonten's didactic materials kept growing over the years in response to exchanges with students, new courses, seminars, workshops, and retreats, scientific collaboration and conferences, and clinical findings. This notwithstanding, care was equally taken to not stray too far away from the classics; the underlying rationale was to grasp their essential meaning, to revise and elaborate, not to contradict. Western European society and modern medicine have definitively influenced and enriched his expertise, but Tibetan sources—foremostly the *Four Tantras*—have remained the central frame of reference.

This balanced yet innovative approach is reflected in the content of *New Light*'s *Foundations*, of which I will now briefly list some of the more significant features. Sowa Rigpa's Buddhist foundations permeate this book and are discussed at in the chapters that provide traditional historical context (1 and 2), as well as in Chapter 4 on the mind, and Chapter 21 on ethics. I would also like to draw the reader's attention to the concise Medicine Buddha *sādhanā* found in the Appendix, which was composed by Genla based on *Gyüzhi*'s ethical code and has since been recited by his students for numerous years. Tantric perspectives on the body have furthermore been incorporated where more strictly somatic sources fall short, particularly in Part 6 on the channels and Chapter 18, which lays out the subtle *la* body, channels, and chakras. This tantric integration equally clarifies, amongst others, the activities of the brain and sense organs through the five minor winds (*yenlak gi lung nga*, see Section 6.3). Explicit but at times admittedly tentative links between biomedical and Tibetan medical terms and concepts, where traditional explanations are interpreted through the lens of pragmatic scientific observation, are repeatedly made. One pertinent example is the consideration of hormones by means of the neologism *kham kyi dangma* (Section 11.2), which play an incontrovertible part in bodily vitality and radiance (*dang*) as well as in female reproductive physiology (Chapter 12)—a topic which has also been given special attention. Other examples of this creative adaptation of tradition are the identification of *sinbu* as microorganisms (11.4), and the more precisely drawn distinctions between veins and arteries, and the lymphatic, endocrine, and nervous systems (17.5). Explanations on the solid and hollow organs have also been newly elaborated in Chapters 14 and 15, mentioning intriguing correspondences between the organs and particular emotions that are partly derived from clinical observations.

Overall, *Foundations* consist of seven parts and 21 chapters. Meticulously referenced, packed with specifically designed illustrations and tables, and with a glossary of more than 600 Tibetan terms, this book offers a solid theoretical foundation for understanding Sowa Rigpa's gross and subtle physiology of the body-mind while also providing essential links with Buddhist philosophy and practice. As the editor, I have strived to maintain Dr. Pasang's simple yet profound way of writing as much as possible, aiming to keep the text easily comprehensible. This equally applies to the quotations, which were checked together but kept as free translations. Although the actual content of this volume is not mine, and even though I cannot always vouch for its historical accuracy from a contemporary academic perspective, I apologize for any remaining inconsistencies. Finally, I would like to thank our dedicated team at Bedurya Publications for the amazing collaboration so far. Genla, Sylvie, Christine, Tiana, and Alexandre: *Merci*!

Dedicated to the flourishing of Sowa Rigpa, we are excited to continue the journey of making these precious teachings available worldwide. The story has only just begun. Look out for the next volumes of this series on diagnosis, treatment, and pathologies in due time. May a new light shine on the science of healing, reflecting wellbeing to all 10 directions!

Jan M. A. van der Valk, PhD
Editor in chief
Bedurya Publications
October 25, 2021

PREFACE

New Light on Tibetan medicine is not a traditional commentary on the *Gyüzhi* (the *Four Tantras*), nor a translation. It is a comprehensive textbook series based on educational materials and insights accumulated over decades of study and instruction, realized through practical experience, and inspired by long-term interactions with biomedical doctors, psychologists, and patients in Asia and Europe. I have dedicated my entire life to Sowa Rigpa, the "knowledge of healing." First, I taught in India in a traditional manner, but most of my teaching ended up taking place elsewhere. Bringing experiences from these two worlds together presents opportunities for progress as well as dilemmas. In the East faith and devotion play a central role (even though Sowa Rigpa is a science), while the West is ruled by rationality. Although the *Gyüzhi* remains the same, I was forced to adapt the way of teaching to the students and their cultural backgrounds, which in turn influenced my own understanding. This journey, this transition, helped me to clarify doubts and gain additional insights, shedding new light on Tibetan medical theory and practice.

Serious students should study the foundational treatises and main commentaries in their own right. The *Four Tantras*, however, is a rather concise synthesis of a much larger body of knowledge. Only memorizing its content is not sufficient to fully understand the complexity of the body-mind and its disorders. Memorization undoubtedly has many benefits, but weaknesses as well. It is certainly not the case that one cannot practice without being able to recite long passages. Some aspects, for instance cold bile (*drang-tri*) pathologies, are only mentioned in a few lines, but in fact these words cover a vast topic requiring much elaboration. I am convinced that looking at modern physiology, anatomy, and pathology through the lens of Sowa Rigpa is an exciting opportunity for practitioners to deepen and expand their own medical tradition. Nowadays, scholars can gain understanding of the physical body and material phenomena with the help of advanced technology and surgery. In this way, we can for instance discover the relationship between brain hemorrhage in the right hemisphere, paralysis on the left side of the body, and ancient etiological concepts such as "channel contamination" (*tsadrip*). Nevertheless, Tibetan medical works attempting to learn from biomedicine, such as Dr. Samten's *New Dawn* (*Skya reng gsar pa*), are not always highly praised by traditionalist scholars even though they are pioneering achievements. Sowa Rigpa is a science, and His Holiness has always encouraged mutual exchange between East and West in this regard. In medicine, the body and material reality are of foremost importance. This is also why Yutok the Younger composed the *Gyüzhi* to cure the body-mind, while his *Yutok Nyingtik* (*G.yu thog snying thig*) lays down a swift path towards liberation—the goal of all Dharma.

Such insights made me appreciate my life journey more. I have never been overly conservative, proclaiming the superiority of my own tradition. An open mind leads to deeper awareness. Both science and religion should live within human society, otherwise they cannot survive. Even 500 years ago, societies were vastly different than today. The tradition should continue, but it can only flourish through constant renewal. The *Four Tantras* are the foundations, but these also deserve and need to be elaborated. Practitioners should uphold and expand their knowledge and be ready to enter the global medical arena. The transformation of Chinese medicine and Ayurveda into providers of contemporary healthcare which are at least partly supported by governments, instructed at universities, and applied in hospitals, could serve as an example. We should, however, also learn from their experiences and recognize the limitations of these modern institutions, in order not to lose Sowa Rigpa's soul: its unique identity and features, historically deeply rooted association with Buddhist philosophy, and its unbiased compassionate heart towards all patients. In this respect, it seems important to avoid the extremes of overly commercial treatment methods on the one hand, as well as rigid conservatism on the other. Giving new life to traditional wisdom boosts its value as well as the confidence of practitioners. Even with profound changes, tradition should not be adulterated or lost. Shining light on the trees of Tibetan medical knowledge gives life once again to this precious science.

Looking at the future, it appears that Sowa Rigpa's vitality depends on several factors. First of all, a thriving intellectual community should be fostered which engages in and publishes original research on topics such as Tibetan medical history, theory, pharmacy, and especially clinical practice in reports, books, and journals. Secondly, a range of high-quality medicinal products must be made widely available. This provides an essential physical basis for survival in and beyond its homelands. Books alone do not guarantee the continuation of practice, whereas restricting treatment to diet, behavior, and external therapies would remain partial. Medicines are in fact at the core of Sowa Rigpa's arsenal. This is also why I have long taken interest in the herbs growing locally in the Alps, comparing them to Himalayan medicinal plants and experimenting with their uses according to Tibetan medical principles. It is of utmost importance that ingredients are collected in a sustainable manner. Traditional practices such as asking the mountain spirits for permission and burning incense ought to prevent carelessness and unscrupulous overharvesting. Both the *Gyüzhi* and *terma* texts related to medicine stress that destruction of the environment brings about natural calamities and epidemics. In the past, medicines were manufactured by *amchi* in small amounts and dispensed for free or at minimal cost to the surrounding population. This local scale facilitated direct, pragmatic, and ethical relationships between practitioners, patients, and nature. Nowadays, industrial mass production seems inevitable to satisfy global demand, which means that biodiversity conservation and ecology become even more important. Yet, the pharmaceutical industry can and should also be a driver of innovation and modern quality standards. It would not be beneficial to restrict authentic pharmacy to manually prepared powders and pills only, which have their own drawbacks, while the rest of the world is producing convenient capsules, extracts, and so on.

Besides an intellectual community and effective medicinal products, a third success factor concerns the professional education of practitioners. It is no longer acceptable for *amchi* to practice in today's globalized urban environments without at least a basic understanding of biomedicine and the legal frameworks in which it operates. In this regard, one promising development is the cultivation of practitioners with dual training, that is, who are also biomedical doctors (or nurses, pharmacists, etc.) or naturopaths. This grants certain professional rights and opens spaces of collaboration, integration, and scientific research on an international level. If we want our voices to be heard and have an impact on the medical sphere, cooperation with other health professionals is a must. At the same time, however, Sowa Rigpa should also be sustained through independent associations that unite, educate, and support practitioners, upholding and transmitting traditional teachings, values, and lineage. Although important, the intrinsic worth of Sowa Rigpa does not depend on its acceptance by external authorities. Many patients are still suffering from disease, and many are looking for alternatives where treatment has failed. Each medical system has its own specialisms and contribution to health and wellbeing. Through our collective clinical experience, we witness for instance how helpful Tibetan medical treatment—including diet and lifestyle advice, as well as ritual techniques—can be for chronic digestive and rheumatic disorders, auto-immune diseases, psychosomatic complaints, post-chemotherapy convalescence, and much more. The phytotherapeutic products we use are generally less harsh on the body than highly concentrated chemical drugs and therefore ideally suited for long-term treatment of complex systemic imbalance. All this implies that we need more *amchi* or *menpa* in the future, both rural family lineage-based physicians and academics: to preserve different aspects of the tradition, to teach and to do research, to make medicine, and—most of all—to treat patients. It is my hope that *New Light on Tibetan Medicine* marks a significant step in this direction, so that Sowa Rigpa may flourish in this world to heal the sufferings of humankind.

My heartfelt gratitude goes to my parents who brought me up in difficult circumstances in Tibet and as refugees. It was their efforts, together with the kindness of Gowo Lopzang Tendzin and other great masters, which helped transform my karma into this path. Furthermore, without the blessings of His Holiness the 14th Dalai Lama, all this would not have been possible.

I am deeply grateful to Dr. Walburg Marić-Oehler and Sonja Marić (Institut für Ost-West Medizin) for promoting my teaching career in Germany, and to Sylvie Béguin for her unwavering assistance in making the teachings of Sowa Rigpa and *tsalung* available worldwide through TME. Sylvie's support and dedication is overwhelming; she also spent great effort proofreading the manuscript of this publication. I also take this opportunity to sincerely thank Prof. Dr. Paolo Lazzaro, Drs. Victorine Cumero and Simona Nicolai, Angela Furfaro, Daniele Vinci, Adele Tencani, Dario Tesorino, Roberto Potocniak, Claudia Bottazzi, and Corine Colette, as well as the many friends and students who nourished TME and the New Yuthok Institute over the years. I also pay homage to my wife, Dr. Chungla Yonten, for her lifelong love and care.

From the bottom of my heart, I extend my sincere thanks to Dr. Jan van der Valk. Jan's extensive editorial work was not only crucial for this series to see the light of day, but he has also succeeded to understand and reveal the fruits of my lifelong study. Without his help, this textbook would not have materialized.

Finally, I wish to express thanks to everyone who directly or indirectly contributed to the completion of this project and which I failed to mention here by name.

PART 1

INTRODUCTION

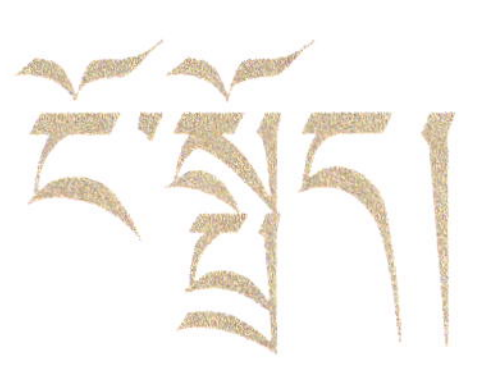

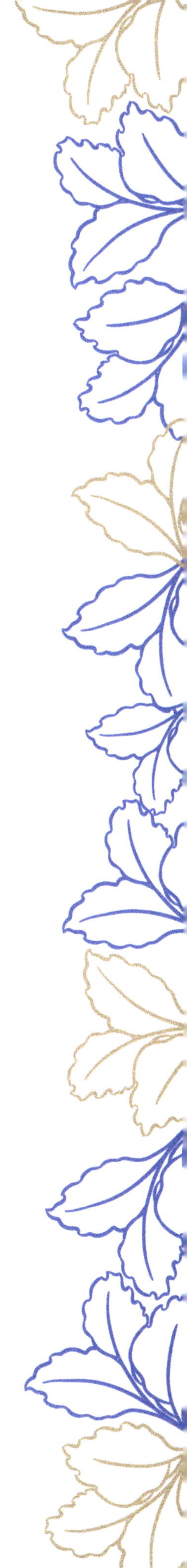

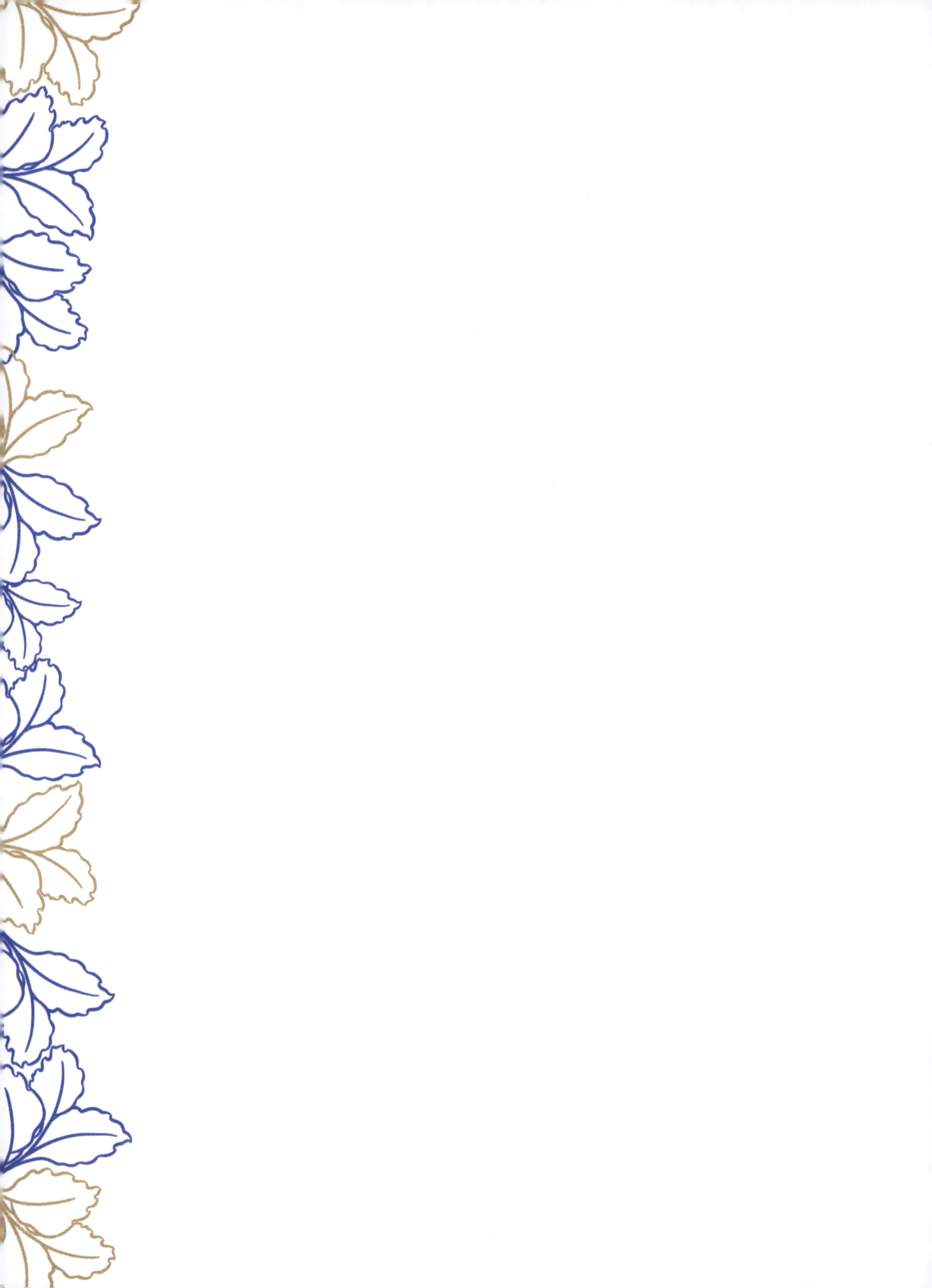

CHAPTER 1

MEDICINE AND RELIGION

To study Sowa Rigpa, the "science of healing," it is essential to first have some historical background. It is common practice for scholars to trace the origins of a science to better understand its concepts and cultural context. To practice medicine, however, it is sufficient to have access to a simple overview. We therefore provide an outline of Sowa Rigpa's connection to religion, along with traditional historical perspectives, as the two introductory chapters of this volume.

We can start off by acknowledging that from before the seventh century CE, there are scant material sources available. Buddhism is the spiritual heart of Tibetan medical practice as described in the *Four Tantras* (*Gyüzhi*) and its commentaries. To understand the context of the *Gyüzhi*, we should thus begin with the arrival of Buddhism in Tibet. In the seventh century, King Songtsen Gampo united disparate factions to form a Tibetan empire. From that time onwards, Buddhism and medicine developed together, yet we can also observe that the Dharma did not influence the technical details of medical theory and practice at that time. There is evidence of a stronger religious influence beginning in the 10th century. Tantric concepts and practices became more prominent in medicine with the advent of Padmasambhava's revealed treasure texts (*terma*). From then onwards, the science of healing was framed within the sphere of Buddhist ethics, with great moral responsibility accorded to "bodhisattva doctors" (*menpa jangchup sempa*); those who become doctors out of the highest altruistic intent: the wish to guide all sentient beings to enlightenment. In this way, the final goal of medical practice was to fulfil the six perfections (*pāramitā*) of the Mahayana tradition. What precisely is the relationship between Buddhism and medicine? Besides Tibetan history, it is equally important to read about the Buddha's life and his connection to healing. As we shall see, Prince Jīvaka and Medicine Buddha Bédurya are amongst the most salient figures of Mahayana Buddhist medicine.

1.1 THE ROOTS OF BUDDHIST MEDICINE

The body of Sowa Rigpa is the *Gyüzhi* and its soul is Buddhism. Therefore, it is important to know about the relationship between medicine and the Dharma. In the *Vinaya Sutra*, for instance, the following anecdote can be found. A monk who suffered from fistulae was avoided by others, remaining without help. Buddha Śākyamuni went there with Ānanda—one of his closest disciples—and relieved the monk's suffering. He washed and cleaned his body, and amended the monastic code of conduct to ensure ailing monks would receive help. According to the *Vinaya*, the Buddha allowed monks to visit physicians and take medicines. However, many continued to suffer from disease. Ānanda thus asked the Buddha to teach which medicines are permitted to be taken daily, over a period of seven days, and so on, and to explain their ingredients and preparation. This is noted in the *Dülwa Menzhi* ('*Dul ba sman gzhi*), the *Vinaya Sutra on Medicine*.[1]

In one of his commentaries, Sumtön Yéshézung reports the Buddha as saying:[2]

> Whoever harms a patient, harms me,
> and who helps a patient helps me.
> Whoever respects the law of cause and
> effect must know this with certainty.

This quote reiterates that if a person accumulates non-virtue vis-à-vis a patient, they must know there is no difference between the patient and the Buddha. Conversely, collecting merit vis-à-vis a patient is identical to collecting merit toward the Buddha. This point is also made clearly in the 31st chapter of the *Explanatory Tantra*, which describes the physician's moral code (see Chapter 21). Physicians who wish to become bodhisattvas must be dedicated to their

---

1 Sde srid sangs rgyas rgya mtsho, 1982, 42–51.

2 Sum ton ye shes gzung, 1999a, 303.

profession and show loving-kindness to all. Their patients should be cherished like their closest relatives, their actions towards them being as respectful as their actions towards the Buddha.

Kumāra Jīvaka

The life story of Jīvaka is another example of the relationship between medicine and Buddhism. The source of this story is again the *Vinaya Sutra*.[3] He was a great physician who eradicated his egoism and pride, illustrating how the Buddha cures the mind and its afflictions. Jīvaka was an illegitimate son of King Bimbisara of Maghada, India. King Bimbisara had had an affair with the wife of a rich merchant in Varanasi. While the merchant was away, his wife became pregnant. In order to recognize his illegitimate child, the king gave his mistress a ring and a white cloth, instructing her to bring these to the door of the palace if the child was a son. She acted accordingly and another illegitimate child of the King, a prince called Abhaya, adopted the child and named him Jīvaka. He was brought up by Prince Abhaya, becoming a celebrated physician, surgeon, and pediatrician, specializing in cranial operations. He studied under the great physician Atreya for seven years in Taxila (in present-day Pakistan). Prince Jīvaka was crowned three times as king of physicians because of his extraordinary skill in craniotomy (surgical incision into the skull) and laparotomy (surgical incision into the abdominal wall). King Bimbisara also sent Jīvaka to Ujjain (in present-day Madhya Pradesh, India) to oversee the medical treatment of King Tumpo Rapnang of Avanti. By curing the king from insomnia, Jīvaka once more achieved great fame.

In the middle of his life, Jīvaka was at the peak of his fame. He became highly ambitious and proud of his achievements, thinking: "I am the supreme king of physicians, able to treat all physical diseases. The Lord Buddha's teachings are said to cure the mind; I should verify this." He went to the place where the Buddha was teaching and sat among the disciples listening to the Buddha's discourse. He did not find the teaching meaningful. Afterwards, the Buddha called Jīvaka and asked him to go collect medicines in the mountains. A disciple called Lakna Dorjé (Vajrapāṇi) escorted him, and they brought numerous plants and minerals back. Jīvaka demonstrated his knowledge about these substances. When he had finished, some herbs were still left unexplained. The Buddha asked

Jīvaka what they were and he replied, "Omniscient One, they also possess medicinal values but I do not know these at the moment." To the great surprise of Jīvaka, the Buddha then explained them to him one by one. He then asked the Buddha, "Do you also know medicine?" Buddha replied:

> Yes, Kumāra Jīvaka, I know medicine and I am an expert in its four branches: (1) examining the disease, (2) discovering its origin, (3) curing the disease, and (4) prevention.
>
> The person who knows these four branches of medicine has the qualification to be court physician to the king. Therefore, I, the Tathagata who has defeated and destroyed the four demons and who possesses the knowledge of the four branches of medicine, am a supreme healer in the three worlds.[4]
>
> Kumāra Jīvaka, I also know the following four supreme healing truths which are beyond somatic medicine: (1) the truth of suffering, (2) the truth of the cause of suffering, (3) the truth of its cessation, and (4) the truth of the path to that cessation.
>
> Ordinary physicians do not know the right method to treat the root causes of a patient's disease, nor how to prevent aging, sickness, death, lamentation, sadness, sorrow, unhappiness, and disharmony of the mind. Only the Tathagata knows the medicine for the disease caused by aging that leads to death.

At that moment, by the Buddha's blessing, Jīvaka clearly understood the teaching as if reflected in a stainless mirror held in his hand. He saw all of existence without obscuration and gained the insight of hearing directly from the master. He deeply experienced interdependence and lost all fear. No doubts remained in his mind about the Buddha's teaching. Through this understanding, he achieved direct realization and became an arhat. He stood up from his seat, put his shawl on his shoulder, folded his hands towards the Buddha in a gesture of profound respect and said:

---

3 What is written here is based on the *Vinaya Sutra* of the Tibetan Buddhist *Kangyur* (*Bka' 'gyur*). Different versions may be found in Pali, Chinese, and other languages.

4 The three worlds are heaven, earth, and the underworld.

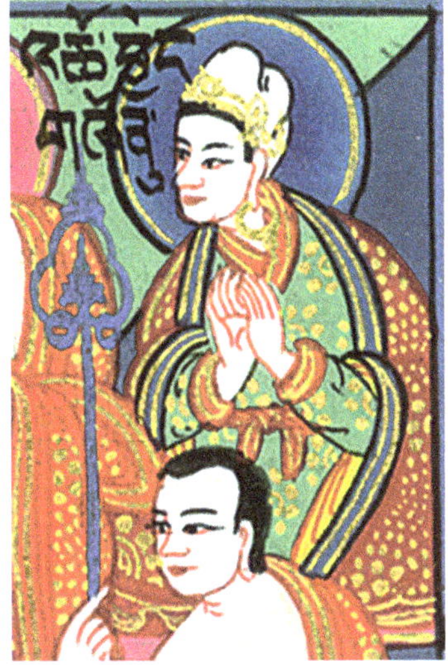

FIGURE 1.1 Jīvaka (Tsojé Zhönu)

Jīvaka offered his life and later a mango grove to the Buddha, who lived there for many years.[5] Jīvaka spent the rest of his life with the Buddha and his community, the Sangha. He visited monks and cured many people through his skillful practice of the art of healing. He also treated the Buddha several times. One such time, when staying in the Himalayas, Buddha had a digestive problem. He also treated the Buddha's foot upon injury by a catapulted stone by order of Devadatta. In this manner, he became the chief lay disciple of the Buddha and main holder of the medicine lineage, especially the tradition of the *Four Tantras*. He achieved a rainbow body upon death, and it is believed that his presence is still in this world.

1.2 THE *GOLDEN LIGHT SUTRA*: BUDDHA'S DIRECT TEACHING ON MEDICINE

When Buddha Śākyamuni visited Vulture Peak, he gave teachings to the Great Hearers and a sublime audience of monks, nuns, bodhisattvas, gods, and spirits. As part of the last turning of the Wheel of Dharma, he taught the *Supremely Victorious Golden Light Sutra* (*Gser 'od mchog tu rnam par rgyal ba'i mdo*). The 24th chapter of this sutra is entitled "The Noble Thorough Pacification of Illness" (*'Phags pa nad rab tu zhi bar byed pa*). In this section, Buddha tells the Goddess-Bodhisattva Rikyi Lhamo about how he learned the art of healing from his father in one of his previous lives:[6]

Countless eons ago, a Buddha called Rinchen Tsukpüchen came to this world. During his time, there was a rich merchant named Tsongpo Chudzin who was also an expert in the eight branches of medicine. He treated many patients and saved many lives. He had a son called Chubep (Skt.: Jalavahana), who was handsome, good-hearted, intelligent, well-learned, and an expert in scripture, art, astrology, and grammar. He was much beloved by his people. An epidemic broke out and thousands of people died. The merchant's son Chubep was distressed, and compassion arose in his heart. He realized that his elderly father was not able to perform many treatments because he was aged and weak, so he became determined to learn medicine. He went to his father and, prostrating before him, said in verse:

The father replied:

---

5 Jīvakāmravaṇa, Jīvaka's mango grove, still exists at Kumrahar in Amravati, Central India.

6 The quotation below is from the Tibetan translation of the Chinese version of The *Golden Light Sutra*, as described by Sde srid sangs rgyas rgya mtsho, 1982, 45–50.

The first two months are the time of
flowering (early spring),
three and four are the hot season (late
spring),
five and six are the rainy season (summer),
seven and eight are autumn,
and nine and 10 are the cold season (early
winter).
The last two are the time of snow (late
winter).
By knowing the different seasons,
you will learn to administer medicine
without mistake.

By prescribing food and beverages
according to the law of seasons,
digestion will be smooth,
and disease will not arise.

If the *dütsik* are disturbed and the four
elements are changed,
and if the body remains without proper
medication,
it will suffer from disease.

Therefore, the physician should know the
four seasons as well as the six *dütsik*,
and he should know the nature of the body.
Then, he will be able to administer diet and
medicine without mistake.

If disease has entered via *dangma*,
into the blood, muscles, bones, bone
marrow, and brain,
one should know if the disease is curable
or not.

Diseases are of four types:
wind (*lung*), bile (*tripa*), phlegm (*béken*),
and all three combined in one.[7]
One should know their manifestation times.

Béken manifests in spring,
summer [monsoon] increases *lung*,
tripa manifests in autumn,
and all three manifest in winter.

Admit pungent, rough, and warm tastes
and qualities in spring,
oily, warm, and salty qualities in summer,
cooling, sweet, and oily qualities in autumn,
and rough, oily, sour, and sweet qualities in
winter.

If during these four seasons,
medication, diet, and beverages are
followed according to seasonal law,
no disease will be produced.

Pain after meals indicates *béken* disorder,
during digestion, it indicates *tripa* disorder,
after digestion, it indicates *lung* disorder.
One should know these related times and
symptoms.

Knowing the root of the disease,
administer the medicine accordingly.
Despite different disease characters
and types,
one should reveal its origin.

Administer oily medicine for *lung*
disorders,
purgatives are better for *tripa* disorders,
for *béken* disorders one should apply
emetics,
and combined disorders require all three
of these.

Combined means that the three humors
equally manifest their symptoms.
One should know the times of disease
manifestation,
but also the patient's constitution.

A wise physician learns through
examination,
treats the patient at the right time by means
of medicine, therapy, food and drinks,
giving advice without being mistaken.

The eight branches are the synthesis of all
medical sciences.
Know these and cure the ailments of
sentient beings:
(1) bloodletting and (2) wounds,
(3) bodily diseases and (4) evil spirits,
(5) poisons and (6) pediatrics,
(7) rejuvenation and (8) geriatrics.

Diagnose the patient's complexion first.
Listen to their words,
and then ask about their dreams.
You will know the three humors and their
distinctions.

---

7   The condition in which the humors are equally combined is
known as brown phlegm (*béken mukpo*).

A thin, skinny body, poor hair,
having an unstable mind,
being talkative and dreaming of flying
indicate a *lung* constitution.

Grey hair at middle age,
much sweating and diarrhea,
intelligence and dreaming of fire indicate a
tripa constitution.

A stable mind and a large upright body,
diligence, an oily and moist head and body,
and dreaming of water and white objects
indicate a *béken* constitution.

The three humors together produce
combined constitutions.
There are double and triple constitutions.
If there are multiple characteristics,
one should know the dominant humor.

After knowing the constitution,
administer the medicine for the disease.
If there are no signs of dying,
the patient is curable.

If the patient's eyes perceive wrongly,
and if they humiliate their master and the
physician,
as well as being angry with relatives,
it is a sign of dying.

The left eye becoming white,
the tongue becoming black,
the nose turning to one side,
the ears becoming bluish,
and drooping lips are all signs of dying.

A chebulic myrobalan fruit possesses the
six tastes,
and cures all disease.
It is harmless and the king of medicine.

The three fruits[8] and three hot ones,[9]
easy to obtain amongst medicines,
as well as molasses, honey, milk, and butter
can cure many disorders.

Administer other medicines as well,
according to the disease.
First cultivate love and compassion,
and do not look for wealth and benefit.

Thus, I have told you how to heal disease.
This precious teaching is the synthesis of
medicine.

Then, Chubep became an expert in the art of healing and cured many people.

This teaching can be seen as the heart of Buddhist medicine, and as such it is also the essence of Tibetan medicine.

1.3 MAHAYANA BUDDHISM AND THE PHILOSOPHICAL VIEW OF THE *GYÜZHI*

The Buddha advised his disciples that bodhisattvas should learn the art of healing to help others and to liberate them from suffering. Saving lives is a great act of generosity and an especially important work of love and compassion; it is even more powerful than curing disease and is a principal cause of enlightenment.

Bodhisattvas should strive for and gain the merits of the six perfections: moral discipline, patience, effort, generosity, meditative concentration, and wisdom. Yet, the most important element in Mahayana Buddhist practice is that of developing *bodhicitta*. This focus was re-established in Tibet by Atiśa Dipamkara Shrijnana, a prince of Bengal and crown abbot of Vikramśila monastic university. He stated that "serving a tired traveler who has come from far, one's aged parents, caring for patients, and meditating upon emptiness collect the same merit."[10] In this context, medicine became a special instrument of Buddhist practice, expressing the bodhisattva's altruistic perfection in practice. Numerous stories about the historical Buddha's life and previous incarnations—recounted in the *Jātaka Tales* and *Vinaya*—confirm this.

In the *Four Tantras* in particular, Medicine Buddha Bédurya is presented as the original teacher of both the medical and religious concepts related to the body-mind's development, together with the Five Buddhas. Explanations regarding the psychology of human ignorance, the mental poisons, the ethical code of conduct, and so on, are directly based on Buddhism. The *Gyüzhi* also contains tantric knowledge regarding the subtle body, psychic states, channels, chakras, and essence drops (*tiklé*). These are known as *tsalung* teachings, which lead to yogic body-mind transformation. Along these lines, one can see glimpses of *Gyüzhi*'s underlying structure, which scholar-practitioners say is "externally medicine and internally tantra."

---

8 *Terminalia chebula, Terminalia bellerica* and *Emblica officinalis.*

9 Ginger (*Zingiber officinalis*), long pepper (*Piper longum*), and black pepper (*Piper nigrum*).

---

10 'Gos lo gzhon nu dpal, 2002, 313.

In these body-mind topics in particular, we can see that the backbone of Sowa Rigpa is Buddhist philosophy, and it is this which forms the moral foundation for the medical profession. As we have seen, the concept of the cause of disease and its symptoms, its diagnosis and treatment, correspond to the Four Noble Truths that underlie the *Four Tantras*. Buddhism and medicine are two sides of the same coin, having the same fundamental motivation and goal: that of liberating the body-mind from suffering. Buddha expounded medicine and declared that the ultimate source of disease is the mind. Therefore, to be fully cured means to be liberated from samsara—the cycle of birth, old age, sickness, and death. Accordingly, Dharma is the supreme medicine for the mind and mental disorders, which also encompass physical disease as there is no rigid separation between mind and body.

Sowa Rigpa belongs to the realm of the secular sciences, but is set within a Tibetan Buddhist framework. This includes the *ta gom chö sum*: right view, meditative concentration, and the dharmic ethics of physicians. The *Explanatory Tantra*'s 31st chapter lays these out as follows (see again Chapter 21). Firstly, doctors and their medical knowledge should adhere to the right view of Nāgārjuna's Middle Way. Secondly, doctors should meditate on and cultivate the Four Immeasurables: the practice of loving-kindness, compassion, rejoicing, and abiding in equanimity in relation to patients and all sentient beings. Thirdly, physicians must avoid the 10 negative actions when practicing their profession, instead undertaking the 10 positive actions.

The Medicine Buddha

The Medicine Buddha, Sangyé Menla in Tibetan, is well-known throughout the world of Mahayana Buddhism: in Tibetan regions, Nepal, Bhutan, Mongolia, China, Korea, Vietnam, and Himalayan areas such as Ladakh and Arunachal Pradesh (India). He has different names in different languages. A more extensive name for the Medicine Buddha is Bhaiṣajyaguruvaiḍūryaprabhārāja, which is known in Tibetan as Sangyé Mengyi Lha Bédurya Ökyi Gyelpo. The longer Sanskrit name can be translated as Medicine Guru, King of Aquamarine Light. Sangyé Menla is the central figure of Sowa Rigpa, with the Five Buddhas surrounding him acting as teachers of the *Four Tantras*. As Sumtön stated in his *Indispensable Lineage Biography*:[11]

> Spontaneously arisen from the Five Buddhas:
> the healing science of the Great *Tantras*.

———————
11 Sum ton ye shes gzung, 1999b, 690.

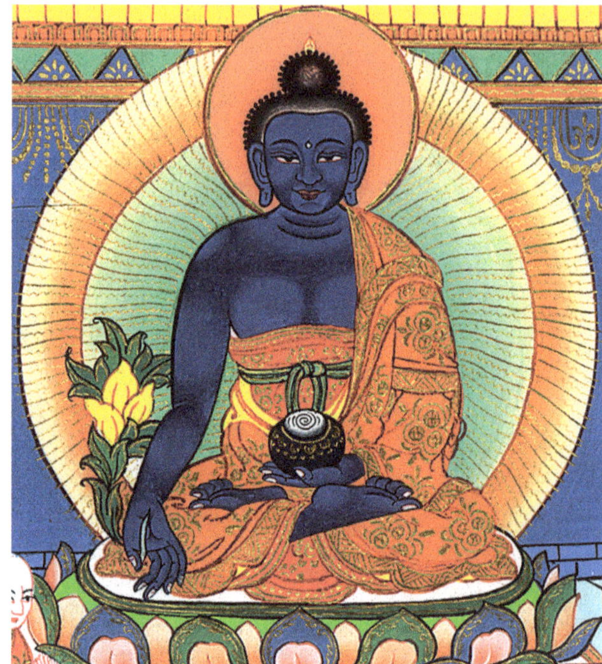

FIGURE 1.2 Bhaiṣajyaguru (Sangyé Menla)

Sangyé Menla in the sutras

What is commonly referred to as the *Medicine Buddha Sutra* is a major spiritual reference for the *Gyüzhi*. Its full title is:

Āryabhagavānbhaiṣajyaguruvaiḍūryaprabhasya pūrvapraṇidhānaviśeṣavistāranāmamahāyāna sūtra

ༀ༔ འཕགས་པ་བཅོམ་ལྡན་འདས་སྨན་གྱི་བླ་བཻ་ཌཱུརྱའི་འོད་ ཀྱི་སྨོན་ལམ་གྱི་ཁྱད་པར་རྒྱས་པ་ཞེས་བྱ་བ་ཐེག་པ་ཆེན་པོའི་ མདོ༔

The Noble Great Vehicle Sutra "The Detailed Account of the Previous Aspirations of the Blessed Bhaiṣajyaguruvaiḍūryaprabha"

This Mahayana sutra was expounded by Buddha Śākyamuni to an assembly of 36,000 bodhisattvas, kings, ministers, humans, gods, Asuras, nagas, *gandharva*, and so on. It also describes 12 *yakṣa* generals, 10 worldly protectors, and four heavenly guardian kings who guard the Medicine Buddha and his sutra, taking care that its environment is a place of peace, harmony, health, and prosperity. The text is said to have arrived in Tibet in the eighth century, brought by the abbot Śāntarakṣita. Based on the sutra, Śāntarakṣita composed *The Greater and Lesser Medicine Buddha Sutra in 800 Verses* (*Sman mdo brgyad brgya pa che chung*).

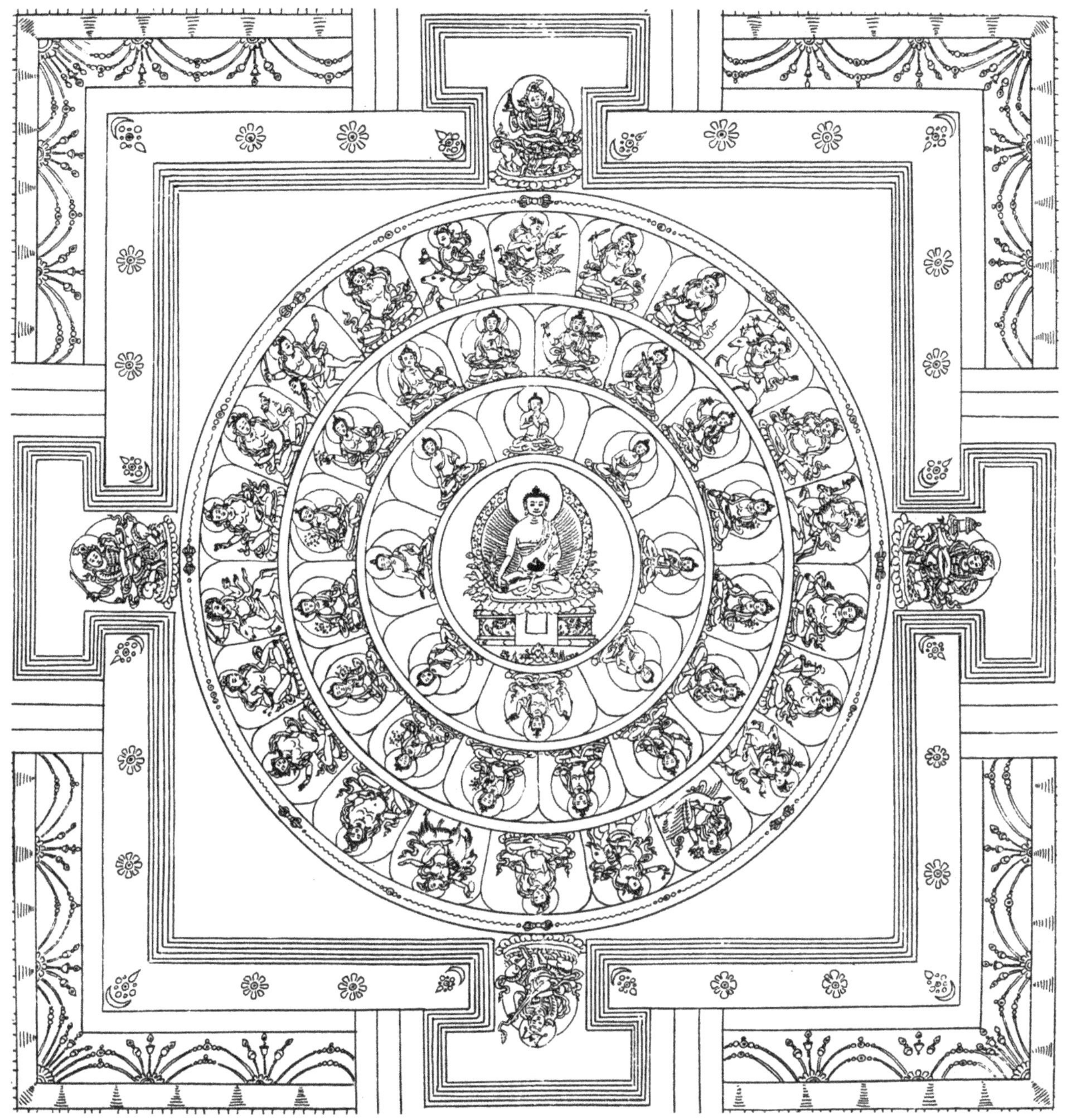

FIGURE 1.3 Sangyé Menla's Great Mandala of 51 Deities, with seven medicine buddhas and Prajñāpāramitā (inner circle), 16 bodhisattvas (middle circle), 10 worldly protectors and 12 *yakṣa* generals (outer circle), and four guardian kings

Medicine Buddha is often depicted with two chief disciples or attendants: Chandraprabha (Dawatar Nangjé) and Sūryaprabha (Nyimatar Nangjé). Buddha Bédurya took 12 vows or commitments, and also appears together with six other medicine buddhas—excluding Buddha Śākyamuni—in the text along with their different gestures (*mudrā*), vows, pure lands and healing practices. Masters of all Tibetan Buddhist schools have composed Medicine Buddha *sādhanā* as well as powerful ritual healing practices for the living and the dead. It appears that these healing rites did not exist in ancient India, but only in Tibet as stated by Taktsang Lotsawa Shérap Rinchen.[12] An incomplete manuscript of the Sanskrit *Medicine Buddha*

____

12 Stag tshang lo tsa ba shes ra brin chen, 2007, 238.

Sutra was unearthed from a ruined stupa in Gilgit (now in Pakistan) during the 1930s. It could be one of the earliest versions, dating back as far as the sixth century CE.[13]

The Medicine Buddha's iconography in paintings and the like differs from country to country. In the Dunhuang cave in Xinjiang, for example, he wears blue Chinese-style clothing, is accompanied by his two chief disciples, and holds a pill in his right hand. In the Japanese tradition, the Medicine Buddha may be depicted seated on a throne and holding a vase in one hand. In Tibetan-style representations, he is of a blue color, seated in meditation posture, and holding a stem of *arura* (*Terminalia chebula*) in his right hand and a vase of nectar in his left. The King of Medicine, together with his countless emanations, is the healing light of the universe. The founders and eminent physicians of all healing traditions are his emanations. His energy manifests without discrimination in the form of masters, physicians, nurses, healers, medicines, therapists, patients, and their assistants. His light rises every day from the east, healing diseases of the body-mind and bringing health and wealth on a universal scale. In the Tibetan tradition, the Medicine Buddha heals patients' diseases and purifies negative karma, especially that which may manifest as disease. The rituals of the *Medicine Buddha Sutra* are performed in the name of patients and the deceased, aiding terminally ill patients as well as bardo beings.

1.4 BÖN MEDICINE AND ANCIENT TIBETAN RULERS

The Bön shamanic tradition is a living religion that propitiates local protector deities and spirits. Native healers such as the Döl Bön (Rdol bon) may be thought of as shamans. Also called "Black Bön" (Bon nag), they may perform animal sacrifice and chant rituals to heal. They believe that evil spirits and misfortune are the source of all disease. In their eyes, spirits govern human society. If these spirits become unhappy—due to, for example, offerings not being fulfilled to their satisfaction—they torment human beings. These ancient healers developed rituals to propitiate local or ancestral spirits, to prevent unfavorable actions and to request protection. Ancestor spirits sometimes possess mediums to communicate with family members and those who are ill. According to the spirit's desire, shamanic healers use animal souls and blood as ransom for their patients' health and prosperity. A long time ago, these types of rites were widespread throughout Tibet and central Asia. Black Bön

traditions are believed to have disappeared from central Tibet after Buddhism developed, sometime in the eighth century. However, sacrificial rituals are still performed in remote areas of Tibet, Nepal, in some parts of the China-Tibet borderlands, and in Indian tribal communities. Such methods are an indirect source of the central Asian and Tibetan religious and medical traditions. Eminent scholars such as Zurkhar Lodrö Gyelpo (1509–1579)[14] and Déumar Tendzin Püntsok (1672–?) quote aspects of Bön medical practice as reliable information.

Tönpa Shenrap Miwoché is a legendary Bön master. He is believed to have come to Tibet from Zhangzhung Ölmolungring (Zhang zhung 'ol mo lung ring) more than 18,000 years ago.[15] This mystical land is located in Tazik (Ta zig, possibly referring to Persia or Tajikistan), and is also said to be situated on the western side of Mount Kailash. Tönpa Shenrap reformed the Black Bön native shamanic culture, creating the "White Bön" religion. Bön followers believe that all of shamanism in Siberia and Central Asia—or even in the whole world—originated in this legendary country, the seat of ancient Bön civilization. The White Bön tradition is more moderate and scholarly, and does not practice animal sacrifice. It may even be an ancient form of Buddhism. Intermarriage with people from the cultures and faiths of West Asian regions such as Persia, Afghanistan, Xinjiang, and Kashmir occurred in Tibet before the seventh century, facilitated by contact through the Silk Road. White *Bönpo* believe that Tönpa Shenrap expounded a medical text called *Bumzhi* ('Bum bzhi) to his son Chébu Trishé, who succeeded him as lineage holder. The banner of Sowa Rigpa rises for the first time with his name, which would establish it as one of the earliest medical systems in the world.

Tibet's first king was Nyatri Tsenpo, who probably lived in the third century BCE. The ninth king, however, was Pudé Güngyel. His minister was called Rulékyé, which means "born from animal horn." It was this minister who allegedly discovered metallurgy and developed irrigation systems for crops. At that time, Tibetans treated health disorders using hot and cold fomentation, bloodletting, and heat therapies, and they treated wounds and injuries using hot melted butter. Many natural therapies had already developed to heal disorders and relieve pain. The knowledge gained by these elders was passed down through the generations in an unbroken oral tradition. The skill of Tibetan healers thus became legendary even in ancient times.

<hr>

13 Hassnain and Sumi, 1995.

14 Zur mkhar blo gros rgyal po, 2000, 280–81.

15 Bstan 'dzin rnam grags, 1962, 24.

According to traditional sources, eye surgery was first recorded in the life of the sixth-century Tibetan King Takri Nyenzik, who was blind from birth.[16] Following his father's advice, ministers invited a physician called Hazhajé from Hazha (a western principality of ancient Tibet), who "opened the eyes" of the young king.[17] In fact, the name of the King is said to derive from the first thing he saw after surgery: a wild sheep (*nyen*) in the mountains (*ri*), which he mistook for a tiger (*tak*).[18] Despite this story, in subsequent centuries very few historical records on surgery have come to light. Tibetan traditional eye cataract operation (re) appeared and was supported during the life of the Fifth Dalai Lama (1617–1682). He invited a surgeon called Drachi Töluk Nélukpa to teach and preserve this technique in Chakpori during the 17th century.

---

16 Sa skya ba bsod nams rgyal mtsan, 2002, 61, and Sde srid sangs rgyas rgya mtsho, 1982, 149.

17 Blo bzang rgya mtsho, 1981, 19.

18 Sde srid sangs rgyas rgya mtsho, 1982, 149.

CHAPTER 2

TRADITIONAL HISTORY

2.1 THE FIRST WAVE (7–10TH CENTURY)

Songtsen Gampo

By the seventh century CE, Buddhism had already spread from India and Kashmir across Central Asia, especially to Gilgit, Swat, and Taxila (in present-day Pakistan). These places themselves became important centers of learning. The Tang dynasty of China was also eager to import Buddhism via the Silk Road. The Indian emperor Harsha's empire was at its height, and supported the Mahayana teachings. King Likmicha ruled the Zhangzhung kingdom on the northern side of Central Tibet, while in the south Ansu Verma ruled as the king of Nepal. This was the time of the Yarlung dynasty in Central Tibet, which was a rather small kingdom.

The young Tibetan king Songtsen Gampo (617–649?), the son of King Namri Songtsen, was expanding his kingdom. Thanks to his intelligence and the support of his devoted ministers, he founded the Great Tibetan Empire, expanding his rule east to China, south to India, west to Taklamakan, and north to Xinjiang. Once he became emperor, Songtsen Gampo's fondest wish was to transform the aggressive warrior nature of his people to create a peaceful and civilized country. With this objective, he is remembered to have introduced Indian Buddhism as an antidote capable of healing and transforming the passions of a warring people. He sent the young minister Tönmi Sambhota to Kashmir to learn Sanskrit and Buddhism. As a result, Sambhota invented the first Tibetan official script, brought Indian Buddhism to Tibet, and started to translate the Buddha's teachings from Sanskrit into Tibetan.

Emperor Songtsen Gampo had five queens: three Tibetan queens, the Nepali princess Brikuti (Belza Tritsün), and Chinese princess Wencheng Kongjo (Gyaza Kongjo). The foreign queens helped to establish Buddhism in Tibet, which spread rapidly inside the country. The Nepali Princess Brikuti had the Potala and Jokhang temples built, and the Chinese princess the Ramoché temple, where statues of the young Buddha are housed. The Tibetan queens also had their tutelary temples built. In addition, Wencheng Kongjo provided astrological guidance for the flourishing of the Dharma and the construction of its monasteries. During the emperor's reign, many temples and religious centers were built, including the Potala which is dedicated to the Bodhisattva Avalokiteśvāra, known in Tibetan as Chenrézik. The Potala Palace served as the seat of Tibet's government. Songtsen Gampo conquered the kingdom of Zhangzhung, the Taklamakan desert, parts of Xinjiang and other Chinese territories, and several small Himalayan kingdoms. He also established friendly relations with the neighboring countries of China, Nepal,[1] and India. Due to the strong military power of Songtsen Gampo's reign, he had great success in establishing harmony through the introduction of Buddhism. However, there was some resistance from the public and amongst the king's ministers.

Songtsen Gampo is said to have invited physicians from India, China, and Persia to participate in a first conference gathering the different medical systems of that time. The foreign physicians to come were: Bharadwaja from India, Henwen Hangte from China, and Galéno from Tazik.[2] These three physicians translated various medical texts, which were subsequently collected into seven volumes called *Fearless Weapon* and offered to the ruler. This is traditionally known to be the first scholarly medical work composed in Central Tibet. The Indian and Chinese physicians returned to their countries with great respect and gifts

---

1 The *White Annals* describe how Nepal was a suzerainty of Tibet under Songtsen Gampo's reign, and remained so for 100 years. Dge 'dun chos 'phel, 2004, 69.

2 Both the Indian and Chinese physicians are legendary personas.

from the emperor, whereas Galéno stayed in Lhasa as a court physician. He translated Persian (Galenic) works such as *Gongön Düpa* (*Mgo sngon bsdus pa*), and *Cock, Peacock, and Parrot* (*De pho rma bya ne tso*). Three treatises were probably about surgery.

To properly understand these legendary events from a modern historical perspective, it is useful to distinguish between two figures with the name "Galéno." The original Galen was the second-century court physician from the Hippocratic medical tradition, serving at the court of the Roman emperor Marcus Aurelius. Galen was a celebrated physician, who was born in 129 CE in Pergamo (today 's Bergama, in Turkey) and died in Rome in 199 CE. His tradition travelled from Europe to Far Eastern countries such as Syria, Persia, and Iraq. The second Galéno is the one Songtsen Gampo invited to Tibet in the eighth century, who came from Persia or Takzik. This Galéno was awarded the title "Prince of Physicians" by Songsten Gampo in recognition of his skill. Although the name Galéno shines brightly in the history of Tibetan medicine, no record of Hippocrates is to be found.

Songtsen Gampo created the infrastructure of Buddhist imperial civilization, hence Tibetans pay their respects to him until this day. Unfortunately, the emperor was assassinated in his thirties.

Trisong Detsen

The eighth century that follows was equally a golden period for the Tibetan people. The great emperor Trisong Detsen (742–798) continued the efforts of his grandfather Songtsen Gampo: to expand the kingdom, to develop Buddhism, and to promote peace and prosperity. Tibet soon became a center of scientific, cultural, and economic development.

To stimulate the flourishing of Dharma in Tibet, Trisong Detsen invited several great Indian Buddhist masters, such as Abbot Śāntarakṣita from Nālandā, the Swatian tantric Guru Padmasambhava along with Bimalamitra, and more. The great Samyé (Bsam yas) Monastery was constructed in 764 CE, developing a library of science, philosophy, and religious texts. For the preservation of Dharma and the propagation of secular sciences in his kingdom, Trisong Detsen formed a committee to translate Buddhist texts from India, Nepal and China. For the first time, seven monks were ordained in Tibet to test whether the passionate Tibetan people could practice the celibacy and self-control required for a religious life. Most of the Tibetan people welcomed the Dharma, the peaceful religion of Buddha Śākyamuni, which took ever-stronger root in Tibet.

Along with developing the Dharma in Tibet, Emperor Trisong Detsen also desired to improve the lives of his people through developing different medical systems. The emperor pretended to be sick and invited many expert physicians to treat him. These came from India, China, Persia, Nepal, Kashmir, Dolpo (Mustang, now in Nepal), Mongolia, and Minyak (Mi nyag, a small kingdom in the eastern part of Tibet). An international conference on medicine was held at the Samyé Monastery in central Tibet. The Indian, Chinese, and Persian foreign medical traditions were accorded official recognition in Tibet and all contributions were translated into Tibetan and collected in a text called *The Brown Treatise for His Majesty's Healing* (*Rgyal po'i bla dpyad spo ti smug po*). The emperor offered the physicians precious jewels and many other gifts, conferring upon them the honorary professional title *Lharjé*. From that time onwards, many physician family names bear this title. Trisong Detsen laid down the 13 codes of conduct, regulations concerning the relations between physicians and patients (see Section 21.1).

He is also said to have invited famous foreign physicians such as Dharmarāja from India, Hashang Mahakyinda from China and Tsampashila from Trom (Khrom, referring to Rome or Persia). They translated many works from their countries and wrote a collective treatise (*Gso dpyad rin chen spung pa'i skor*) as tribute to the emperor. Tsampashila remained in Tibet for a long time, where he composed a work known as *Bébum Nakpo* (*Be bum nag po'i skor 'jal tshad*), which was dedicated to his son and probably about pharmacy. He also translated Caraka's *Drang srong rnying rgyud mgo byang khog yan lag gi pra 'khrid skor*, probably a work concerning anatomy and physiology, and the *Mgo byang khog yang lag 'du ba thor bu dang bcas pa'i bcos thabs man ngag don brgyad pa* on surgical treatment. He collected and printed these works together as *Biji Puti Khaser* (*Bi ji'i pu ti kha ser*), the last text in this volume being *The King's Shining Treatise* (*Rgyal po'i bla yig 'od 'bar*).

Tibetan medical schools were established under the auspices of Trisong Detsen, and their different medical traditions became widespread. From these, nine schools eventually emerged. Three arose from the upper part of Tibet: (1) Chéjé Zhikpo (Che rje zhig po), (2) Biji Lekgön (Bi ji legs mgon), and (3) Ukpa Chözang (Ug pa chos bzang). Three arose from the middle or central part of Tibet: (4) Yutok (G.yu thog), (5) Drangti Gyelnyé Kharpuk (Brangti rgyal mnyes mkhar phug), and (6) Minyak (Mi nyag). And three arose from the lower or eastern part of Tibet: (7) Nyapa Chözang (Gnya pa chos bzang), (8) Tongpa Drakgyel (Stong pa grags rgyal) and (9) Tazhi Darpo (Mtha' bzhi dar po). Amongst these family traditions, Yutok (the Elder), Drangti, and Tazhi became long-standing medical

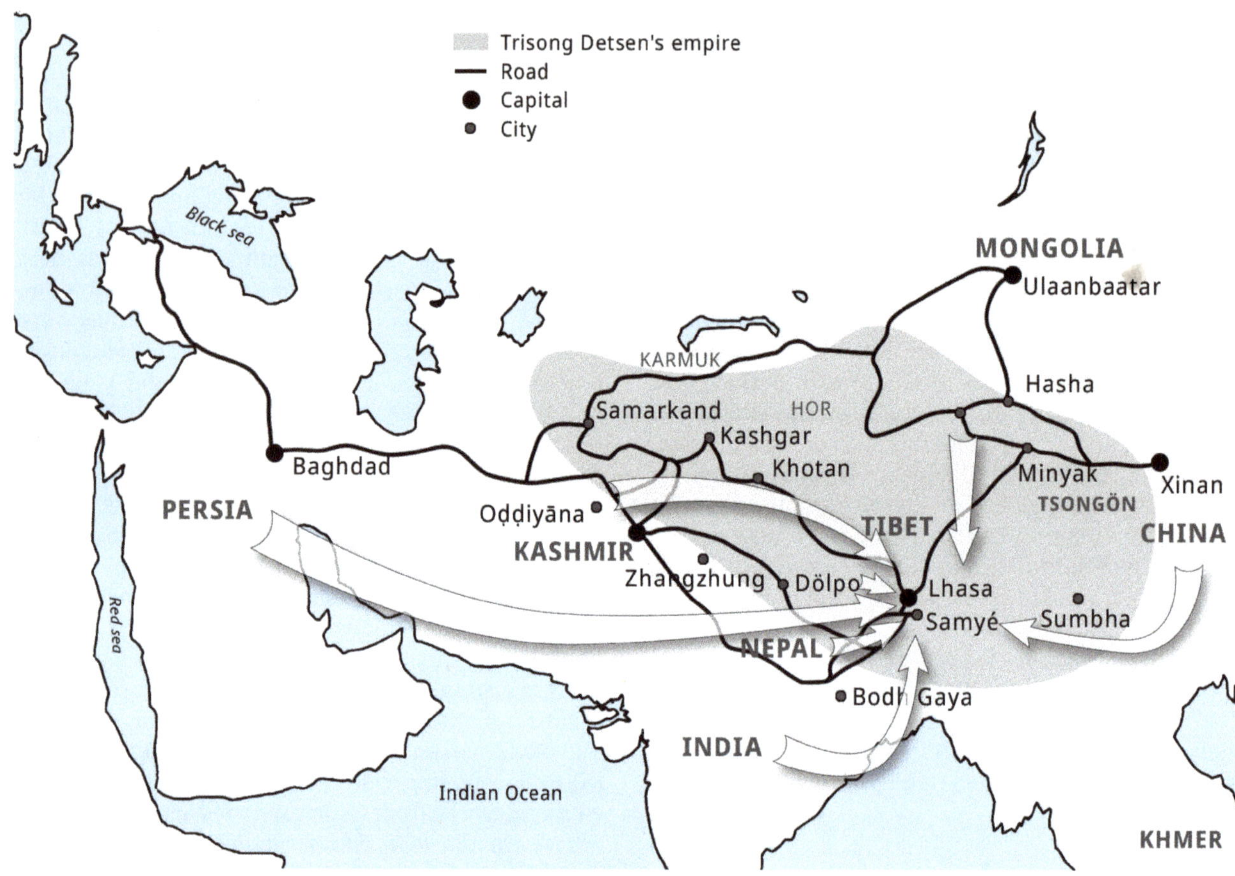

FIGURE 2.1 Routes of the nine physicians who were invited by the Tibetan emperor in the eighth century. Three came from China.

schools. During the following centuries, Tibetan medicine was practiced, developed, and passed down to younger generations. Family lineages of physicians emerged in Tibet. One of these great-grandfather figures is Yutok the Elder, who may have lived for 125 years (708–833?). He is revered as the founder of the Kongpo Medicine Valley School (Kong po sman lung) in southeast Tibet, renowned for establishing the four-level medical study curriculum that is still largely followed up to this day.

According to the author's understanding, the medical systems which developed during the Songtsen Gampo and Trisong Detsen era were secular scientific traditions. Religion was not that influential on medical theories. Some traditions, such as that of the Indian master Śāntigarbha, were religiously oriented. However, Sowa Rigpa remained primarily a somatic system until the 10th century.

Indian Buddhist medicine in Tibet

The Dharma Kings who established Buddhism in Tibet invited the Indian master Śāntigarbha, Guru Padmasambhava, Bimalamitra, as well as Nepali master-physicians who translated medical texts and gave many instructions. Many of their works disappeared during the ensuing dark period. There is no question that these works should be considered part of Sowa Rigpa, even though direct Buddhist influences on medicine only became evident after the 10th century. Most of this body of medical texts, except for rare works such as Guru Rinpoché's *Vase of Ambrosia* cycle (*Bdud rtsi bum pa*, a treatise on epidemics and *nyenrim* disease), remain hidden treasures.

During the late 10–11th centuries, Tibet became ever more renowned for its medical sciences and spiritual authority. Gradually, over a period of approximately 300 years, the Tibetan people embraced Buddhist concepts and practices. According to Indian histories of medicine, a Buddhist medical system was practiced in much of the South Asian subcontinent. This brought forth (veterinary) hospitals, hospitals specializing in fevers or infections, and the planting of medicinal plant gardens in different regions. The improvement of public health and building of public rest rooms and sanitary systems were promoted by Jīvaka, Emperor Aśoka the Great, Nāgārjunācarya, and so on.

The great monastic universities such as those at Nālandā, Vikramaśīla, Bodh Gaya, Taxila, Kashmir, and Varanasi became centers for the study and practice of an ancient Buddhist medical system. Unfortunately, Buddhism gradually declined as Indian royal dynasties turned to the services of Hindu Brahmins, and as Islamic invasions (10th–12th centuries) swept away monasteries and sacred sites. As the practice of Buddhist medicine declined in India, it traveled along with Mahayana teachings to new homes in Tibet, Nepal, Mongolia, Bhutan, and China.

2.2 THE SECOND WAVE (10–16TH CENTURY)

A dark period followed the collapse of the monarchy, lasting for about four centuries (842–1247). During these times, the Sakyapa (Sa skya pa), Pönchenpa (Dpon chen pa), Pakmodrupa (Phag mo gru pa), Rinpungpa (Rin spungs pa), and Tsangpa (Gtsang pa) clans ruled the Tibetan plateau. Religious and secular life suffered considerably and deteriorated. It is evident from Zurkhar Lodrö Gyelpo's biography the Yutok lineage and the Drangti, Jangpa, Zurkhar, and Gongmen traditions were declining like rainbows in a stormy sky. Priceless texts perished or were scattered. The teachings survived within a few family lineages.

During this dark period of revolutions and civil war, gangs and warlords ruled large tracts of Tibet. Like a lotus flower growing from the mud, the great master Lotsawa Rinchen Zangpo (958–1055) was born in Gugé, in the upper part of Tibet. He was especially gifted. While he was a teenager, he was chosen by Gugé kings Lha Lama Yéshé Ö and Jangchup Ö, who were descendants of the old Tibetan kings. Rinchen Zangpo was sent to Kashmir to study Buddhism. He subsequently became a master of sutra and tantra, translating many texts from Sanskrit that started a new wave of Buddhist teachings in Tibet. These included Ayurvedic treatises such as *The Eight Branches of Medicine* (*Sman dpyad yan lag brgyad pa*), as well as Chandrānandana's commentary *Padarthachandrika*, and Shalihotra's *Asvayursaṁhitā* (on veterinary medicine, particularly for horses). Rinchen Zangpo taught medicine in Toling (Mtho lding, capital of Gugé) to many disciples, four of whom became eminent scholar-physicians. This tradition is now called Töluk (Stod lugs): the Upper Tradition of medicine. Sowa Rigpa was resurrected and once again spread throughout the Land of Snow to benefit the health of its people. Lotsawa Rinchen Zangpo met Atiśa in the later part of his life. Following his advice, he went into retreat for 12 years, eventually achieving the state of *parinirvāṇa*.

Atiśa Dīpaṃkara Śrījñāna (982–1055) was also invited by the Gugé rulers, reaching Tibet in 1038. He brought the light of Dharma back to Tibet once again, giving teachings of love, compassion, and karma-dharma. People were finally able to breathe freely after the sufferings of civil unrest. He was venerated as a living buddha, staying in Tibet for more than 17 years. His *Path of the Bodhisattva* (*Byang chub lam sgron*) became the foundation of the Kadampa tradition of Tibetan Buddhism.

2.3 THE ORIGINS OF THE *GYÜZHI*

According to traditional Tibetan history, the *Gyüzhi* dates back to the eighth century. The young Pagor Bérotsana (Vairocana) had been sent to India by Trisong Detsen and Guru Padmasambhava to become realized. It is said that Vairocana and the Kashmiri Buddhist physician Candrānandana together translated the *Gyüzhi* from a Sanskrit source, after which it was brought from Kashmir to Tibet. The tradition is said to have come through an unbroken ear-whispering lineage (*nyengyü*) from the Buddha to Jīvaka, Nāgārjuna, Vāgbhaṭa, Candrānandana, and then to Vairocana, as described in the first chapter of the *Root Tantra*. Spiritual transformation through the practice of Sangyé Menla is the secret path of this lineage. The *Exploratory Tantra* states:[3]

> Physicians will achieve the highest state of
> the realization of Buddhahood, as was said
> by the King of Bédurya Light.

This lineage is known as *kama*, which refers to it being a direct and blessed teaching (*jinlap kyi ka*) from the Medicine Buddha. According to more contemporary historical methods, it is difficult to trace this unbroken line from Vāgbhaṭa back to the Buddha. Vāgbhaṭa's *Aṣtangahṛdayasaṁhitā* and Candrānandana's commentary are considered authentic Indian sources of the *Gyüzhi*.

Vairocana returned to Samyé and offered the translation to the emperor. Trisong Detsen presented it to Guru Padmasambhava and, according to his advice, the *Gyüzhi* was hidden in a pillar on the monastery's middle floor. Padmasambhava ordered Shing Jachen to be the chief protector of this hidden treasure text. The time was not ripe for the *Four*

---

3   G.yu thog yon tan mgon po, 1993, 101.

Tantras to be disseminated. It is also possible that Padmasambhava knew the demise of the monarchy in Tibet was at hand through his clairvoyance, and that a dark period would follow. He hid the text to avoid the destruction of the *Gyüzhi*, preserving it for future generations. It remained there in the pillar as a hidden treasure for more than 150 years. Finally, it was revealed by the treasure revealer Drapa Ngönshé.

Terma literature

Terma means "hidden treasure." It could be anything, for example a precious stone or a buried text. It is popular in Tibetan society, particularly in relation to religious circles and especially in the Nyingma and Bön traditions. Much literature is available regarding tantra, medicine and astrology.[4]

The first origin of *terma* is that during the reign of Trisong Detsen, there was persecution of indigenous ritual practices. Much Bön literature was burnt or thrown into rivers. Many of these texts were copied by Bön scholars such as Drenpa Namkha and hidden in various mountain caves, rocks, and huts. They kept these locations secret, which began to be revealed from the 10th and 11th centuries onwards. The first *terma* revealers (*tertön*) are *Bönpo* scholars. A second origin is Guru Rinpoché. He and his consort Yéshé Tsogyel hid many Buddhist, medical, and astrological texts to avoid their destruction during the revolutions and unrest in the 10th century. These texts were then later rediscovered. Many *terma* revealed by Bonpo and Buddhist scholars were merged, and literature was exchanged between groups of practitioners. The influence of such *terma* literature on medicine is considerable. Future research on *terma* medicine could provide fascinating insights into the development of Sowa Rigpa.

Drapa Ngönshé (1012–1090) was an eminent scholar with a powerful capacity to study, who constructed hundreds of monasteries. His existence was foretold by Guru Padmasambhava:[5]

> These times one people is worse than the other: the Jing[6] and the Chinese are fighting like ants in disturbed anthills. At this time, the hidden medicine treasure of Samyé Pagoda and the hidden treasure in the Three Sisters' Mountains will come to be revealed by a man called Drapa Ngönshé.

Tertön Drapa Ngönshé was born in the water-bird year of 1012 and became an important historical figure. He studied medicine with his uncle. He had a vision of Zhanglön, the protector deity of the *Gyüzhi*, who implored him to reveal it. According to Khétsün Rinpoché's work, Drapa Ngönshé revealed the *Gyüzhi* in the year of the earth tiger at midnight of the full moon (corresponding to 1038 CE), from the central pillar at Samyé Monastery.[7] Tibetan medical histories also indicate that Drapa Ngönshé composed a summary of the *Gyüzhi* that was passed on to Üpa Dardrak, and then to Tsalungpa Tsojé Könchok Kyap. The latter composed a text called *The Wheel of Pacifying and Repulsing Critics* (*Rtsod bzlog gegs sel 'khor lo*) to clear up points raised by followers of the *Aṣṭāṅgahṛdaya* translation. Yutok the Younger composed 18 works, which were mostly supplementary (including *Sman gzhung cha lag bco rgyad*). He propagated these in the later part of his life, giving instructions to Sumtön Yéshézung and his own son Bumseng. Soon his teachings began to flourish all over Tibet.

The age of Yutok the Younger

In the early renaissance, Tibetans took up the idea of going to India to study Buddhism and medicine. Some became great translators (*lotsawa*) and masters. After over three centuries of turmoil, many parents sent their young sons to India, via Nepal and other routes. One of them was to become the enlightened master-physician Yutok Yönten Gönpo, otherwise known as Yutok the Younger.

Yutok was exceptional from an early age. He was born to his father named Khyungpo Dorjé and mother Péma Öden in the fire-horse year of 1126 at Nyangtö Gozhi Rétang (Sgo bzhi re thang). He came from a family of physicians. His birthplace lies at a distance of approximately 20 kilometers from Gyangtsé city in the upper part of Tibet.[8] He is believed to have been an emanation of the Medicine Buddha, and he acknowledged himself to be a manifestation of Bodhisattva Mañjuśrī. He studied medicine with his father from an early age, beginning when he was only eight years old. He also studied various medical traditions under the Nine Experts (Mkhas pa mi dgu). However, Yutok was not satisfied with the knowledge available in Tibet at the time. To study more deeply, he traveled to Persia and China,

---

4   Arya pa sangs yon tan, 2021 (1989), 85–94.

5   Sde srid sangs rgyas rgya mtsho, 1982, 202.

6   The Jurchen people, a Chinese ethnic minority.

7   Mkhas btsun bzang po, 1973, 275.

8   The author visited Yutok's birthplace in 2004, following instructions from Jampa Trinlé, director of Lhasa Mentsikhang. Dr. Trinlé had constructed a small temple there in Yutok's memory, but the land seemed different from what can be inferred from Yutok's biography.

and undertook trips to India via Nepal no less than six times. Details of his travels and of his extraordinary powers can be found in his biographies.[9] For example, once he is said to have returned to Tibet from India via Nepal in just one day, bringing fresh *arura* leaves to show to his disciples.

Yutok became a great expert on Vāgbhaṭa's *Aṣṭāṅgahṛdayasaṃhitā* and the *Chandrika*, from which his teachings are derived, as well as the whole of the ayurvedic tradition as it existed at that time in India and Tibet. He brought many treatises to Tibet, which were to become the essence of the ocean of Indo-Tibetan medical science. He gathered many disciples and wrote numerous works. More than 30 titles claim his authorship, but the *Gyüzhi* remains the essence of all his efforts.

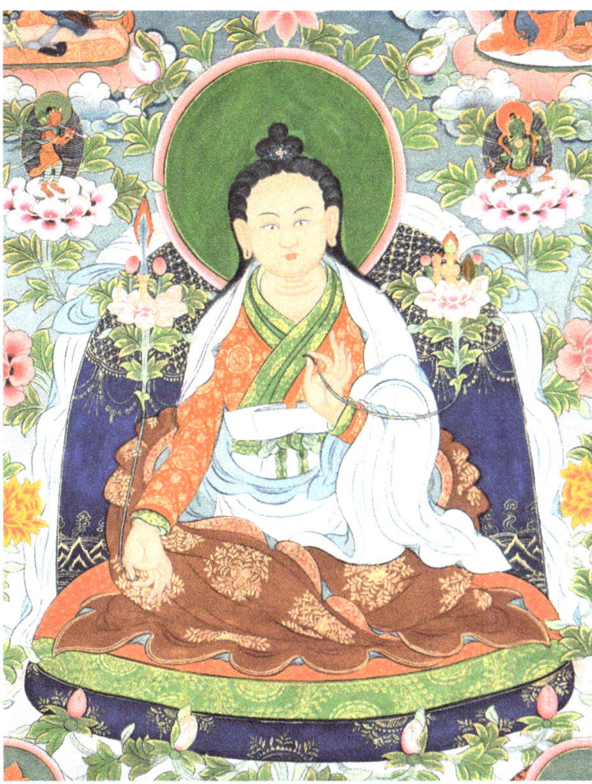

FIGURE 2.2 Yutok the Younger

The authorship of the *Gyüzhi*

The *Gyüzhi* is like all Mahayana teachings: it is considered by its proponents to be part of a lineage extending back to Buddha Śākyamuni. On the other hand, scholars attribute the composition of the *Gyüzhi* to the Younger Yutok. Many scholars avoid the dispute,

attempting to properly acknowledge and retain both views of the work's origins, without discarding any vital aspects. From the author's point of view, both sides have validity, their differences being more a matter of interpretation. Some scholars have interpreted the origins of the *Four Tantras* as follows:

- Externally (generally), it was taught by the Buddha (as the Medicine Buddha)

- Internally, it is the work of a pandita (cf. Vāgbhaṭa's *Aṣṭāṅgahṛdayasaṃhitā*)

- Secretly, it is the work of Yutok the Younger

Both Yutok the Elder (Yutok Nyingma) and the Younger (Yutok Sarma) are highly respected and recognized by all schools of Tibetan Buddhism as emanations of the Medicine Buddha. They have similar biographies, full of mystery and miracle powers. However, the Elder Yutok's story is difficult to situate. Hence, the Younger Yutok's biography may well be more historically accurate. Yutok Sarma made two different annotations of the *Four Tantras*. The first, dedicated to his sons and written with golden ink is called Serchen (Gser mchan). The second, dedicated to his disciples and written in black ink, is called Zongchen (Zong mchan). The first is said to be more detailed than the second. The earlier part of Yutok's life was devoted to becoming an expert on the *Aṣṭāṅgahṛdaya*, and the latter part was dedicated to instructing his heart disciple Sumtön Yéshézung and his son Bumseng.

The true story of the origins of the *Gyüzhi* is described in Yutok the Younger's medico-spiritual practice, in the history chapter of the *Yutok Nyingtik* (*G.yu thog snying thig*) that was written down by Sumtön following Yutok's instructions:[10]

> Having achieved the two *siddhi* in one in
> this life, and after having a vision of the
> *yidam* and receiving their blessings,
> I finished composing the medical treatise,
> which is not different from the highest
> tantras.

After completing this composition, Buddhas and bodhisattvas appeared in the sky from the 10 directions, who proclaimed:

> *A LA LA!* Well done my son. In the future,
> your work will be of great benefit to all
> sentient beings.

---

9 Dar mo sman ram pa blo bzang chos sgrags, 1984.

10 G.yu thog yon tan mgon po, undated blockprint published by Bkra shis g.yang 'phal, 8.

Yutok structured the *Gyüzhi* as a teaching by Sangyé Menla and the Five Buddhas. Zurkhar Lodrö Gyelpo, in his *Root Tantra* commentary, correlates the four medical traditions of Tanaduk with the four directions of Yutok's Gozhi Rétang School and with his four disciples. Dési Sangyé Gyatso agreed with Zurkharwa in saying that Yutok was a fully enlightened yogi-physician and an emanation of the Medicine Buddha, but his authorship remains somewhat hidden. Nevertheless, both stated that there was no reason to doubt his words. According to this generally held point of view, the Medicine Buddha was ultimately the one who taught the *Gyüzhi* and initiated the Tibetan medical tradition, which has come down in an unbroken lineage to the present day. Yutok accepted that he was the reincarnation of Jīvaka of Buddha's time, who subsequently reincarnated as Nāgārjunacarya, Vāgbhaṭa, Kyébu Mélha, Gampopa, and finally as Yutok the Younger himself.

Yutok Nyingtik, the tantric medical lineage

Yutok Sarma's biography tells us that in the later part of his life, he and about 300 of his disciples left for Kyirong (Skyid grong), where he had been invited by the local king. There, he performed a great offering to the Jowo Rangjungwati Zangpo, the Avalokiteśvara statue that was brought from Nepal during King Songtsen Gampo's reign. One day, while Yutok was sitting in front of this statue, a bright light radiated from it accompanied by the sounds of the mantras of Avalokiteśvara and the Medicine Buddha. The statue spoke to Yutok and prophesized the future. After that, Yutok transmitted his "heart essence" cycle, the *Yutok Nyingtik,* to his chief disciple Sumtön Yéshézung.[11] Master and disciples came back to Gozhi Rétang, and instructions were given to Yutok's sons, daughters, and other important disciples.

Yutok left for Tanaduk, Medicine Buddha's pure land, at the age of 76 (1202 CE). Sumtön and Bumseng later passed on the *Gyüzhi* and Yutok's other teachings to their disciples. This remains the living tradition of Sowa Rigpa. Sumtön held the main medical transmission as well as the *Yutok Nyingtik,* while Bumseng, continued his father's tradition at home, holding the seat of the Gozhi Rétang house. Sumtön's lineage became the main transmission of these simultaneously medical and spiritual teachings. Through his effort, the tradition spread like a Banyan tree all over Tibet, across the Himalayan regions, and beyond.

---

11 He is considered an emanation of Avalokiteśvara.

2.4 TIBETAN MEDICAL SCHOOLS

During the reign of the Tibetan kings and emperors and due their influence in neighboring countries, many masters and scholars came to Tibet like swans gathering on a lake. Buddhism and the secular sciences developed. During the reign of Songtsen Gampo, Indian, Persian, Chinese, and other sources were introduced. Three medical schools were officially propagated: (1) Indian medicine via Bharadwaja, (2) Chinese medicine via Henwen Hangte, and (3) the Upper Tradition (Töluk) related to Galéno.

Nine foreign physicians were invited in Trison Deutsen's time. He requested them to teach local students and pass on their knowledge and expertise. Their main disciples were nine Tibetan scholar-physicians. They became the roots of Sowa Rigpa. Among them, the lineages of Yutok, Drangti Gyelnyé Kharbu, and Nyapa Chözang have been blessed with many disciples. The abovementioned three and nine schools can be summarized into three traditions based on their time of development:

1. Galenic and Indian medicine-based ancient medical schools (7–8th centuries onwards)

2. Rinchen Zangpo's *Yenlak Gyépa* tradition (10th century onwards)

3. Yutok Sarma's *Gyüzhi* lineage (12th century onwards)

Later on, the two earlier traditions integrated further with *Gyüzhi* medicine, emerging as a single dominant medical system. However, some important historical works strongly affiliated to these other lineages are still available.

The Jangpa tradition

Jangpa Namgyel Drakzang (1395–1475) was born in the city of Ngamring (Ngam ring). During his life, Namgyel Drakzang was recognized as an incarnation of Dharma King Sucandra of Shambala. He oversaw the construction of a complete three-dimensional Kālacakra mandala alongside many other enlightened activities and the composition of Dharma treatises. He founded a local monastic community, yet excelled in particular in the science of medicine. His medical contributions—more than a dozen titles, including commentaries on the *Gyüzhi* and the *Aṣṭanga*—led to a renaissance of Sowa Rigpa and laid the foundation for the Northern or Jangpa Tradition. He and his many followers invented numerous new formulas and were experts in the treatment of infectious disease. Their identification of herbs is slightly different, but has been kept a living tradition up to this day.

The Zurkhar tradition

Zurkhar Nyamnyi Dorjé (1439–1475) was a great yogi-physician from the southern part of Central Tibet. Born into a family medical lineage, he received teachings from his father as well Shara Rapjampa, Taklung Ngawang Drakpa, and others. At the age of 10, he had a vision of Yutok Sarma. Yutok transmitted oral instructions on his medical and tantric works, requesting Nyamnyi Dorjé to correct the interpretation mistakes made by later scholars. Nyamnyi Dorjé taught physicians in the Dakpo (Dwags po) and Kongpo valleys, and authored the extensive *Relic of Millions* (*Bye ba ring bsrel*, with more than 400 sections) as well as *Gyüzhi* commentaries. He was also an expert in the alchemical process of mercury purification, with many precious pill formulas coming from his texts. Even though he passed away at the young age of 37, the Zurkhar tradition continues to flourish across the Himalayas. His nephew, the monk-physician Zurkhar Lodrö Gyelpo (1509–1579), later composed the detailed historical reference work *Oral Instructions of the Forefathers* (*Mes po'i zhal lung*).

The Gongmen tradition

The brilliant scholar Könchok Pendar (1511–1577) was initially encouraged to study medicine alongside his monastic training by his mother to support his financially strained family. Könchok Pendar first learned Sowa Rigpa from his brother, and the medical master Gongmen Könchok Délek (1477–1506) was his maternal uncle. He then became the personal physician of the regent of a town in the Sakya (Sa skya) area, receiving instructions from Drangti Chögyel Tashi at Sakya Medical College (Sa skya sman grong). Könchok Pendar composed a comprehensive three-volume collection known as *Fulfilling All Needs Within the Science of Healing* (*Gso rig dgos pa kun 'byung*), gaining fame throughout the Land of Snow and attracting many disciples. His teachings and those of his uncle constitute the Gongmen tradition, which later became especially adept in tantric and yogic healing techniques.

Chakpori and later medical colleges (17th century–)

The ensuing centuries, the lineages of Sowa Rigpa succeeded to survive and flourish in changing times. Fortunately, the Fifth Dalai Lama (1617–1682) became a great patron of medicine, although his work was unfinished when he passed away. To fulfill his aims, his regent and chief disciple Dési Sangyé Gyatso (1653–1705) founded Chakpori Medical College in Lhasa in 1696, on Iron Hill (Lcags po ri) next to the Potala Palace. Traditionally, Tibetans respect this place as the abode of the deity Vajrapāṇi, who is important for the Potala's stability. The Dési was a genius: an extraordinary scholar well versed in secular sciences, sutra and tantra, and especially in the sciences of healing and astrology. He printed a re-edited edition of the *Gyüzhi* at Dratang (Gra thang) and wrote an extensive commentary on it titled *Blue Beryl*.[12] He attempted to clarify the concepts and practices of the *Gyüzhi* and keep them pure by means of his commentary and the direct teachings he gave at Chakpori. He distributed his *Blue Beryl* to contemporary physicians for them to review it. To the Dési's disapproval, hardly any critique of his work was provided.

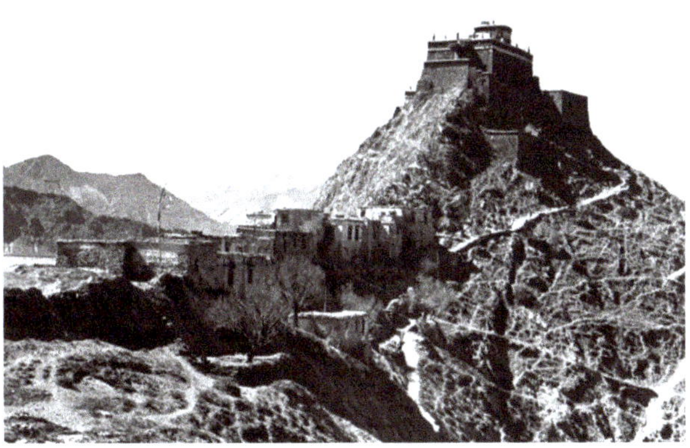

FIGURE 2.3 Chakpori Hill with the old medical college at its top (1938/1939)

Sangyé Gyatso also oversaw the production of 77 excellent medical *tangka* paintings, engaging numerous artists. His idea to create illustrations appears to have been developed based on the Lhündingpa Tradition (Lhun lding lugs). To update pathology and medical practice, he composed the *Mengak Lhentap* (*Man ngag lhan thabs*), which contains 133 chapters. The *Mirror of Beryl*, in which he traces the origins of

---

12 Sde srid sangs rgyas rgya mtsho, 1994.

Sowa Rigpa up until the 17th century, was the crown on his work.[13]

The Dési further composed the *White Beryl* (*BaiDUr dkar po*), which laid the foundation for Tibetan astrology and the almanac, combining astronomy, astrology, and the Indian zodiac. He distributed this work amongst scholars as well, receiving 208 questions from critics in return. He was extremely pleased with this, and composed the two-volume *Bédur Yasel* (*BaiDUr dkar po las 'khrul snang g.ya' sel*), in order to fully clear up the points raised. These works have since guided Tibetan astrologers in theory and practice without any hindrance.

Dési Sangyé Gyatso inaugurated Chakpori as a medical monastery, a center for the study and training of physicians. Thanks to the government's support, Chakpori became a successful institution for the teaching and preservation of the Tibetan art of healing. Sangyé Gyatso invited many scholars to teach their ancient traditions, thereby preserving valuable heritage for the benefit of younger generations. He collected many young monks from different regional monasteries, providing them training as physicians. The Dési personally administrated the institute, transmitted the *Gyüzhi*, gave teachings on his commentaries, and set up a curriculum. After their graduation, the young physicians were sent back to their monasteries—which were often in remote villages—to serve local people. They received an official graduation certificate and the authorization to practice medicine. Chakpori soon became known as a city of physicians. It was the greatest center in history for the study of Sowa Rigpa and its medico-spiritual practice. Hundreds of great physicians were trained there. Dési Sangyé Gyatso's legacy revitalized Tibetan medicine. Unfortunately, he was assassinated in 1705, at Tölung, perhaps by Lhasang Khan's wife. His remembrance stupa still stands at the place he met his end. This unforgiveable episode was a great loss, especially for the intellectual community. After his demise, the pace of Tibetan medicine slowed down due to political instability and economic fluctuations. Although the Chakpori College became a permanent facility for monks to reside, the study of medicine and astrology strongly declined, like a lamp consumed by water.

Tibetan medical colleges in the 20th century and beyond

Over 200 years later, in 1916, the Venerable Khyenrap Norbu (1883–1962) founded Mentsikhang (Sman rtsis khang) during the reign of the 13th Dalai Lama. His aim was to bring about a new elan for the study of medicine by training physicians. He taught medicine, astrology, and all the other secular sciences as Mentsikhang's first director. Monks and nuns as well as laypeople were accepted without restrictions to become professional physicians and astrologers. In a short period of time, Mentsikhang was overwhelmed by students coming from Tibet and neighboring countries.

In the wake of the Chinese communist invasion, many Tibetans fled to India. The Indian government not only hosted the refugees but also supported efforts to preserve and develop their culture, arts, and religion. In 1961, in the Indian hill town of Dharamsala, His Holiness the 14th Dalai Lama re-established Men-Tsee-Khang as a college for Tibetan medicine and astrology. His Holiness gathered eminent doctors to teach Sowa Rigpa to younger generations. The aim of this institute was and is to preserve the traditional Tibetan medical system. Sowa Rigpa is now also taught in other colleges across India, including the Central Institute of Higher Tibetan Studies in Sarnath, the Central Institute for Buddhist Studies in Ladakh, and Chagpori Tibetan Medical Institute in Darjeeling. In 2010, the Indian government officially recognized Sowa Rigpa as a traditional medical system under the Ministry of AYUSH (Ayurveda, Yoga, Naturopathy, Unani, Siddha, Sowa Rigpa, and Homoeopathy).

Sowa Rigpa has indeed been practiced for centuries in the Indian Himalayas (especially in Ladakh), as well as in the highlands of Bhutan and Nepal. It also spread and developed greatly across the Mongolian steppes, and into the Buddhist republics of Russia (Buryatia and Kalmykia). In these countries, a number of medical colleges has been established with varying support from governments. Over the past few decades, Tibetan medicine in China has become a booming industry with large specialized drug factories and hospitals, and university-level education for practitioners.

---

13 *Sde srid sangs rgyas mtsho*, 1982. This volume is a precious jewel of ancient Tibetan medicine, especially concerning anatomy (*rotra*) and surgery (*turché*).

CHAPTER 3

THE STRUCTURE OF THE *GYÜZHI*

Before studying the content of the *Four Tantras* (*Gyüzhi*), one should know its structure and the relationship between its parts. The *Gyüzhi* consists of four volumes and has 156 chapters, containing in all about 5,900 stanzas (Sanskrit: *śloka*). There are several reasons for why there are four volumes.

Firstly, the *Four Medical Tantras* were composed according to the different capacities of pupils, with the aim of leading them on a gradual path towards an ever-higher level of understanding. The text therefore starts with the smallest volume, the *Root Tantra*, which is a synopsis of the entire *Gyüzhi* in six chapters. The second volume, the *Explanatory Tantra*, deepens the engagement with medical theory and praxis over its 31 chapters. The third *Oral Instruction Tantra* is the largest, with 92 chapters covering pathologies, whilst the *Subsequent Tantra*—spanning 27 chapters—concludes with more concrete diagnostic and therapeutic practices. The *Gyüzhi* thus contains 156 chapters in total.

Secondly, the relation between the *Tantras* is like the structure of a tree. The first tantra provides the root and is therefore called the *Root Tantra* or *Tsa(wé)gyü* (*Rtsa ba'i rgyud*). The root grows a trunk and branches that form the body of the tree; this is the *Explanatory Tantra* or *Shé(pé)gyü* (*Bshad pa'i rgyud*). The leaves and flower buds on the branches of this tree represent the *Oral Instruction Tantra* or *Mengakgyü* (*Man ngag rgyud*). The buds blossom, becoming flowers and producing fruits, which correspond to the *Action* or *Subsequent Tantra* (*Chimagyü*, *Phyi ma rgyud*).

The *Tsagyü* is suited to students of the highest intelligence; those who are capable of understanding and practicing after only a brief period of study. It is very succinct yet profound, like an ocean or like the sky. It presents the foundation of Sowa Rigpa, the essence of knowledge about the physiology, etiology, pathology, diagnosis, and treatment of the three humors. At the end, there is a summary in the form of an allegorical medicine tree, which synthesizes the essential points. Such medicine trees are a unique characteristic of the Tibetan medical tradition. The *Root Tantra* acts as an antidote to hatred and its resultant disorders and symptoms (such as bile and fever, being angry, and holding grudges) in particular. The *Subsequent Tantra*'s 27th chapter, the entrustment, states:[1]

> The *Root Heart Tantra* is like a seed:
> there is no healing science not born from it.

The *Shégyü* was taught for pupils with an intermediate level of intelligence; those who are interested in gaining detailed knowledge on anatomy, physiology, etiology, disease classification, dietetics, behavior, materia medica, surgical instruments, therapeutic and diagnostic methods, and the ethical code of conduct of physicians. It shows the knowledge of the body-mind like the sun and moon that expel darkness. On a more spiritual level, it is said that the *Explanatory Tantra* is chiefly an antidote to ignorance. It cures diseases manifesting from closed-mindedness (such as phlegmatic diseases, often involving feeling heavy). The *Subsequent Tantra*'s entrustment chapter states:[2]

> The *Body Explanatory Tantra* is like the sun
> and moon shining in the sky:
> it clearly teaches terms and meanings
> without obscuration.

The *Mengakgyü* is for students who need more detailed and direct instructions, being tailored to students of third-level intelligence. This treatise describes pathogenesis, disease classification, diagnosis, and therapies extensively, as well as humoral pathologies, chronic internal diseases, fevers, the head, the organs, and genital, miscellaneous and congenital diseases, pediatrics, gynecology, psychiatry, wounds, poisons, geriatrics, and rejuvenation. The *Oral Instruction Tantra*

---

1 G.yu thog yon tan mgon po, 1993, 664.

2 Ibid.

is an antidote to pride, greed, and miserliness. It is a wish-fulfilling treasure vase that cures the manifestation of physical and mental disorders. The *Subsequent Tantra*'s entrustment chapter says:[3]

    The *Qualities Oral Instruction Tantra* is like a jewel:
    it contains all necessities without lacking any.

The *Subsequent Tantra* is for students who focus more on practical application than on philosophical and theoretical aspects of medicine. It is for the fourth level of intelligence, including direct practical teachings on pulse and urine diagnosis, the 10 different ways of making medicines, and therapies such as purgatives, emetics, nasal therapies, clysters, vein cleaning, venesection, moxibustion, fomentation, medicinal baths, oil therapy, and surgery. The last two chapters give advice to all students on how to keep the tradition and best ensure its continuation. The *Chimagyü* is known as an antidote to jealousy, fear, desire, and obsession. It cures all diseases derived from these mental states. Chapter 27 states:[4]

    The *Activity Subsequent Tantra* is like a diamond:
    there is no obstruction to the treatment of disease.

The fifth chapter of this volume also concludes:[5]

    The complete assemblage of the *Tantras* is like a soaring *garuḍa*,
    fearlessly flying over the cliffs of disease.

A third reason behind the structure of the *Gyüzhi* is related to the Five Buddhas as transmitters of the *Four Tantras*, which provides an important link between the traditions of medicine and spiritual healing. Everything manifests from mind and mental states. Disease is connected to negative emotions, so its cure necessarily involves healing and purifying the body-mind. Although these Buddhas are an integral part of the *Gyüzhi*, it is important to remember that the meaning of the word "tantra" (*gyü*) in its title is not identical to its use in the context of Vajrayāna teachings. In the *Four Medical Tantras*, tantra refers to continuity: the continuation of the knowledge system and practices that preserve and transmit the tradition that protects the lives of beings.

All *Four Tantras* explain the eight branches of Sowa Rigpa, the science of healing. They are like the ground from which the medicine trees grow. The treatises are in fact themselves referred to as "the eight branches of medicine." The *Oral Instruction Tantra* in particular describes each branch systematically from the perspective of pathology. These eight branches are also the main subjects of specialization for advanced medical studies.

---

3   Ibid.
4   Ibid.

5   Ibid., 665.

TABLE 3.1 The Five Buddhas and the *Gyüzhi*

Five Buddhas	Four *Tantras*	Chakras (colors)	Buddha qualities	Transmuted emotions and disorders
Akshobhya, Mikyö Rikpé Yéshé	*Root Tantra* (*Tsagyü*)	Heart chakra (blue)	Mirror-like wisdom	Hatred, anger, and bile disorders
Vairocana, Nangta Rikpé Yéshé	*Explanatory Tantra* (*Shégyü*)	Crown chakra (white)	Absolute wisdom	Ignorance, closed-mindedness, and phlegm disorders
Ratnasambhava, Rinjung Rikpé Yéshé	*Oral Instruction Tantra* (*Mengakgyü*)	Navel chakra (yellow)	Wisdom of equanimity	Miserliness, greed, pride, and combined disorders
Amoghasiddhi, Jadrup Rikpé Yéshé	*Subsequent Tantra* (*Chimégyü*)	Secret chakra (green)	Wisdom of accomplishment	Jealousy, lust, desire, wind and psychological disorders
Amitābha, Sortok Rikpé Yéshé	Questioner of the four Rikpé Yéshé	Throat chakra (red)	Wisdom of discernment	Attachment, wind and bile disorders

TABLE 3.2 The eight branches of medicine

	Eight branches	Translation (corresponding modern subject)
1.	*Lü*	The body (internal or general medicine)
2.	*Jipa*	Children (pediatrics)
3.	*Mo né*	Women's diseases (gynecology)
4.	*Dön*	Evil spirits (psychiatry)
5.	*Tsön*	Wounds (traumatology)
6.	*Duk*	Poisons (toxicology)
7.	*Gépa*	The aged (geriatrics)
8.	*Rotsawa, bümé tselwa*	Aphrodisiacs and fertility (infertility)

3.1 THE DISCOURSE

Traditionally, teaching on the *Gyüzhi* starts with the five virtuous factors (*géwa nga*), which are explained in a similar fashion to other teachings of the Buddha. This indicates that the subject being taught is perfect in every detail; that there is nothing misleading about it. The *Gyüzhi* can be taught in accordance with the following five factors: (1) excellent teaching, (2) suitable place, (3) good disciples, (4) right time, and (5) supreme teacher. In the context of the dharma, all five must be present. However, in this volume we start with the title of the *Four Tantras*, proceeding with a simpler way to understand its contents. The treatise's title is given in Sanskrit and Tibetan at the very beginning, after which homage is paid to the Medicine Buddha (Sangyé Menla) with verses attributed to the translator Vairocana. The title of the *Gyüzhi* is:

Amṛta hṛdaya aṅga aṣṭa guhya upadeśa tantra nāma (Sanskrit, transliteration)

༄༅། །བདུད་རྩི་སྙིང་པོ་ཡན་ལག་བརྒྱད་པ་གསང་བ་
མན་ངག་གི་རྒྱུད་ཅེས་བྱ་བ་བཞུགས་སོ།

(Tibetan script)

Bdud rtsi snying po yan lag brgyad pa gsang ba man ngag gi rgyud ces bya ba bzhugs so (Wylie transliteration)

Dütsi nyingpo yenlak gyépa sangwa mengak gi gyü chéjawa zhuk so (phonetics)

Quintessential Ambrosia of the Eight Branches: The Secret Pith Instruction Tantras

Word-by-word meaning:

- *amṛta*: nectar, immortality-granting ambrosia
- *hṛdaya*: heart essence
- *aṅga*: branch, limb, or division
- *aṣṭa*: eight
- *guhya*: secret (for the three types of unqualified students)
- *upadeśa*: pith instruction, direct (oral) transmission
- *tantra*: continuity of lineage, keeping alive; treatise
- *nāma*: "(it is) called," respectful indication of a text's title

First the translator pays homage to the Sangyé Menla, Bhaiṣajyaguru-vaiḍūryaprabhārāja:

I prostrate to the King of Aquamarine Light, Buddha Bédurya Ökyi Gyelpo, the Master of Medicine and Awakened One who acts to benefit living beings, protects them from the miseries of inferior realms, and dispels the three mental poisons and their resulting ailments, merely by hearing his name.

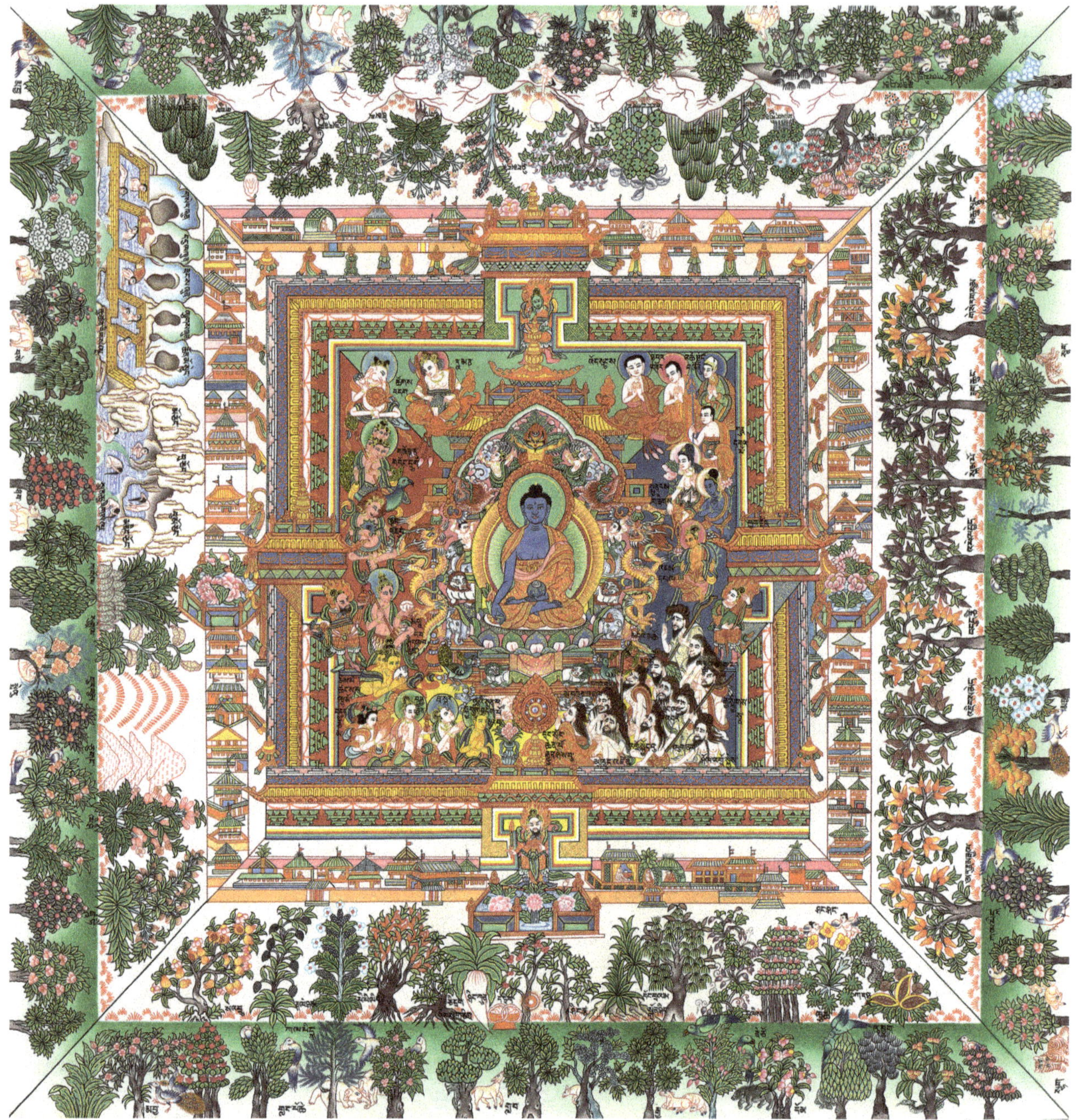

FIGURE 3.1 The mandala of Sudarśana (Tanaduk)

Tanaduk, the city where the *Four Tantras* was expounded

Then, Buddha Bédurya begins to expound the *Root Tantra*:

> In the land of sages, Tanaduk, the City of Medicine, was spontaneously accomplished from five precious materials, with a palace decorated by various kinds of healing gems.

This sentence can be considered the beginning of the *Gyüzhi*, which describes where the *Gyüzhi*'s discourse takes place. Because Varanasi (Bihar, India) is known as "the place where a sage fell" (*Drang srong lhung ba ri dags kyi gnas*)—which refers to an ancient legend—this area might be the right location for the origins of *Gyüzhi*'s story. Generally, *Gyüzhi* followers accept that the text was expounded by Buddha Shakyamuni in the form of the Medicine Buddha, from the city of Tanaduk (Skt. Sudarśana). Tanaduk (Lta na sdug) means "beautiful to behold."

There are different opinions amongst scholars regarding the precise location of Tanaduk. The Fifth Dalai Lama, Lozang Gyatso (Blo bzang rgya mtsho) believes it lies in Oḍḍiyāna.[6] Zurkhar Lodrö Gyelpo (Zur mkhar blo gros rgyal po) described it as being in the Medicine Forest, which is somewhere in India, probably in Varanasi. Jangpa believed it to be in Bodh Gaya (also in Bihar). The author's personal interpretation is that it is a pure land that is not visible to the ordinary eye. The ability to see it depends on spiritual experience and insight. Therefore, it cannot be revealed by scientific research or by any other material means such as archeological findings.

Wherever it may be, Buddha Shakyamuni instantaneously accomplished its transformation into Tanaduk, the pure land of the Medicine Buddha: a miraculous paradise of healing surrounded by four mountains. Shakyamuni then transformed himself into Medicine Buddha Bhaiṣajyaguruvaiḍūryaprabhārāja, a buddha of a deep blue yet translucent beryl color, seated on a bejeweled teaching throne. Four heavenly guardian kings and 12 *yakṣa* generals guard the palace together with their retinues. Tanaduk is a spacious medicine city. Four great medicine mountains, located in each of the four directions, surround the city. It is rich in medicinal plants, flowers, fruits, minerals, and animals. Buddha Bédurya's palace stands at the center, made of five precious substances (gold, silver, white and red pearls, and blue beryl). Its walls, pillars, and roof are made from gems of the human realm. Deva and bodhisattva gems with 14 qualities turn the palace transparent and luminous. The human gems have seven qualities: they have the clear color of pureness, they cure poisoning, expel evil spirits and darkness, heal swelling, relieve fever, ease pain, and fulfill wishes. The deva gems have four additional qualities: they accompany one wherever one goes in this land, they are perfectly pure, have the ability to speak, and they emit a wonderful light. Bodhisattva gems have three more qualities than the deva gems: enabling one to know the time of the death of beings, to predict life-changing events, and granting knowledge about the end of life and liberation. By the power of these gems and Medicine Buddha's blue-colored rays, there is no difference between day and night. The gems and medicines become cooling in power for hot diseases, and warming against cold diseases, effortlessly curing all disease. They cure all diseases manifested from *lung*, *tripa*, *béken*, and combined disorders (*düpa*). They also pacify the 404 diseases and the 1080 obstacle makers (*gek rik*, types of evil spirits which can cause disease). Occasionally, gems, medicinal trees, herbs, religious banners, and flags produce the beautiful sounds of the Dharma: the Buddhist teachings that have the power to heal the diseases of body, speech, and mind. The breeze and even birdsong whistle mantras. These medicinal gardens and mountains exist in serene eternal peace, gem trees and flowers blossoming profusely around the palace. There are no seasonal changes here. Birds, bees, and countless animals enjoy their life without fear or hunger. There is no sorrow caused by the four sufferings of rebirth, aging, sickness, and dying. In short, this is a pure land, the sacred abode of King of Aquamarine Light.

There are multiple interpretations of Tanaduk. In the biography of Yutok Yönten Gönpo the Elder, for instance, Buddha Bédurya states that outer, inner, and secret cities of Tanaduk coexist:[7]

> There are three medicine cities: outer, inner, and secret.
> The Outer Tanaduk is found in India, and Oḍḍiyāna in the west,
> O'g min,[8] or at the top of Mount Sumeru.
> Wherever you pray, fortunate son, you will get a vision of this pure land.
>
> The Inner City of Tanaduk is wherever you are, you yourself are Buddha Bédurya.
>
> The Secret City called Tanaduk is the great blissfulness chakra at the crown (center).
> Think that your mind is *bédurya* light, and that the throat enjoyment chakra is Malaya Mountain (Ma la ya, west),
> the dharma heart chakra is Pöngéden Mountain (Spos ngad ldan, east),
> the navel manifestation chakra is Bikjé Mountain ('Bigs byed, south),
> and the secret bliss-sustaining chakra is Gangchen Mountain (Gangs can, north).
>
> Go to these four mountains.
> Observe their qualities and the places where medicines grow.
> Collect the important teachings from India, and light the lamp of medicine in Central Tibet.
> To protect the people of the Land of Snow, stay there for 125 years.
> Then, return to Tanaduk, the City of Medicine, to lead the assembly of heroic lineage holders,
> without doubt or hesitation.

---

6 A sacred, mystic place of tantric Buddhism that has several names. It is believed to be an ancient kingdom situated in the Swat Valley of modern-day Pakistan.

7 Dar mo sman rams pa blo bzang chos grags, 1984, 168–69.

8 Akaniṣṭha or "Heaven Beneath None," is a miraculous heavenly place where bodhisattvas will take rebirth to complete their paths to enlightenment.

The four mountains listed above can also be identified externally. Gangchen, for example, directly refers to the Himalayas, whereas Bikjé is also a name for the Vindhya Range of Central India.

Medicine Buddha Bédurya Ökyi Gyelpo

In the center of the palace, the Supreme Healer, Medicine Buddha Bédurya[9] Ökyi Gyelpo is seated on a throne facing east. He holds a branch of chebulic myrobalan (*arura*) in his right hand as a symbol of the antidote to all physical ailments, and a bowl of ambrosial nectar (*dütsi*) in his left hand that stands for the spiritual awakening that cures ignorance and mental afflictions. The throne is made of red, white, yellow, and blue gems and covered by heavenly silks. It is flanked by eight lions and phoenix birds, all in vibrant colors.

Sangyé Menla's body is transparent and of a deep blue beryl color. Like all other buddhas, it is adorned with the 80 signs of perfect beauty and the 32 great marks. Dressed in a maroon silk robe, he is peaceful in appearance, sending healing light to samsara that liberates sentient beings from disease and suffering. The surroundings consist of medicinal ingredients, religious banners and bells, nectar water springs and rivers, and so on. The beauty and qualities of the Tanaduk palace are beyond that of the human and deva realms. The wish-fulfilling trees, flowers, and religious objects are moved by a gentle wind carrying a splendid fragrance along with the sound of cosmic harmony, Medicine Buddha's healing mantra:

ཨོཾ་ན་མོ་བྷ་ག་ཝ་ཏེ། བྷཻ་ཥ་ཛྱེ་གུ་རུ་བཻ་ཌཱུ་ཪྻ་པྲ་ར་ཛཱ་ཡ།
ཏ་ཐཱ་ག་ཏཱ་ཡ། ཨ་ཪྷ་ཏེ་ས་མྱཀྶཾ་བུ་དྡྷཱ་ཡ། ཏ་དྱ་ཐཱ།
ཨོཾ་བྷཻ་ཥ་ཛྱེ་བྷཻ་ཥ་ཛྱེ། མ་ཧཱ་བྷཻ་ཥ་ཛྱེ་བྷཻ་ཥ་ཛྱེ། ཪཱ་ཛཱ་ཡ་ས་མུ་དྒ་ཏེ་སྭཱ་ཧཱ།

OM NAMO BHAGAVATE BHAIṢAJYAGURU VAIḌŪRYAPRABHARĀJĀYA TATHĀGATĀYA ARA-HATE SAMYAKSAMBUDDHĀYA TADYATHĀ OM BHAIṢAJYE BHAIṢAJYE MAHĀBHAIṢAJYA BHAIṢAJYA RĀJĀYA SAMUDGATE SVĀHĀ
(Sanskrit transliteration)

OM NA MO BHA GA WA TÉ BÉ KHA DZÉ GU RU BÉ DUR YA PRA BHA RA DZA YA TA THA GA THA YA AR HA TÉ SAM YAK SAM BU DHA YA TÉ YA THA OM BÉ KHA DZÉ BÉ KHA DZÉ MA HA BÉ KHA DZÉ BÉ KHA DZÉ [BÉ KHA DZÉ] RA DZA YA SA MUNG GA TÉ SO HA
(Tibetan phonetics)

The four medical traditions

The masters and followers of the four ancient Asian medical traditions are gathered in the four corners of the Tanaduk palace (see Figure 3.1). All are waiting for the Buddha's discourse on medicine. The deva physicians are on the front right side of the Medicine Buddha, led by Indra, the Ashwin twins, and Lhamo Dütsima (Lha mo bdud rtsi ma). The non-Buddhist physicians are seated at the back right side of the throne, including Brahma, Shiva, Vishnu, Kartika, and many more. The rishi physicians are seated on the front left side, led by Rishi Punarvasu Ātreya, Dhanvantari, Kaśyapa, Agnivesh, and Jatukarna. The Buddhist medicine group, headed by the bodhisattvas Avalokiteśvara, Mañjuśrī, and Vajrapāṇi, the Great Hearer Mahākāśyapa, Ānanda and Kumāra Jīvaka, is seated on the left side to the back of the Medicine Buddha. These lineage holders are accompanied by thousands of disciples on each side. All four schools are awaiting Sangyé Menla's teaching:

1. Sojé Bumpa (Gso byed 'bum pa): the healing vase medical system, practiced in the heavens

2. Wangchuk Nakpö Luk (Dbang phyug nag po'i lugs): the Black Shiva tradition (This is probably a Siddha system of non-Buddhist medicine)

3. Drangsong gi Luk (Drang srong gi lugs): the Indian Rishi medicine, corresponding to the eight branches of *Carakasaṃhita* (Ayurveda)

4. Riksum Gönpö Luk (Rigs gsum mgon po'i lugs): the Buddhist medical system which Avalokiteśvara, Mañjuśrī, and Vajrapāṇi spread to India and Tibet, China, and Oḍḍiyāna respectively

As the Buddha's discourse was completed, each school of medicine heard teachings according to their own tradition.

Buddhist medicine

Dési Sangyé Gyatso recounts that the Buddhist medical system was heard by bodhisattvas, who further developed this lineage in three principal countries: via emanations of Avalokiteśvara in India and Tibet, Mañjuśrī in China, and Vajrapāṇi in the Swat valley. The Dési quotes from Rinchen Pungpa (Rin chen spungs pa):[10]

---

9 *Bédurya* is the Tibetan variant of the Sanskrit term *vaiḍūrya*.

10 Sde srid sangs rgyas rgya mtsho, 1982, 86.

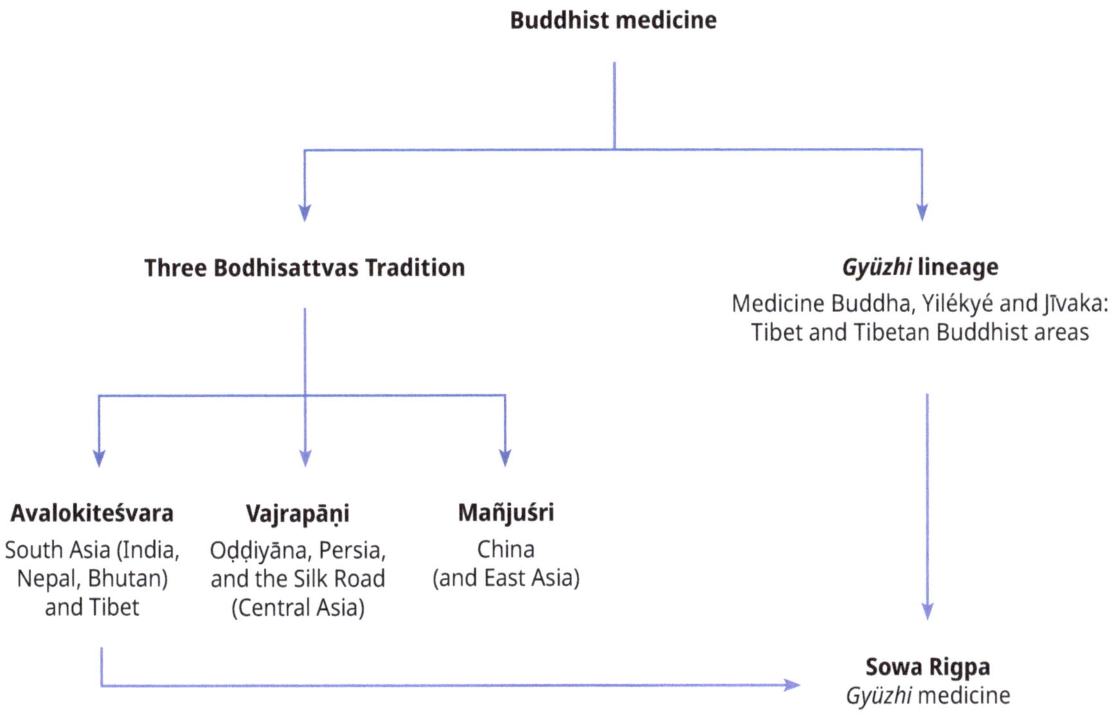

FIGURE 3.2 The Buddhist medicine lineage

In the manifestation land of Mount Wu Tai Shan (Rtse lnga) in China, Mañjuśrī emanated as a parrot and expounded medicine.

In Bodhgaya and on Jakang (Bya rkang) Mountain, medicine was expounded by Avalokiteśvara, who manifested as a rishi.

In Goshanting (Go shan ting) in Oḍḍiyāna, it was taught by a *rākṣa* emanation of Vajrapāṇi.

Such a story is hard to evaluate based on our modern way of thinking. Nevertheless, this piece of ancient history lays down a trajectory, giving the names of countries in which scholarly medical traditions developed. Considering the roots of medicine in Tibet before the 10th century, this description highlights intriguing connections in the history of Asian medicine. In ancient India and the countries of the Indian sub-continent, Buddhist doctrine and medicine flourished. When this knowledge travelled along the silk roads, it became known as the Upper Tradition (Stod Lugs) in Tibet. This lineage was later absorbed into the *Gyüzhi*, which is believed to be translated into Tibetan by Vairocana in the eight century CE. A related section in the *Subsequent Tantra*'s concluding chapter reads:[11]

Buddha expounded pharmacy in India.
In China, he taught moxibustion and *tsajong* (channel cleansing therapy).
In Dölpo (Mustang, Nepal), principally bloodletting.

In Tibet, he transmitted pulse reading and urine analysis.
To the retinue of heavenly gods, he expounded Sojé Bumpa.
To the sages, Caraka's Eight Branches.
To non-Buddhists, the Black Shiva Tantra.
To Buddhist disciples, the teachings of the Three Bodhisattvas.
In this medical tantra (the *Gyüzhi*), all are expounded: there is no medical science not included here.

____

11 G.yu thog yon tan mgon po, 1993, 660.

Buddha's blessing has no prejudice,
even though it appears differently
according to one's faith.
Like the moon shining in the sky,
reflected differently in each ladle of water.
One teaching is expounded, but it is heard
differently.

These mystical lineages go back centuries. They are a Tibetan Buddhist way of understanding the origin of medical systems. Karma and Shakyamuni's manifestation as Medicine Buddha are beyond ordinary human thought. The existence of all other medicines and their practitioners are thus included and validated: Atreya and Kumara Jīvaka of India, Huang Fu Mi in China, Hippocrates and Galen of Greece, Zakariyā Rāzī and Avicenna of Persia, and many more throughout the world.

The origins and authorship of the *Gyüzhi* is disputed, and has become more so in recent times. However, it is not that crucial to be able to trace the historical development of the body of *Four Tantras* and whether it was composed by Yutokpa or others. What is far more important, is to uphold *Gyüzhi*'s whispering lineage (*nyengyü*), and not to cut the spiritual connection to the Medicine Buddha. Like all other Mahayana tantras, the ultimate origin of the teaching is traced back to Vajradhara, the primordial Buddha. In this sense, it is crucial to receive the unbroken oral transmission (*lung*) from a true lineage holder.

It is said that the *Gyüzhi* was only heard by Yilékyé, the speech manifestation of the Medicine Buddha who was reborn as monk. He transmitted the *Gyüzhi* to Kumara Jīvaka (Tsojé Zhönu), who passed it on to Nāgārjuna (probably in a vision). It then reached Vāgbhaṭa (Lopön Pawo), Chandranandana (Dawa Ngönga), and Vairocana. The *Gyüzhi* is considered to be the nectar essence of all medical knowledge, which was secretly passed on from person to person and eventually reached Tibet. This is what is known as *nyengyü*, the secret hearing transmission. If we observe the chronology, there are about 1,200 years between Buddha Shakyamuni and Vairocana to account for. This is difficult due to the lack of historical material. Nevertheless, there are many legendary stories related to this lineage that remain a fascinating subject of study and contemplation up to the present day.

3.2 INTRODUCTION TO TIBETAN MATERIA MEDICA

The palace of the Medicine Buddha lies in the center of the city of Tanaduk, surrounded by four great mountains in the east, south, west, and north. All important and precious medicines including plants, herbs, fruits, trees, minerals, gems, stones, flowers, and animals thrive there. The mountains correspond to the directions of the palace mandala and to the body, along with the five aspects of consciousness and the five elements. They can be differentiated from each other based on the materia medica concept of cooling, warming, and neutral potency.

These are termed the external four mountains, but there are also four internal mountains.[12] Yutok once had a vision of Tanaduk. In the center of the palace, he saw the blue-colored Medicine Buddha Akṣobhya, Medicine Buddha Ratnasambhava in yellow in the south, the red Medicine Buddha Amitābha in the west, the green Medicine Buddha Amoghasiddhi in the north, and the white Medicine Buddha Vairocana in the east. Their colors were brilliant, and they were all surrounded by a retinue of bodhisattvas, arhats, great hearers, devas, asuras, humans, and other beings.

The Southern Mountain

The Southern Mountain is called Riwo Bikjé (Ri bo 'bigs byed), "Piercing Mountain," referring to its warming nature nourished by sunshine. Many medicines including roots, trunks, branches, leaves, flowers, and fruits that belong to the warming group of ingredients, grow there. Examples are pomegranate (*sendru*), black pepper (*nalésham*), long pepper (*pipiling*), *Plumbago zeylanica* (*tsitraka*), *Clematis rehderiana* (*yimong*), *Kaemferia galanga* (*dongdra*), nutmeg (*dzati*), and *Ferula asafoetida* (*shingkün*). All have pungent, sour, and salty tastes, with hot and sharp properties that alleviate *béken* and *lung*. Riwo Bikjé is covered with beautiful flowers and pleasing fragrances that protect from and cure all types of cold disorders.

The Northern Mountain

The Northern Mountain is called Riwo Gangchen (Ri bo gang can): "Snowy Mountain." It is very high, covered by a white blanket of snow. An icy wind blows across its slopes. Riwo Gangchen has a cold lunar energy, and a healing forest where cooling medicines grow. These include white sandalwood (*tsenden karpo*), camphor (*gabur*), eaglewood (*agaru*), neem (*nimpa*), different types of gentians, and *Swertia chirata* (*tikta*). All these substances possess bitter, sweet, and astringent tastes with a cold and blunt power that

---

12 See for instance Elder Yutok's biography, Rechung Rinpoche, 1973, 237–38 and 243–46.

cures bile (*tripa*), hot disorders (*tsawa*) and infectious fevers (*rimtsé*). Medicinal plants of superb beauty grow there which prevent and cure sicknesses even by means of their splendid fragrance.

The Eastern Mountain

The Eastern Mountain is called Riwo Pöngéden (Ri bo spos ngad ldan): "Fragrant Mountain." It is covered with majestic forests where five types of chebulic myrobalan (*arura*) and many other medicinal trees grow. The roots of these *arura* trees cure bone disorders, their trunks cure muscle disorders, their branches cure ailments of the channels and tendons, while their barks cure skin disorders. Their leaves cure the hollow organs, their flowers cure the senses, and their fruits cure diseases of the vital organs. These trees carry the five types of myrobalan fruits. *Aru namgyel*, the superior quality of *arura*, possesses all six tastes, eight powers, three post-digestion tastes, and 17 qualities; it is a universal panacea. The other types of *aru* have similar qualities, which also promote life energy, increase the digestive fire, and provide wholesome energy to the body-mind. They cure all kinds of diseases manifested from the three humors. The five types of *arura* are:

1. *Aru namgyel*: This superior type is said to have "double fruits," the secondary fruit being contained inside a larger one. It is considered the sacred king of medicine. This type is held in the right hand of the Medicine Buddha as a panacea for all bodily illness. It cures all 404 humoral disorders and brings auspiciousness, wealth, and prosperity. *Aru namgyel* rarely exists in the human world, growing only in the heavens.

2. *Aru jikmé*: The fruits of this myrobalan have five vertical lines or furrows. It cures eye disorders and protects from negative spirit influences.

3. *Aru düdtsi shatuk*: This myrobalan has a thick, fleshy skin. It increases weight and rejuvenates the body.

4. *Aru peljé*: This myrobalan is shaped like a vase and has thick flesh which heals wounds and physical trauma.

5. *Aru kempo*: This myrobalan has a thin skin and a yellow color. It cures children's bile disorders.

Besides the types of *aru* mentioned above, there are also others such as *aru nakchung*: a small, seedless, black *Terminalia chebula* fruit that improves the voice and heals the throat. *Aru churing* is a long fruit that looks like a kingfisher's beak. It cleans the intestines and heals bile disorders.

Other medicinal fruit trees include *barura* (*Terminalia bellirica*), which cures *béken* and lymph disorders, and *Emblica officinalis* (*kyurura*), which cures excessive heat disorders of bile and blood. *Arura*, *barura* and *kyurura* are together called the three fruits (*drébu sum*). Their combination balances the three humors, curing chronic fever, chronic liver disorders and bile in the stomach, regulating the intestine and cleansing the skin. Many other medicinal trees and bushes also grow on the eastern mountain. All are of the highest quality, stunning beauty, and ward off countless diseases.

The Western Mountain

The Western Mountain is called Riwo Malaya (Ri bo ma la ya), "Rosary Mountain." On it one can find the six superlative medicines (*zangpo druk*), five types of calcite (*chongzhi rik nga*), five types of mineral pitch (*drakzhün rik nga*), five types of medicinal waters (*menchu rik nga*), and five types of hot springs (*chutsen rik nga*).

The six superlative medicines, which balance the vital organs, are:

1. *Dzati* (*Myristica fragrans*), which calms the mind and cures heart disorders

2. *Lishi* (*Syzygium aromaticum*), which cures life channel disorders and cold wind in the intestines

3. *Chugang* (*Bambusa textilis* / kaolin), which cures the lungs and heals wound inflammation

4. *Gurgum* (*Crocus sativus*, substitute: *Carthamus tinctorius*), which cures liver diseases, and stops bleeding

5. *Kakola* (*Amomum subulatum*), which heals cold spleen and stomach

6. *Sukmel* (*Elettaria cardamomum*), which treats the kidneys and cold wind disorders (*dranglung*)

The six superlatives for the six hollow organs (*nö kyi zangpo druk*) are:

1. *Sendru* (*Punica granatum*), which treats all cold stomach disorders, improves the digestive fire, and cures *béken* and cold diseases

2. *Dukmonyung* (*Holarrhena pubescens*), which cures small intestine disorders

3. *Ruta* (*Saussurea lappa*), which cures large intestine disorders, gastritis, shoulder and back pain caused by high blood pressure, chronic lung disorders, throat infection and chronic wounds

4. *Sergyi métok* (*Herpetospermum pedunculosum*), which cures bile and gallbladder inflammation

5. *Gyatsa* (sal ammoniac), which kills germs, is an antidote to poisoning, and clears bladder and urinal tract disorders

6. *Wangpo lakpa* (*Dactylorhiza hatagirea*), which increases bodily strength, rejuvenates, and produces reproductive fluids

The five types of calcite (*chongzhi rik nga*)

Calcite stone is an important substance in the Tibetan medical tradition that can be found in some ancient mountains. It has a fat-like appearance, and its divine masculine energy is praised in pharmacological texts. *Chongzhi* strengthens all the paternal white components of the body such as the bones, spinal cord, ligaments, fat, brain, nerves, and sperm. There are five types: male, female, son, daughter, and neutral *chongzhi*. Generally, processed calcite cures phlegm as well as chronic stomach acidity caused by *bétri* disorders (disorders caused by the bile and phlegm humors combined), and hidden fever. It is also used for the purpose of rejuvenation.

The five types of mineral pitch (*drakzhün rik nga*)

Mineral pitch is another principal medical ingredient. It is called *drakzhün*, which literally means "rock liquid." It is found in a semi-liquid form similar to melted dark chocolate. The sun's heat melts the rocks and draws out this rich mineral solution. It oozes like honey from a honeycomb, having a beautiful smell but a bitter taste. *Drakzhün* is attributed divine feminine energy as it is blessed by female deities. It thus

regenerates the energy of the maternally derived parts of the body such as blood, liver, flesh, menstruation, and skin. Five types are described, deriving from rocks rich in gold, silver, copper, iron, or lead ore. The type and quality of *drakzhün* depends on its origin. If the rock is silvery, it is known as silver *drakzhün*, and so on. All *drakzhün* are coffee-colored. They are rich in minerals and have a cooling power that cures all chronic kidney inflammations, minor skin disorders, and especially chronic inflammations of the stomach, liver and blood. In short, *drakzhün* is widely used to counteract chronic inflammations and gastritis, for blood purification, and hepatic complaints.

The five healing waters (*menchu rik nga*)

Due to their different minerals, natural or spring water has different qualities that assist in curing disease. All are drinkable, with a particular taste and effect, and thus are known to Tibetan medicine as medicinal waters. The following *menchu* can be found in many countries:

1. Water with a sour and salty taste cures *béken* and *lung* disorders, especially stomach diseases

2. Water with a sour and sweet taste cures *béken* and *tripa* disorders

3. Water with a sour and bitter taste cures *béken* and blood disorders

4. Water with a sour and astringent taste cures *béken mukpo* (brown phlegm, a chronic gastric disorder)

5. Water with a sour and pungent taste cures single *béken* disorders

The five types of hot spring (*chutsen rik nga*)

Hot springs are known as *chutsen*. They are places where heated water naturally emerges from underground. Varying due to the mineral composition of the bedrock, five main types of hot springs are mentioned in the *Root Tantra*. This number is elaborated upon in the Dési's *Blue Beryl* commentary, as well as in Déumar Tendzin Püntsok's *Crystal Orb and Garland*. They are generally indicated for conditions such as rheumatism, arthritis, osteoporosis, various skin and neurological disorders, as well as chronic phlegm and wind imbalance. The five main type of hot springs are:

1. Coal and calcite hot springs, which cure chronic inflammation, hidden fever and bone and articulation disorders

2. Coal and sulfur hot springs, which cure cold and *chuser* disorders (including dermatological conditions), but bathing in these waters tends to increase *lung*

3. Coal and mineral pitch hot springs, which cure bile-phlegm disorders, and are especially good for bile and inflammation disorders of the digestive system

4. Coal, calcite, and sulfur hot springs, which have a neutral quality and cure all chronic diseases, and are especially good for disorders of a cold and damp nature, such as rheumatism and arthritis

5. Coal, sulfur, mineral pitch, and realgar hot springs, which cure cold *chuser* disorders and chronic inflammation caused by combined humors

Besides the raw materials described above, there are many other herbal medicines to be found on Riwo Malaya, including *khenpa* (*Artemisia* spp.), iris (*dréma*), wild rose (*séwé métok*), and lotus (*métok péma*). All kinds of stone medicines (*do men*) and salt medicines (*tsa men*) are also present. Many animals roam freely on Western Mountain, especially animals considered of medicinal value, such as the elephant, bear, musk deer, rhinoceros, peacock, and parrot.

3.3 THE MAIN CONTENT OF THE *GYÜZHI*

Following the title, homage, and description of Tanaduk, we will now begin to cover the actual teachings of the *Root Tantra.* Buddha Shakyamuni transformed into Sangyé Menla and went into a particular state of meditation called "the King of the Medicine which cures all 404 disorders." Immediately, bright rays of light with thousands of colors radiated from his heart chakra into all directions, healing the disorders of multitudes of sentient beings, and then returned to his heart. After this, Medicine Buddha emanated Rikpé Yéshé in an aquamarine color, whose nature is that of Buddha Akṣobhya. He positioned himself at the level of Medicine Buddha's heart, took up a teaching posture, and greeted the gathered audience with the following words:[13]

____
13 G.yu thog yon tan mgon po, 1993, 4.

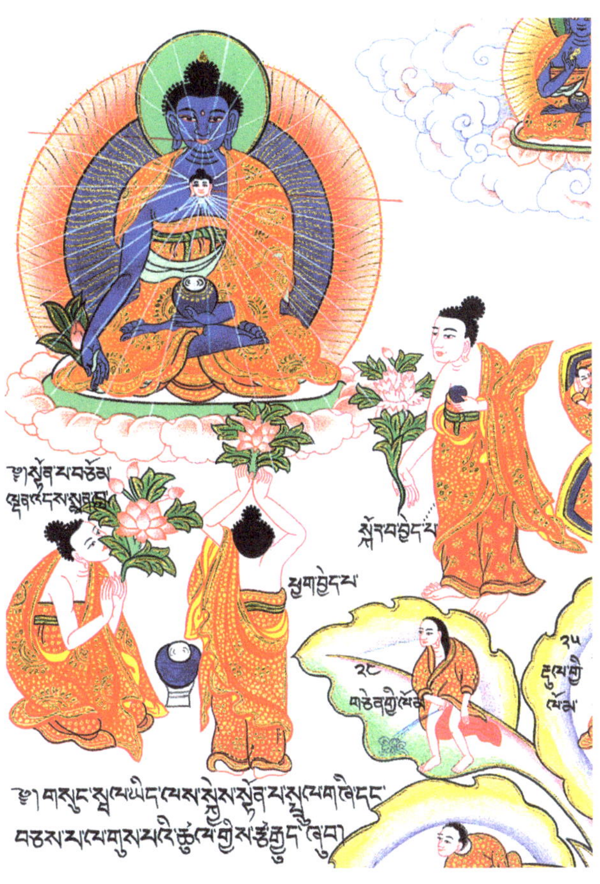

FIGURE 3.3 Medicine Buddha and the three actions of Yilékyé

After Rikpé Yéshé spoke these words, thousands of colored rays of light radiated from the tongue of the Medicine Buddha. These lights healed the diseases caused by wrong speech, resulting in karmic disorders such as speaking and hearing impairments, stammering, muteness, and diseases provoked by evil spirits. The light returned to his tongue, from where a monk called Yilékyé manifested. Yilékyé, "born from the heart-mind," is an emanation of the enlightened speech of Buddha Amitābha. Yilékyé circumambulated the Medicine Buddha three times and then stood in front of him with his hands folded at his chest in the wish-fulfilling jewel mudra. He made prostrations on behalf of everyone, requesting the Medicine Buddha to teach by saying:[14]

O master, sage Rikpé Yéshé!
We, who are gathered here,
all wish to receive the perfect teachings for benefiting others and ourselves.
Please, kindly bestow upon us the oral instructions of Sowa Rigpa.

Rikpé Yéshé responded:
O great sages, listen!
One should study the *Four Tantras*, which are:
the *Root Tantra* and the *Explanatory Tantra*,
the *Oral Instruction Tantra* and the *Subsequent Tantra*.
Thus, the *Gyüzhi* should be understood.

Then Rikpé Yéshé started to teach the *Tsagyü*, the first of the *Four Treatises*, by first giving an outline of all its divisions and chapters.

1. *Tsagyü*

Rikpé Yéshé as emanation of Buddha Akṣobhya expounded the *Root Tantra* in six chapters:

1. The origins of the *Four Tantras*
2. The content of the *Four Tantras*
3. The basis of medicine: health and disease
4. Diagnostic methods
5. Treatments for the three humors
6. The allegorical medicine trees

2. *Shégyü*

Rikpé Yéshé, now as an emanation of Buddha Vairocana, expounded the 31 chapters of the *Explanatory Tantra*.

1. The summary of the *Explanatory Tantra*

Six chapters on anatomy and physiology:

2. Embryology
3. Body similes
4. Anatomy
5. Physiology
6. Constitution
7. Signs of death and dying

Five chapters on etiology:

8. The distant cause of disease
9. The immediate cause of disease
10. Disease entrance gates
11. The symptoms of disorders of the three humors
12. Disease classification

Three chapters on behavior:

13. Daily routine behavior
14. Seasonal behavior
15. Incidental behaviors

Three chapters on nutrition:

16. Dietetics
17. Dietary restrictions
18. The right intake of foods and beverages

Three chapters on materia medica:

19. The tastes of medicines
20. The potencies of medicines
21. Compounding methods

One chapter on surgery:

22. Medical instruments

One chapter on rejuvenation:

23. Ways to maintain health

Three chapters on diagnosis:

24. Direct diagnosis
25. Wise diagnosis
26. An analysis of when to accept or decline a patient

Five chapters on therapeutic methods:

27. General therapeutic techniques
28. Specific and detailed therapeutic techniques
29. Two special therapeutic methods
30. Principal treatments
31. The physician's ethical code

---

14 Ibid., 5.

3. Mengakgyü

Rikpé Yéshé, this time emanating from Buddha Ratnasambhava, expounded the 92 chapters of the *Oral Instruction Tantra*.

1. The request

Four chapters on humoral disorders:

2. Wind disorders
3. Bile disorders
4. Phlegm disorders
5. Brown phlegm (*béken mukpo*)

Six chapters on chronic metabolic diseases (*chong né*):

6. Indigestion (*mazhuwa*)
7. Tumors (*tren*)
8. Initial stage edema (*kyabap*)
9. Second stage edema (*or*)
10. Final stage edema (*muchu*)
11. Consumption (*chongchen zéjé*)

16 chapters on hot disorders (*tsawa*):

12. General fever
13. Deceptive states of heat and cold disorders
14. "Hill meets plain" fever (*tsawa ritang tsam*)
15. Unripe fever (*mamin tsawa*)
16. High fever (*gyétsé*)
17. Empty fever (*tongtsé*)
18. Hidden fever (*gaptsé*)
19. Chronic fever (*nyingtsé*)
20. Turbid fever (*nyoktsé*)
21. Spreading fever (*dramtsé*)
22. Disturbed fever (*truktsé*)
23. Infectious fever (*rimtsé*)
24. Smallpox (*drumpa*)
25. Gastro-enteritis (*gyuzer*)
26. Diptheria (*gakpa*)
27. Flu (*champa*)

Six chapters on diseases of the head:

28. Diseases of the head
29. Diseases of the eyes
30. Ear disorders
31. Nasal disorders
32. Mouth disorders
33. Goiter (*bawa*)

Eight chapters on the vital and hollow organs:

34. Heart disorders
35. Lung disorders
36. Liver disorders
37. Spleen disorders
38. Kidney disorders
39. Stomach disorders
40. Small intestine disorders
41. Large intestine disorders

Two chapters on genital diseases:

42. Diseases of the male genitals
43. Diseases of the female genitals

19 chapters on miscellaneous disorders:

44. Hoarseness (*kézer né*)
45. Anorexia (*yiga chüpa*)
46. Thirst disorders (*kom né*)
47. Hiccups (*kyikbu*)
48. Breathing disorders (*uk mi déwa*)
49. Colic (*langtap*)
50. Parasite disorders (*sin né*)
51. Vomiting disorders (*kyuk né*)
52. Diarrhea disorders (*tru né*)
53. Constipation (*tsagak*)
54. Dysuria (*chingak*)
55. Frequent urination (*chinyi*)
56. Dysentery (*tsétru*)
57. Gout (*drek*)
58. Rheumatism and arthritis (*drumbu*)
59. Interstitial fluid and plasma (*chuser*) disorders
60. Nerve (*tsakar*) disorders
61. Skin diseases
62. Miscellaneous diseases

Eight chapters on congenital disorders (*lhenkyé ma*):

63. Malignant tumors (*dré*)
64. Hemorrhoids (*zhangdrum*)
65. Shingles (*méwel*)
66. *Surya*, a group of severe skin diseases
67. Diseases of the glands and lymph nodes (*menbu*)
68. Hydrocele (*likluk*)
69. Severe leg inflammation (*kangbam*)
70. Anal fistula (*tsenbar dölwa*)

Three chapters on pediatrics:

71. Labor and childcare
72. Pediatric diseases
73. Children's psychiatry

Three chapters on gynecology:

74.　General gynecological disorders
75.　Specific gynecological diseases
76.　Common gynecological diseases

Five chapters on psychiatry:

77.　Possession by wandering evil spirits (*jungpö dön*)
78.　Madness (*nyojé*)
79.　Amnesia (*jéjé*)
80.　Epilepsy (*za*)
81.　Diseases caused by malignant serpent spirits (*lu dön*)

Five chapters on wounds:

82.　General wounds
83.　Head wounds
84.　Neck wounds
85.　Chest and back wounds
86.　Arm and leg wounds

Three chapters on poisoning:

87.　Compounded poisons
88.　Food poisoning
89.　Poisoning from natural sources

One chapter on rejuvenation:

90.　Geriatric disorders

Two chapters on aphrodisiacs:

91.　Aphrodisiacs and infertility
92.　Searching for the right woman

4. Chimagyü

Rikpé Yéshé, emanating from Buddha Amoghasiddhi, expounded the 27 chapters of the *Subsequent Tantra*.

Two diagnostic chapters:

1.　Pulse diagnosis
2.　Urinalysis

10 chapters on medicines:

3.　Decoctions
4.　Powders
5.　Pills
6.　Syrups
7.　Medicinal butters
8.　Ash medicines
9.　Concentrated solid extracts (*khendra*)
10.　Medicinal spirits
11.　Precious pills (*rinchen rilbu*)
12.　Herbal medicines

The five internal therapies (plus two more):

13.　Oil therapy
14.　Purgation
15.　Emesis
16.　Nasal therapy
17.　Mild enemas (*jamtsi*)
18.　Strong enemas (*niruha*)
19.　Channel cleansing (*tsajong*)

Six chapters on external therapies:

20.　Bloodletting
21.　Moxibustion
22.　Fomentation
23.　Medicinal baths
24.　Oil application
25.　Surgery

Two supplementary chapters:

26.　*Gyüzhi*'s concluding chapter
27.　Transmitting the authority to practice the *Gyüzhi* to disciples

The *Four Tantras* contain a total of 156 chapters. Study this text completely and your practice will be powerful, as the *Subsequent Tantra* indicates:[15]

> *Gyüzhi* is like a protection cord without the need for chanting mantra,
> a conqueror whose machinery subdues the Lord of Death's army,
> a hero who conquers the disease enemy,
> a leader that keeps the humors in check,
> a sword that cuts the Lord of Death's noose,
> a hammer that strikes the spikes of pain,
> the hook that pulls one out of the swamp of suffering.
>
> *Gyüzhi* protects life from death, granting the generosity of fearlessness.
> It is the vase of resurrection.
> Sages should regard this healing science as precious.

15　G.yu thog yon tan mgon po, 1993, 665.

PART 2

THE THREE HUMORS

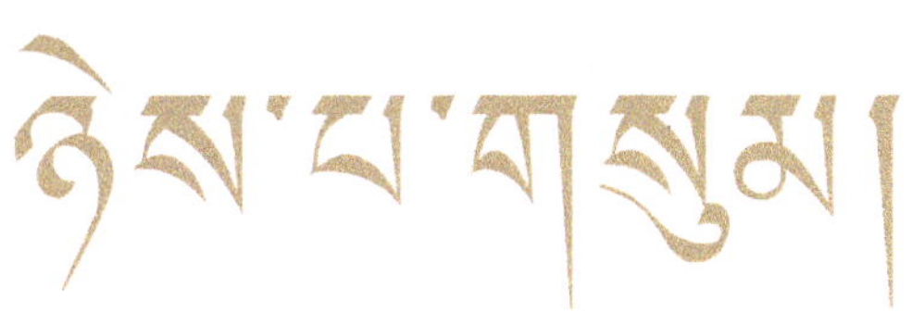

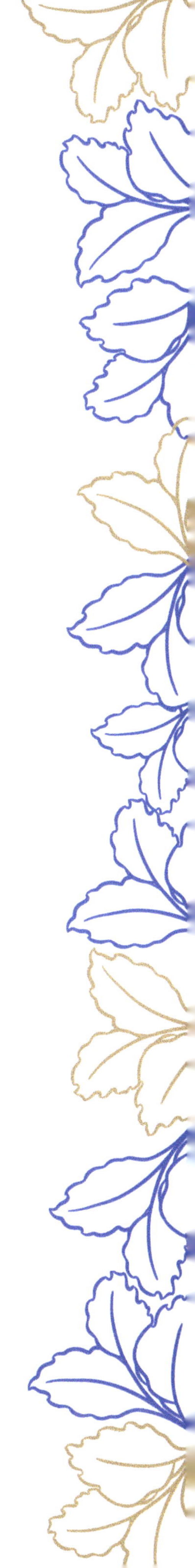

CHAPTER 4

MIND AND EMOTIONS

4.1 THE NATURE OF MIND

Buddhism and Sowa Rigpa share the same central concept of body, mind, and speech (energy). This chapter does not attempt to exhaustively cover Buddhist conceptions of consciousness, instead providing a more medical perspective on the body-mind. Nevertheless, the tantric understanding of mind and matter is closely related to medicine.

The mind is commonly referred to as *sem* in Tibetan, which can be defined simply as "thinking power," "thought," and "the knower." Its fundamental nature is clear light (*ö sel*): immaterial, luminous, pervasive, and boundless. The mind, however, is also the *prima materia*, the original cause of everything. According to Buddhism, all things manifest from the mind. *Sem* is often translated as "mind," but actually refers to the union of mind and subtle wind in Tibetan medicine and tantra. *Sem* is like the buttery essence of milk, the fragrance of white sandalwood, or the brightness of the sky. It is there but cannot be pinpointed. This quintessence of matter is in fact "the essence of Buddha-nature" (*kham déshek nyingpo*).[1]

Ordinary mind appears when the clarity of this natural mind is veiled by ignorance. This is the mystical creator of matter and non-matter, beings and non-beings, love and hate, beauty and ugliness, earth and sky, paradise and hell, emptiness and solidness, cells and microbes, and so on. Everything manifests from mind and subtle wind, which accumulate individual and collective *karma.* Ordinary mind is not enlightened. It is led by mental passions and karmic activities, like a silkworm which tirelessly crafts its own cocoon, thus being enveloped in darkness. This

is what is meant by ignorance in Buddhism, which creates samsara and all suffering.

Mind in the sutras

From the point of view of Buddhist sutra teachings, the mind has no beginning because its past lives are countless. But it has an end. It is like the seed of a banyan tree[2] whose ultimate origin cannot be traced but which will cease to exist when burnt. Similarly, when the fire of wisdom incinerates the ignorance clouding the mind, the cycle of rebirth will end, and suffering will cease.

The mind manifests due to causes and conditions. Without factors, the mind would remain in a state of eternity. This does not mean that the mind does not exist; the mind is there, but it only manifests through conditions. Mind reacts when there is an object to reflect, and the mind ceases its function if no object is there. The mind's nature is clear, luminous, colorless, and formless, but its clarity of knowing and perceiving continues throughout countless reincarnations, changing the shell of its body life after life according to its own karma, crossing the boundary of death.

The mind's qualities or powers are clarity, reflection, and knowing. Mind is not a substance; its nature is beyond duality (*nyi nang*). It is immaterial, and its fundamental nature can never be obscured nor contaminated by ignorance. The nature of mind is immaterial like space: completely void, shapeless, and stainless. Its true appearance is the light of love and compassion. The mind is a sky-like eye that perceives everything through the senses of the body without itself having a solid form. Its nature is without

---

1   *Kham déshek nyingpo* is the essence of the uncontaminated mind of all sentient beings, which can be explained through nine metaphors: a lotus, honey, grain, gold, a treasure in a poor man's home, the seed of a tree, an emperor in an evil woman's womb, and a golden statue covered in mud.

2   An Indian fig tree (*Ficus benghalensis*) whose branches produce aerial roots which later become accessory trunks.
A mature tree may cover several acres in this manner.

obscuration, perfectly clear, and therefore has the ability to reflect. Because of its capacity to know and discriminate things, it is called *rikpa*: "the knower" or "awareness." Other synonyms for *sem* are *lo* (intellect) and *shépa* (consciousness). The sutras emphasize the mind's clarity but do not elaborate much on its relationship to subtle wind energy.

Mind in tantra and medicine

According to Sowa Rigpa and Tibetan Buddhist tantra, mind is comprised of two elements: a nonmaterial aspect, and a material aspect consisting of subtle wind (*trawé lung*). "Nonmaterial" refers here to the mind's clarity (*ö sel*), which is the causal energy of mental development. Yet, the material subtle wind energy is with the mind from the very beginning. The inseparable union of mind and wind energy is described as *lung sem yer mé*. This union is the driving force behind the world as well as the nature of living and nonliving beings that manifests through the five elements, the six consciousnesses, the three humors in our bodies, and as disease.

Subtle wind is the vehicle and sustainer of the mind and its functions. It provides the capacity for thoughts to change and for the thinking process to continue. From a philosophical viewpoint, the union of mind and wind is like that of man/woman, sky/earth, sun/moon, method/wisdom, and *vajra*/bell. Like the body-mind, mind and subtle wind are one in two aspects, interdependent like a flower and its fragrance. The immaterial mind's clarity reflects sense objects with the help of material wind energy, which allows it to perceive and experience. Tantra states that without the power of this wind, mind alone cannot react to the outer world. Therefore, all mental characteristics, functions, constitutions and personality, and thoughts, are determined by the functioning of subtle wind. There are 72,000 channels in which the same number of winds flow, regulating the emotions, determining the quality of people's lives, and their mental passions.

Buddha-nature

The clarity of the mind is, by its very nature, free from the contamination of delusions or ignorance. It is light, true compassion, primordial wisdom, peace, unconditional love, the ultimate union of the body-mind.[3] This "essence of Buddha-nature" (*kham déshek nyingpo*) is shared by all beings as they all have love and compassion in their hearts. This fundamental love is itself free from the dualism that spontaneously arises from subtle wind. When this contamination is purified, ordinary mind becomes enlightened mind (*dharmakāya*), while purified subtle wind becomes the enlightened body of the buddhas (*nirmāṇakāya*). Unenlightened beings have not yet completely purified their mind streams and attained the state of boundless compassion. Ordinary unenlightened mind is like the seed of a flower that has not yet blossomed, a crystal covered by dust, or impure gold ore.

Ignorance (*marikpa*)

The *Explanatory Tantra* expounds:[4]
> There is one cause for all disease:
> ignorance, not realizing the meaning
> of selflessness,
> like a bird soaring in the sky that cannot
> separate from its own shadow.
> For all wandering beings, even when
> living happily,
> it is impossible to separate from disease
> because of ignorance.
> The particular causes arise from ignorance:
> the three mental poisons; attachment,
> hatred, and closed-mindedness,
> resulting in the three humors; wind, bile,
> and phlegm.

Ignorance is lack of knowledge, lack of awareness. It is a negative mental attitude that mistakenly clings to self and phenomena, wrongly holding them to be independent, permanent, and stable. This mental attitude forms the *künzhi* mind,[5] on the basis of which the "I" or "self" is fabricated, which consequently produces all mental afflictions the illusory self suffers from. This process prevents the mind from recognizing its true nature and realizing that external phenomena are its own projections. The mind "drugged" with ignorance is like a blind old grandmother who cannot even recognize her own family. It is like a muddy crystal. The mud, born with the crystal, covers and imprisons its light, and continues to do so until mud and crystal are separated. Similarly, mind and ignorance have two entirely different natures, therefore they can be separated. Ignorance can be washed away to reveal the

---

3 Some Buddhist traditions refer to it as primordial Buddha (Ādibuddha), Samantabhadra, or Vajradhāra.

4 G.yu thog yon tan mgon po, 1993, 34–35.

5 The *künzhi* is one of the eight consciousnesses in the Cittamatra or Semtsampa School of Buddhist philosophy, which is closely related to tantra and Tibetan medicine.

true clarity of the purified mind. Ignorance can only temporarily dim and obscure the light of consciousness. Tibetan medicine and tantra share the following interpretation: the dirt of ignorance manifests through the subtle wind of the mind, which in its unpurified state is a material energy that dims awareness. This in turn causes confusion, leading to a cloudy mind and selfishness. Ignorant mind is like the sun temporarily hidden by clouds; the clouds cannot obscure the spacious nature of the sky. Or like a lotus seed in the mud: even though the mud is unclean, the lotus growing from it is not contaminated by it. Or like murky water, which when left undisturbed, reveals the transparent nature of water as the sediment settles. In the same way, the self-clinging of ignorance can be removed. If self-clinging is released and the negative emotions pacified, the mind becomes like clear water again. So, even if the mind is temporarily veiled by ignorance, its natural state can never be contaminated by ignorance. When the right conditions are present, they will separate, leading to awakening. In this manner, the Buddha reached enlightenment. In Tibetan, such a person is called *sangyé*, a fully awakened being.

The creative cleverness of the ignorant mind

Ignorance in the ordinary minds of sentient beings is the foundation for complicated collective systems and whole worlds as well as the turmoil found in individual lives. *Marikpa* is actually very clever, like a patient in a mental ward who experiences complex hallucinations that are rich in detail but void of reality. In other words, ordinary mind produces delusive mental passions that in turn lead to sensual pleasures and the search for worldly success but, at the same time, these are never detached from the shadow of suffering. This mind sustains the phenomenal world and leads to rebirth, creating the body, gods and demons, love and hate. Without ignorance, the wheel of samsara would cease to turn. If all the beings in the world were to become enlightened, the world as we know it would end, revealing the perfection of nirvana and the end of all suffering.

In the Buddhist sense, the word "ignorance" has a philosophical and spiritual meaning. It is not just a synonym for stupidity. Even though *marikpa* may bestow us the temporary pleasures of life (like cheese in a mouse trap), it will eventually bring us the four inescapable sorrows of samsaric existence: rebirth, aging, sickness, and death. Buddha taught that suffering has its causes and that those who seek complete freedom from suffering and dying must be mindful of the trickery of ignorance. Ignorance produces the body, emotions, the humors, and the results of suffering and

disease. This is why the humors are called *nyépa* or "faults," as they are derived from our mental poisons.

4.2 MIND BEFORE NEW LIFE

Künzhi

The mind and all emotions arise from the all-ground (*künzhi*): the basis and container of mind that holds consciousness, karma, memory, and the mental poisons. *Kün* refers to "all," *zhi* means "base." According to tantra, the *künzhi* is located in the center of the heart chakra, where all six or eight consciousnesses reside.[6] The *künzhi* stores the imprints of all positive and negative experiences collected by the mind. It opens its doors in the morning, activates the six sense consciousnesses throughout the day, and closes in the evening during sleep. As a subtle karmic memory bank, it records all deeds throughout each life. Memories in the mind and karma are not very different in this matter: both are *bakchak*, recorded residues or impressions. The heart is the seat of the subtle ignorant mind, where subtle winds and memories block and obscure the mind, preventing awakening. In this way, all unenlightened beings dwell in a deep slumber. The heart chakra is comprised of five hundred channels. It is known as the *dharmacakra* or "chakra of phenomena" because one can reach omniscient Buddhahood by purifying the gross and subtle ignorance it houses.

"I" (*nga*)

Ignorance forms the world of the body-mind through the *künzhi*. The first design of the ignorant mind is the mental structure of a sense of self or "I," which then governs the body-mind in a self-centered manner. This sense of "I" is produced by the five aggregates as they gather together during bodily development. Once created, it always dwells with the mind and body, even during sleep and in the bardo. The self's memory starts functioning during the 26th week of fetal growth. This manifestation, the first gross memory of that life, sprouts from the *künzhi* in the center of the heart. The mind continues to develop the self through sensory contact with physical objects: through smells, sounds, touch, and so on. This produces feeling, which leads the mind to develop likes

---

6 Differences in the number of consciousnesses may be found in different philosophical systems.

and dislikes. These then induce the mind to produce more and stronger emotions, which, however, are still underdeveloped in early childhood.

According to Buddhist philosophy, the self is in fact not real or permanent. It is fake, fabricated, and only seemingly unchanging. Its illusory quality is much like a rainbow or the moon's reflection in water. Even though they are just illusions, the mind grasps at these, mistaking them for solid and independent objects. This further induces a feeling of self-importance and egoism, referred to as *dakdzin*: self-grasping. Since ignorance acts as a fundamental cause of the body-mind and its sense of self, it is an organizing principle throughout life. As a result of the feeling of self-importance, attachment begins to develop through contact with external objects and internal thoughts, further evoking the three mental poisons of desire, hatred, and closed-mindedness, and their emotional offspring. This multitude of positive and negative emotions accumulates karma, which is stored in the *künzhi*, and continues to turn the wheel of samsara. After death, the gross sense of self dissolves into the bardo consciousness, which continues its journey to the next life, where it fabricates the gross sense of "I" again. This cycle is repeated for all remaining lives.

The three subtle mental poisons

The subtle mental poisons are attachment, hatred, and closed-mindedness. They are products of ignorance which continue to exist throughout all lives in the *künzhi* of the mind, generating countless positive and negative thoughts and emotions. These subtle

TABLE 4.1 The 12 links of interdependent origination (*tendrel yenlak chunyi*)

	Causes and conditions	Link	Life
1.	Distant mental cause	Ignorance (*marikpa*)	Past lives
2.	Past lives	Karma/Formative actions (*dujé kyi lé*)	Past lives
3.	Mental continuum, conception	Consciousness (*namshé*)	Transition period (bardo)
4.	Fetus development	Name and form (*ming zuk*)	This life
5.	Development of senses and sense organs	Sources (*kyéché*)	This life
6.	Birth	Contact with external objects (*rekpa*)	This life
7.	Experience	Feeling (*tsorwa*)	This life
8.	Generation of desire and attachment	Craving (*sépa*)	This life
9.	Collecting karma	Grasping (*lenpa*)	This life
10.	Searching for one's own security	Existence (*sipa*)	This life
11.	7–10 causes rebirth in samsara	Birth (*kyéwa*)	This life
12.	End and karma for next life	Aging and death (*ga shi*)	This life and transition to the next

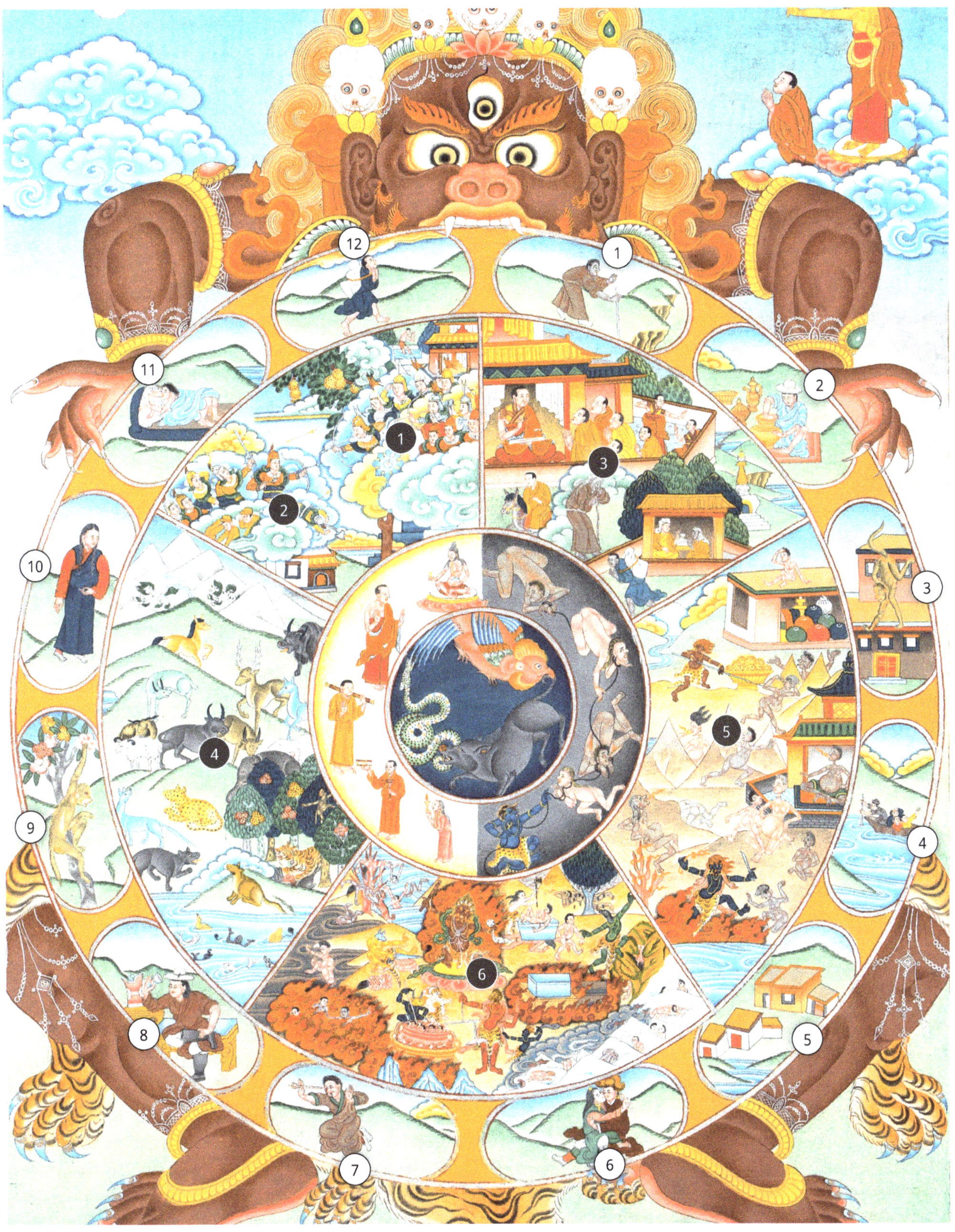

FIGURE 4.1 The wheel of life (*bhāvacakra*), ruled by the Lord of Death

poisons actively cause karma and turn the wheel of cyclic existence, leading to rebirth, health, happiness, and joy, as well as sorrow, ageing, suffering, and death. The Buddha taught that ignorance and the three poisons create the 12 interdependent links that constitute the chain of samsara as well as the six realms of existence (Figure 4.1). The six realms of existence where beings are reborn as a result of their individual karma are: (1) the realm of gods, (2) demi-gods, (3) humans, (4) animals, (5) hungry ghosts, and (6) hell beings.

Karma (*lé*): the force behind everything

Karma means "action," referring to the actions of the body-mind generated by subtle and gross desire, hatred, and closed-mindedness, and other related emotions. Karma is a dynamic force that is imprinted on the *künzhi*, continuously generating the energy that moves samsara and one's individual life. This force propels sentient beings to be reborn until they are liberated from dualistic illusion.

Karma is of three types: (1) positive, (2) negative, and (3) neutral. Positive karma is accumulated through positive actions, and gives prosperity and good results in this life and the next one. Negative karma is collected by negative actions and manifests in the form of ill-health and problems. Neutral karma is collected by neutral actions and can be easily influenced to become positive or negative. These three types give two kinds of results: (1) collective karma and (2) individual karma. Collective karma manifests its results within a group of people who share a common environment, for example within a country, city, village, or family.

Individual karma defines one's own life, health, and prosperity, often described as destiny. Karma is collected by oneself or by a group, but each person has their own karmic storage. For example, if during a past life one has been used to harming others through killing, enslavement, stealing, etc., this negative karma could ripen as poverty and poor health in this life or the next. On the other hand, helping others through generosity and healing suffering could bring good health and beneficial effects. Karma is neither a person nor a soul; karma is an energy that accumulates and infuses life like the electric charge of batteries. Buddhists believe that as long as collective and individual karma are not consumed or purified—even without the collection of new karma—samsara will continue to exist. Therefore, samsara will never end unless all sentient beings are freed. Karma gives rise to two sets of causal forces: the psychic and life pillar energies.

4.3 THE TRANSFORMATION OF MIND INTO MATTER

Three natural psychic energies (*sem kyi rangzhin gyi nüpa sum*)

The transition from mind to matter is effected by means of three mental forces. As karma moves the subtle wind of the bardo consciousness, a very subtle psychic force (*nüpa*) is generated that has the ability to transform into pre-material energies carrying the five elements in embryonic form. Three of these psychic energies carry out the transition from mind to matter: *münpa* (corresponding to the wind element), *dül* (fire), and *nyingtop* (water and earth). Once united with the reproductive fluids of the parents, they reactivate the parental elements by acting like a fermenting agent, thus beginning the construction of the physical body, the humors, and gross emotions.

Münpa is a pre-wind energy that has the power to form the empty spaces of the heart, lungs, and colon. It governs physical movement, respiration, the ears, and the skin, and forms the central channel as well as the nervous system. Psychologically, *münpa* manifests desire, attachment, love, fear, interest, and mental instability. It also develops and sustains the neutral wind humor that acts as an interface between body and mind, and produces wind microorganisms.

Dül is a pre-bile or fire energy that has the power to form red blood, the liver, and the eyes. It rules the right half of the body and its channels, the circulatory system, temperature, and metabolism. Psychologically, it manifests hatred, anger, fear, jealousy, pride, ambition, perfectionism, intelligence, and sharp memory. It is a feminine and solar energy. It sustains the bile humor and microorganisms.

Nyingtop is a pre-phlegm or water energy that has the power to form the various tissues of the body, white blood cells, the spleen, the kidneys, nose, tongue, the brain, the spine and bones, and the lymphatic and endocrine systems. It governs the left half of the body. Psychologically, it manifests compassion, gentleness, calmness, melancholy, selfishness, stubbornness, doubt, and confusion. Energetically, it is a lunar and masculine energy. It sustains the phlegm humor and microorganisms.

The three hidden pillars of life (*bépé tsé yi kawa sum*)

During fetal development, the psychic energies introduced above give rise to the following three hidden life-supporting entities housed inside the central

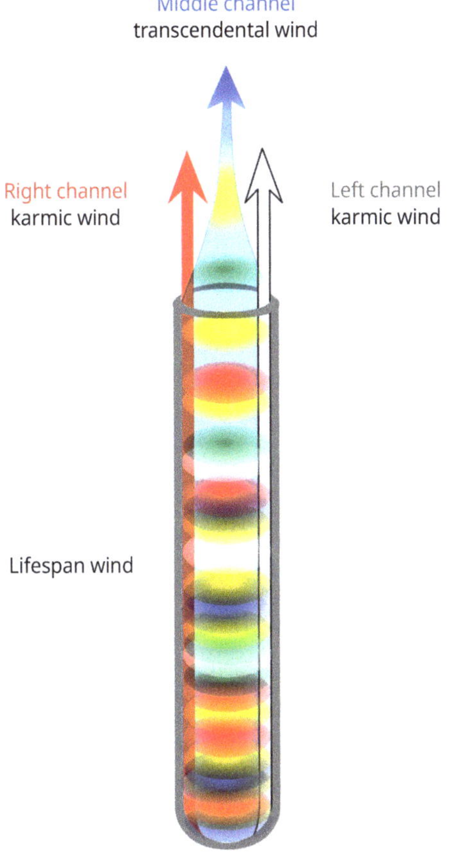

FIGURE 4.2 The three pillars of life

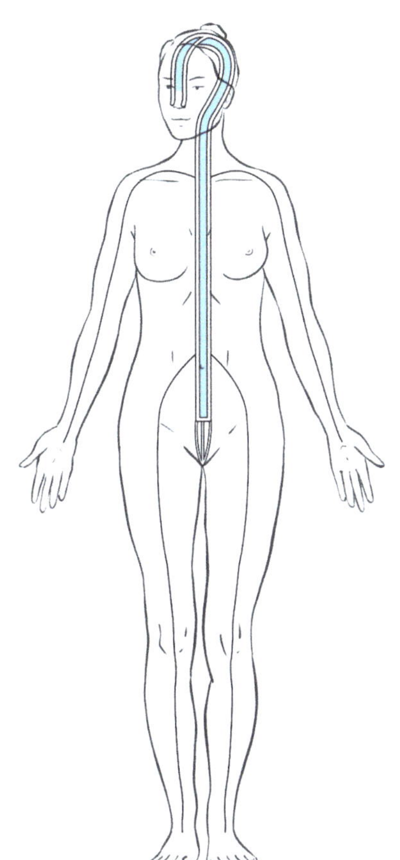

FIGURE 4.3 Lifespan wind in the central channel

channel of the growing body: lifespan (*tsé*), the current life's karma (*lé*), and fortune (*sönam*).

Tsé is the lifespan wind energy that determines the duration of life. Lifespan wind is deposited in the central channel and "colored" by various karmic imprints just like colored sand in a glass tube. This life fuel empowers a person, like gasoline does for a car. Every day of our lives, the breath transports a tiny portion from the central channel through the mouth and nostrils. Each person has a different amount and quality of lifespan energy. A healthy person generally breathes 21,600 times every 24 hours.[7] Each breath consists of two components: the major part is the bodily breath (*lélung* or "karmic wind") whereas the second component is subtler and in a smaller amount. The latter part is the actual lifespan energy, also referred to as life-sustaining wind (*sokdzin gyi lung*). Both come out from the central channel along with general respiration. The

tiny amount of lifespan wind contained in each breath divides into two parts when it reaches the nostril root from the central channel. One part goes to the crown chakra (i.e., the brain) and is consumed there, becoming the life-sustaining wind energy that supports consciousness. The other part of the breath is expelled from the mouth and nostrils. In this way, a small quantity of lifespan energy is lost every time, reducing our remaining lifespan day by day like a burning candle. According to Buddhism, the amount of this life fuel is determined by one's karma accumulated in previous lives.[8] It is nearly impossible for common people to judge its quantity and quality. However, tantric yogic practices of breath retention such as *kumbhaka* (*lung bumpachen*) are said to reduce the loss of lifespan wind.

Lé is the portion of one's karma that has to ripen and be exhausted in this lifetime. The person's accumulated positive or negative karma determines success, health, fame, and so on.

---

7 A healthy person at rest takes about 15 breaths per minute, totaling 21,600 in 24 hours. The same number can be found in sutra and tantra.

8 Detailed explanations can be found in astrological tantras such as the Kālacakra cycle.

Sönam is the fortune and merit of this life, leading to wealth and prosperity or poverty.

These three hidden pillars are the unseen powers that maintain life, keeping the body-mind going until death. They are like the three dimensions of the theatre of one's life. Collectively, these aspects are generally referred to as "karmic results" in Asian countries. Tibetan Buddhists believe that the course of birth and life, whether happy or full of suffering, is the result of these three energies. If the lifespan wind flowing through the breathing is positive for a day, week, month, or years, the individual will obtain positive results and enjoy life for that period. If the flow is negative, negative results will manifest as suffering. In accordance with this conception of karma and relying on Tibetan astrology, a person's life and success can be predicted and constructed in the form of a natal chart. At the moment of birth, the new life cycle is under the influence of the starts and planets, having an effect on the newborn's life and health through the elements. In this way, astrological calculation can be used to measure and analyze the life-force, wealth, and success.

The three pillars are in effect different aspects or functions of the same lifespan energy. They are life-force itself. If compared to fire, their distinction is like fire, heat, and flames. When one, two, or all three decrease or are consumed, misfortune, difficult economic conditions, lack of success, bad health, and relationship problems may arise that could even lead to death. Strong energies, on the other hand, will bring success, power, fortune, prosperity, and health. In short, they are the cause of the whole spectrum of lived experience.

The six consciousnesses (*namshé tsok druk*) and mental development

There are six inner sense consciousnesses that arise from the *künzhi* mind: the eyes (sight), nose (smell), tongue (taste), ears (hearing), body (tactile perception), and mental consciousness.[9] They all stem from the mental clarity of the mind, which develops after birth in the form of the gross sense consciousnesses. According to the *Explanatory Tantra*, "The sense consciousnesses manifest from one's mind." The gross sense consciousness begins to develop its functions after birth through contact with the six outer objects of perception (*kyéché druk*): forms (colors and shapes), sounds, odors, tastes, objects of touch, and external phenomena. The faculty of vision develops when the eyes perceive images. Smells develop the olfactory

consciousness. Hearing sounds develops the ear consciousness. The tongue tastes flavors and develops the taste consciousness. The body feels sensations and develops the tactile consciousness, and the mind perceives all phenomenal objects, developing the mental consciousness. This implies that the functions of the six sense organs are strengthened through experience, producing feelings of like and dislike. Discrimination gives rise to three types of emotions: positive, negative, and neutral. This in turn produces the three gross mental poisons: attachment, hatred, and closed mindedness, as well as numerous related emotions.

4.4 AFTER REBIRTH

The three gross mental poisons or characters

The three gross mental poisons derive from the subtle poisons of attachment, hatred, and closed-mindedness. They are predispositions, hidden tendencies (*bakchak*) in the mental continuum coming from past lives. After birth, they become the three gross mental characters whose development is strongly influenced by physical conditions.[10] This is the causal pathway of rebirth and how the three humors, with their inherent qualities, are produced.

Emotions arise from sensory contact, and give birth to other emotions such as love, compassion, jealousy and hatred, attraction, happiness, joy, pleasure, suffering and sorrow. All these feelings, whether enjoyable or not, coproduce the positive and negative causes of health or disease based on self-grasping. Although some emotions are beneficial in terms of contributing to a positive life, they eventually turn into sorrow and dissatisfaction. That is why, in Buddhism, the three mental dispositions of attachment, hatred and closed-mindedness, whether they are subtle or gross, are collectively called the three mental poisons. This terminology has equally been adopted in Tibetan medical literature, with the added specification that these "poisons" or types of mental states produce the three humors that make the body vulnerable to disease. Wind, bile, and phlegm each rule a particular body-mind system and related organs. Wind governs the nervous system. Bile is in charge of blood circulation and metabolism. Phlegm controls the lymphatic and endocrine systems. When in harmony, these psycho-humoral energies—which manifest both in the body and mind—sustain health and wellbeing. When the balance is disrupted, they are the ground for disease and suffering.

---

9   Some philosophical schools mention eight consciousnesses. The two additional ones are the *künzhi* and the mental affliction mind (*nyönmongpé yi*).

10 In the context of this book, the three mental poisons are often described as "mental characters," as they are natural manifestations of the unenlightened mind.

Attachment (*döchak*)

The Tibetan term for attachment is comprised of two parts: the first (*dö*) referring to "desire," the second (*chak*) means attachment or clinging. As the body grows, this desirous attachment that is present in the mind in subtle form first generates curiosity and subsequently enthusiasm for pleasurable objects. When there is strong longing for an object, attachment increases, leading to various emotions. As pleasure arises through sensory contact, a notion of self-importance and a feeling of need is naturally projected on the object of desire, strengthening the self-grasping mind and further developing mental delusions. The strongest forms of attachment are related to one's sense of I, and to sexual intercourse. Generally, *döchak* is defined as a greedy mind, seeking pleasure and possessions and hungry for power. The gross emotion of attachment produces the wind humor and system of the body-mind.

Hatred (*zhédang*)

The Tibetan term for hatred is also comprised of two words: *zhé*, which refers to deep-seated hatred, and *dang*, which is resentment and anger. Attachment can manifest hatred when desires are not fulfilled, or for instance when jealousy arises. Rage then emanates from the heart, turning the mind wrathful. Hatred is a destructive mental state, with an aggressive energy. It is a psychic fire that can burn the body-mind, leading to loss of judgment and awareness. Anger may also arise from other mental states, including closed-mindedness, jealousy, selfishness, and pride. *Zhédang* is conditioned in particular by the liver, gallbladder, and heart. The gross emotion of hatred produces the bile humor during the body's development. After birth, it governs the bile system and blood circulation.

Closed-mindedness (*timuk*)

Timuk consists of two syllables: *ti* refers to selfishness, and *muk* means obscured, confused, or unclear. The mental state produced by closed-mindedness is a lack of awareness and knowledge. It is like being in an unlit room at night. Strong anger can easily produce closed-mindedness and selfishness. The mind becomes dull, heavy, and cloudy, with feelings of sadness, melancholy, depression, and doubt. The brain and its mental functions become sluggish. The gross emotion of closed-mindedness produces the phlegm humor in the body during the body's development, governing phlegm functioning after birth.

Each mental character or gross emotion gives rises to many other related emotions. In short, the sutras usually describe 84,000 emotions, while tantras mention 72,000. All of these ultimately manifest from the three mental poisons.

The three seats of the mind (*sem kyi né sum*)

The mind is pervasive; there is no specific organ or body location where it is located. It is like butter in milk or the taste of honey. Under certain conditions, however, mind and emotions may be collected and function more actively in particular places. Neuroscientists locate consciousness mainly in the brain, while Eastern philosophies put more emphasis on the heart. Buddhist tantras detail three places where the mind plays different roles according to its nature: very subtle, subtle, and gross.

The very subtle mind (*shintu trawé sém*) is generally dormant. It is active only during the bardo (the intermediate mental state after death and before rebirth), conception, and the dying process. It is the root of the mind and the mental tree, residing in-between the navel and the secret chakra, the lower part of the central channel where jealousy arises. It is the seed of the body-mind that will leave the body after death to germinate again in the next life. *Shintu trawé sem* may be experienced when the thoughts and feelings of the gross and subtle minds are momentarily interrupted, for example during deep sleep, ecstasy, fainting, or meditative absorption. The very subtle mind provides the condition for the development of the central channel, the navel chakra, the subtle mind of the heart, the nervous system, the wind humor, and the psychic tree structure of the mind.

Subtle mind (*sem trawa*) is an intuitive mind that resides in and manifests from the heart chakra of the central channel, which is the seat of the *künzhi* and hatred. It can be experienced when the gross mind becomes less active, such as during sleep. It is the main seat of the mental consciousness and an emotional center. It is the trunk of the mind tree. All positive and negative karmic actions of this life are stored there, joining with the very subtle mind during the dissolution process. After death, these karmic traces are carried to the next life. *Sem trawa* provides the condition for the development of the right channel, and manifests in hatred and anger, the blood circulatory system, and the bile humor.

The gross mind (*sem rakpa*) is a conscious mind residing in the crown chakra, which is the seat of closed-mindedness. It generates the life-sustaining wind function through the brain and sense organs, controlling perception, sensation, memory, analytical thinking, and the physical ability to respond. It is active throughout the day, becoming inactive during sleep. It is a mind conditioned by the brain's mechanical function and by the sensory organs. *Sem rakpa* is the rational mind, the flower and fruit of the mind tree. It provides the condition for the development of the left channel and the lymphatic and endocrine systems, manifesting as the phlegm humor and the psychic energy of closed-mindedness. The gross mind governs the functions of the six consciousnesses.

Mind and memory

From a Tibetan medical perspective, memory can be understood as operating by means of two memory banks that communicate with each other through the funnel of the throat chakra. The first memory bank is in the head (brain), and records experiences of this life through the six sense consciousnesses. Each experience is filtered, analyzed, and labeled in degrees of true and false. Each experience is also imprinted with strong or light interest and emotion. Fleeting feelings and unimportant information may be discarded, while more significant information is retained. This process is called *drenpa* in Buddhist philosophy. To improve memory, this recollecting mind (*drenshé*) needs to be strengthened by revision and repetition.

The strength of memory depends on the quality of the brain,[11] which is strongly influenced by one's body constitution. A wind constitution person is generally more creative but has an instable memory. Bile people have a sharp mind, and are rational and intelligent. Phlegm peoples' mind and memory is slow but profound. The brain memory must develop its power each new life, which requires education and training. In other words, this is what is called the "base of ignorance," what is referred to as gross mind and memory. The gross mind develops from childhood, accumulating experiences throughout life.

The second memory bank is the *künzhi* in the heart. The *künzhi* collects all information passed on via the brain, stores it, and expresses the results in the form of karma, mental latencies (*bakchak*), and thoughts. It is a profound memory, representing the unconscious mind that influences the direction of life, communicating through dreams and intuition.

The third aspect of memory is a conditioning factor that operates from the throat chakra. Rather than being a storage, its role is to provide the conditions for the two memory banks to function well by regulating the life-sustaining and ascending winds. It acts as a filter that stimulates and clears memory , thus increasing awareness.

As described above, the gross and subtle mind mainly manifest in certain locations of the body during different mental states:[12]

- During sleep: the gross mind dissolves into the phenomenal chakra (heart) and enters a deep sleep

- When dreaming: the subtle mind of the heart rises and travels to the enjoyment chakra (throat) to experience dreams

- During the day: the collective concentration of gross and subtle mind is in the manifestation chakra (navel)[13]

- During orgasm: the gross mind concentrates in the crown chakra (head); its functions are temporarily suspended as the subtle *tiklé* of the reproductive organs move up (through *düpé tsa*), resulting in a state of empty blissfulness in which more subtle states of consciousness can be experienced.

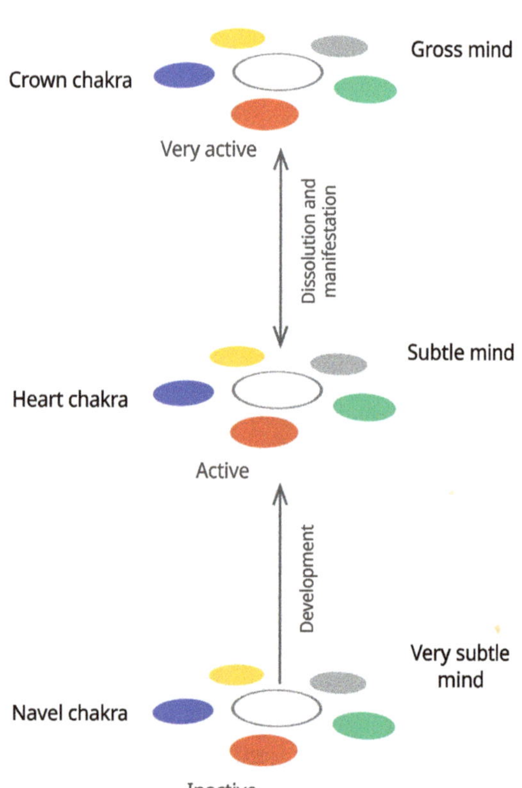

FIGURE 4.4 The three seats of mind: mental consciousness is surrounded by the five sensory consciousnesses

---

11 Seven brain types are described in the trauma chapter of *Oral Instruction Tantra*. Each type has different qualities.

12 In tantra, these states of mind are related to the four *kāya* of Buddhahood.

13 The gross and subtle mind are active in the brain and heart respectively, but during the day, the root of body-mind balance is held in the navel chakra.

The map of the mind

There are countless mental states and emotions. In the sutras, the structure of the mind is explained as follows:

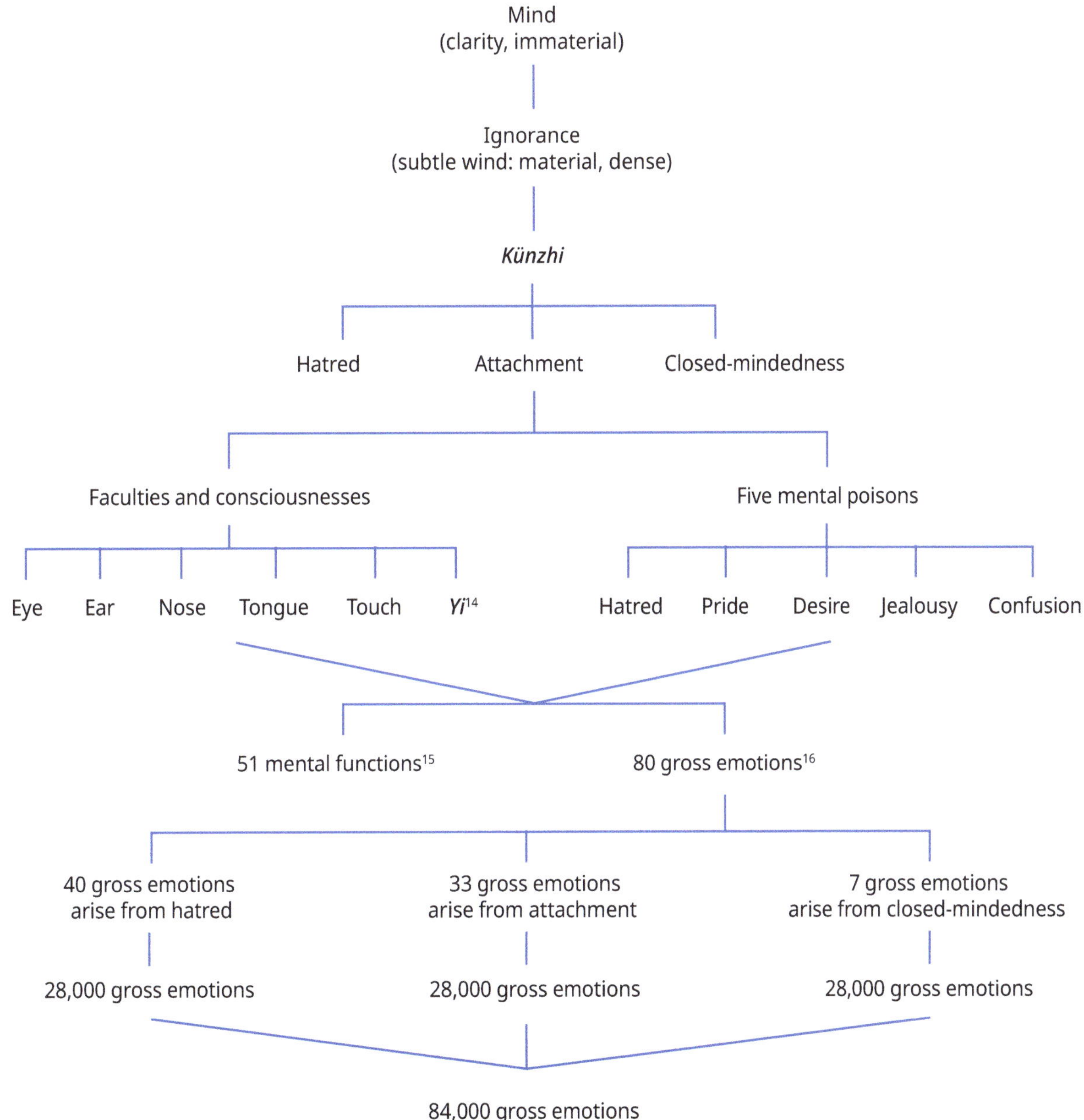

FIGURE 4.5 Mental development according to the sutras

---

14 A synonym for the principal mind.

15 See Rabten, 1992, and Lati Rinbochay and Napper, 2013.

16 See Lati Rinbochay and Hopkins, 1985.

In tantra (especially in the Mother Tantras), 72,000 channels are described where 72,000 winds flow, giving rise to 72,000 emotions. They are divided into three groups: 24,000 emotions manifest from *tsa roma* (the solar energy channels arising from hatred) and 24,000 emotions manifest from *tsa kyangma (*the lunar energy system arising from closed-mindedness*)*. There are also 24.000 emotions which manifest from the neutral energy or attachment from the central channel (*tsa uma*).

During the dying process, the gross mind and emotions dissolve into the subtle mind in the heart, while the very subtle mind rises up to the heart from the two lower chakras. Generally, the complete dissolution of the body elements and consciousness into the central mental consciousness in the heart takes up to three days. Then, the consciousness departs from the physical body and enters the intermediate state (bardo), searching for its next life.

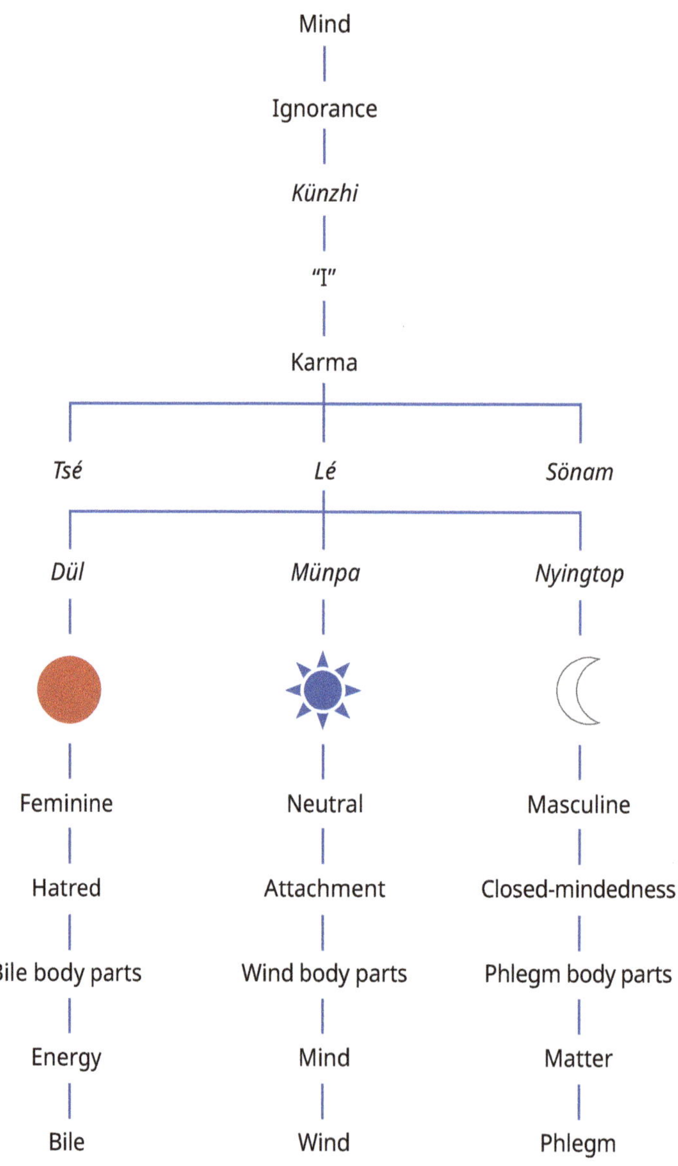

FIGURE 4.6 Schematic synthesis of body-mind development

CHAPTER 5

INTRODUCTION TO THE THREE HUMORS

The fundamental principle of Tibetan medicine is the functioning of the three humors (*nyépa sum*). This dynamic system rules the seven constituents that make up our body (*lüzung dün*) as well as the three waste products (*drima sum*), the impurities which are eliminated from the body. The humors are subjects, and the body constituents and waste products are its objects or bases. The relationship between them is like electricity, machine, and its product. Their interaction causes both health and disease. Medicine Buddha said at the start of the *Root Tantra*'s third chapter:[1]

> Health sustainment or decline is defined
> by the state of the humors, body
> constituents, and waste products.

This phrase summarizes the entirety of Tibetan medical theory. The detailed study of harmonious and disharmonious relations between the *nyépa* is the science of healing called Sowa Rigpa. The humors, more aptly called *nyépa*, can be interpreted as "faults," "defects," or "results of imperfection." Ignorant mind is the origin of the body-mind, which implies that the humoral system is inherently weak, fragile, and delicate, and that the body is inclined to suffer from sickness, old age, and death. It is in this respect that the humors literally can be referred to as "defective," based on the Buddhist conception of ignorance as the ultimate cause of suffering (see Section 4.1). From this perspective, all worldly existence follows the three natures of the humors and their karmic causes, allowing life to evolve naturally. The term "psychogenesis" can perhaps be applied to this process.

How is ignorant mind able to produce the body-mind? This question is addressed in the humors chapter of the *Explanatory Tantra*. It says, Insects on a poisonous tree are nevertheless sustained by it."[2] The impure cause of the three mental poisons produces three delicate, contaminated humors. The impermanent nature of the *nyépa* system could bring disharmony and disorders at any moment in time, given the presence of certain factors. As the *Root Tantra* says:[3]

> There are three causes for disease, and
> four co-emergent factors giving conditions
> for these to manifest.

5.1 CAUSES OF THE THREE HUMORS

There are three mental causes for the humors: attachment, hatred, and closed-mindedness. They compose the mind from birth. The mind's three natures manifest *lung* (from attachment), *tripa* (from hatred), and *béken* (from closed-mindedness). Besides these, subtle material energies are also involved. The movement, hot and cold natures of the body-mind are of the essence of the five subtle elements (*trawé jungwa nga*) and exist interdependently with the three unenlightened mind natures and the parental energies, coexisting as friends or foes. The subtle elements consist of both collective[4] and individual aspects. The *lung* element has mobility, dryness, and life energy (*sok*), and produces the *lung* humor. Fire is hot and produces *tripa*, which gives temperature and the metabolism that transforms the body constituents. Earth and water are together cold and wet, giving *béken*, which provides the solidity and

---

1 G.yu thog yon tan mgon po, 1993, 9.

2 Ibid., 27.

3 Ibid., 9.

4 The collective mind is a shared common sense, including "normal" ways of thinking and being part of a community, society, or a country.

cohesion that binds particles to form larger masses. These three natures or principles underlie the functioning of both the outer world and the human body.

The humoral energies can be understood in terms of the energy of the elements and the interaction between their hot, cold, and neutral qualities. The energies circulate in the body in the form of air, metabolic heat, and as bodily fluids. It is intriguing to compare the subtle nature of this composition to the structure of atoms in modern physics, consisting of protons (+), electrons (-), and neutrons (0), which together form materials.

The mind is the background of all, the pillar of life, the hidden power, the essence of life as well as the cover of the body. It sustains humoral function. The mind is called *sem*, which literally means "thinking" or "thought." *Lung* is the base and vehicle of the mind. Subtle wind (*lung trawa*) produces gross wind (*lung rakpa*) and gross mind, which in turn (re-)produces the three gross mental poisons (*duk sum rakpa*). The ultimate root of the three mental poisons is *marikpa*, meaning "lack of awareness" (Sanskrit: *avidyā*); it is the selfish, unenlightened mind. This impurity of the mind is born with the mind and accompanies it always. It is a subtle wind, a material energy aspect of the mind. In tantra and medicine, it is therefore said that mind and subtle wind are inseparable (*lung sem yer mé*, see again Section 4.1).[5] It is co-produced by and actively functions in the body, especially in the brain (*lépa*).

The subtle mind (*sem trawa*), on the other hand, is more deeply rooted. It gives the sense of "I," and resides in the heart chakra's backside channel that is governed by the mental affliction wind (*nyönmongpé lung*). This affliction wind pushes the mind and emotions to engage in negative actions. The subtle mind and the associated winds in turn produce mental sensations or feelings (*sem tsor*). In short, ignorance is caused by the material power of *lung*, which obscures and afflicts the mind's clarity. This is the prime cause of the physical body and the gross mind and emotions. Therefore, ignorance is called the principal cause. Ignorance is like dust on a perfectly translucent crystal, or oxidation on gold. They go together, but it can be purified.

The cause of the three *nyépa* is threefold. They develop from mind-matter connection, that is, the joining of the bardo consciousness with the parents' two energies. Both mind and the elemental

---

5   In this book, the words "psyche" and "psychology" refer to the gross mind.

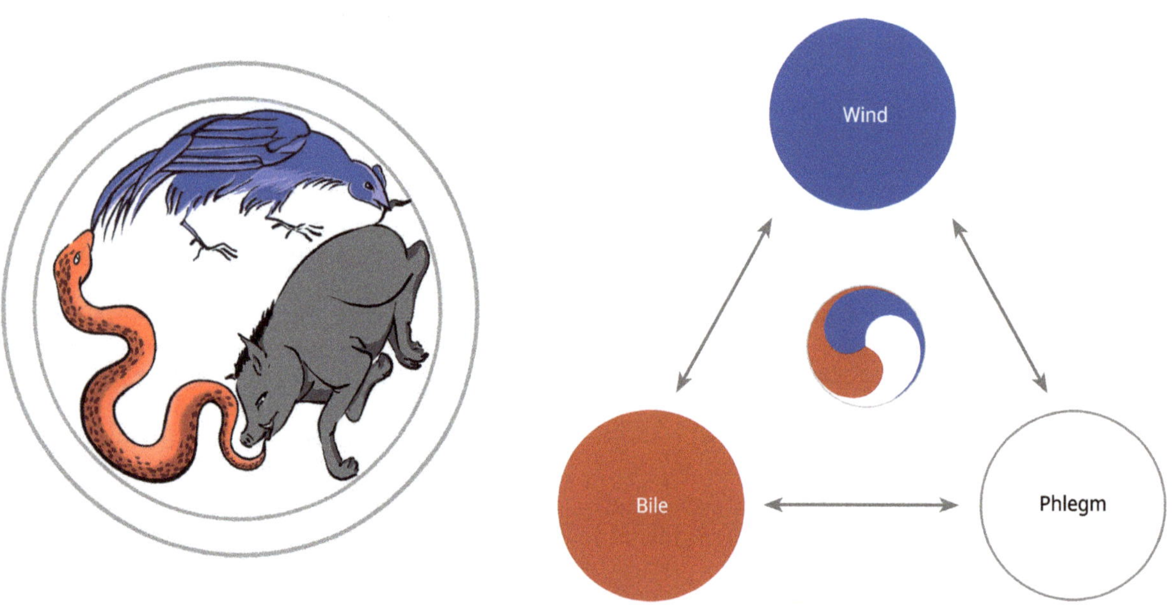

FIGURE 5.1 The relationship between the three mental characters and the three humors

energies produce the *nyépa* after their unification, and the *nyépa* produce the physical body constituents and waste products. These become the body's foundation. The subtle bardo mind produces the gross mind and consciousness. The body and mind develop side by side and jointly produce the three humors. This is the start of new life, as we are told in the *Root Tantra* and *Explanatory Tantra*. After the unification of mind and matter during conception, the subtle mind becomes the cause for the manifestation of the three gross mental poisons or emotions, which in turn develop the three humors.

Secondly, the five elemental energies provide the cause for the three humors to arise: the wind element gives the light and mobile qualities that produce the *lung*, the fire element produces the heat that manifests *tripa*, and the earth gives physical form and the water element moisture that binds together, manifesting *béken*. The ether or space element gives space for this manifestation and contributes to all channels and

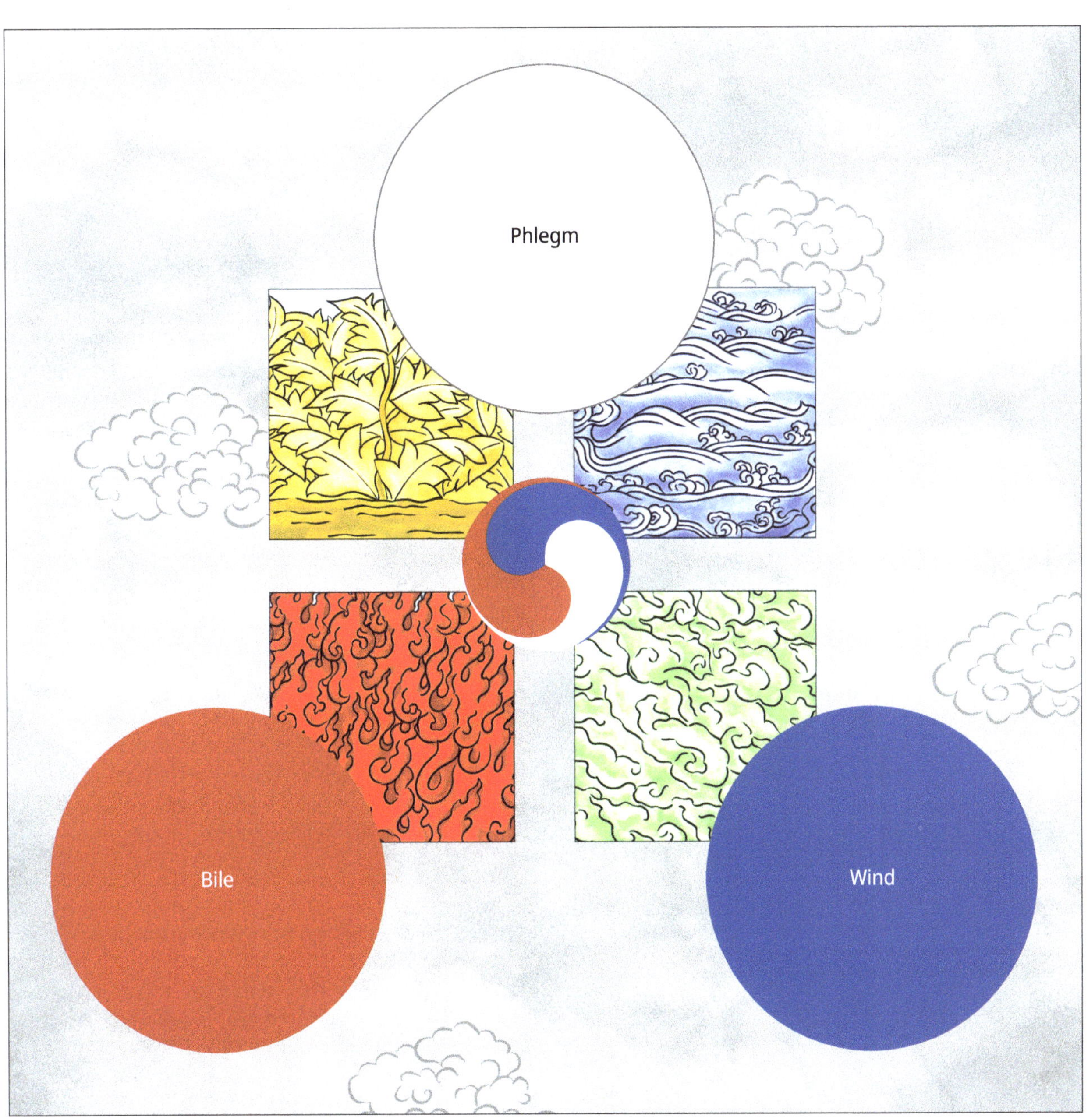

FIGURE 5.2 The relationship between the three humors and the five elements

cavities of the body. These five elements are found in the parents' two physical energies.

Thirdly, the physical or material causes of the three humors are: (1) the father's semen, which is the cause of *béken*, the brain, spinal cord, bones, glands and of the lymphatic and endocrine systems and all white-colored body tissues; (2) the mother's red menstrual blood (including ovum), which is the cause of *tripa*, the blood, organs, flesh and of the digestive tract; and (3) the wind element, becoming the cause of the *lung* humor, respiration, movement, skin, channels, cavities, tubes and pores, and the nervous system and brain-mind.

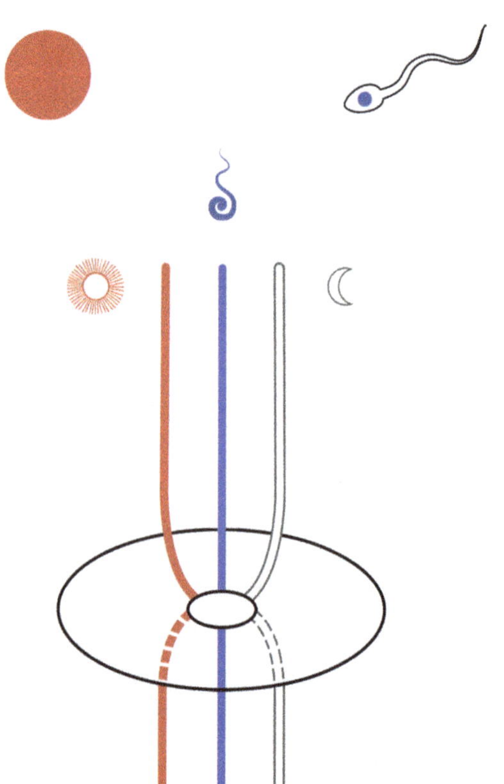

FIGURE 5.3 Symbolic illustration of body-mind reunion, with development starting from the channels of the navel chakra

5.2 DISTINGUISHING FEATURES

The threefold humoral system of the body is derived from the mind, elements, and parental contributions as explained above. The humors develop and build the body-house and govern its physiology, regulating the functioning of the organs and tissues. Balanced humors give positive health and harmony to the body-mind (*lüsem*), providing a good basis for its development and maintenance, and for mental stability and immunity. Loss of balance among the humors causes energetic disharmony and physical and mental disequilibrium, which may manifest at any time and become the cause of disease.

Characteristics of the *nyépa*

Six characteristics of *lung*

The nature of the wind humor is cold, but it functions dual or neutral relative to the other two humors. It has six characters: (1) rough, (2) light, (3) cold, (4) subtle, (5) hard, and (6) mobile. *Lung* balances *tripa* and *béken*.

Seven characteristics of *tripa*

Bile is hot and sharp in nature. It warms *lung* and dries *béken*. It has seven characteristics: (1) oily, (2) sharp, (3) hot, (4) light, (5) malodorous, (6) purgative, and (7) wet (in terms of inducing sweating).

Seven characteristics of *béken*

Phlegm is cold and humid in nature. It cools down *tripa* and moisturizes *lung*. Its seven characters are: (1) oily, (2) cool, (3) heavy, (4) blunt, (5) smooth, (6) stable, and (7) mucus-like (sticky, slippery).

Correspondences of the three humors

The wind humor is neutral and corresponds to wind (element), eclipse (function), the central channel (position), and the nerves (body system). It generally sustains the body-mind. The bile humor is hot-natured and corresponds to the sun and fire, dominates the right side of the body, and generates *tripa*. The phlegm humor is like the moon, earth and water elements, and its nature is cold and humid. Phlegm governs the left side body and raises *béken*.

Roughly, one can say that *lung, tripa* and *béken* activity corresponds respectively to the nervous system, the blood (circulatory system), and the lymphatic and endocrine systems of modern biology.

Three body locations

Phlegm humor location

The humors occupy different positions in the body according to their nature. *Béken* is in the head (brain, glands, and cerebral fluid), like a snow-capped mountain or lake that stores icy water. From there, water flows down along the neck, chest, abdomen, and legs, nourishing the organs in the form of supportive phlegm (*béken tenjé*). This water is heated by *tripa*, rising again to the head like clouds forming in the sky, and eventually becoming snow on the mountain of phlegm again. The glacial water cools down the bile heat and nourishes the body/earth. The spinal column, glands, stomach, spleen, kidney, bladder and reproductive organ, fat, bone marrow and lymph vessels are the channels of phlegm circulation. It is like a river flowing downhill, giving life to the entire valley. The *Root Tantra* says:[6]

> Phlegm is located in brain, the upper part of the body.

Bile humor location

Tripa is concentrated in the center of the body, where its fire is active in the liver, gallbladder, heart, and digestion. It digests and transforms food into nutrition by means of digestive bile (*tripa jujé*). It is the body fire that gives temperature, and which evaporates the phlegm water into steam that rises up into the sky. It warms up, dries, and thus balances phlegm, moving it upward to the chest and head. The blood channels, perspiration, digestive organs, skin, eyes, and heart are of the bile humor. The *Root Tantra* says:[7]

> Bile is located in the liver and gallbladder, the middle part of the body.

Wind humor location

Lung is situated in the lower abdomen, lumbar-sacral area, and colon, and especially in the descendant

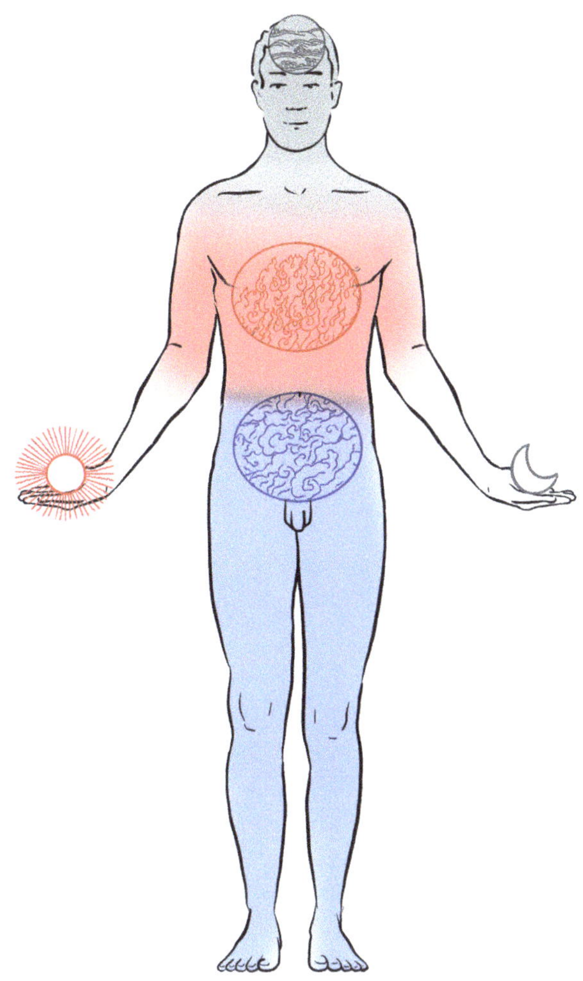

FIGURE 5.4 The general bodily locations of the three humors

colon and reproductive organs. Wind rises up from its lower abdomen base and fans the digestive fire in the form of fire-like wind (*lung ményam*). Wind acts as a fan, blowing the bile flames and increasing bile heat, which in turn warms up the phlegm of the lungs and head. The *Root Tantra* states:[8]

> Wind is based in the pelvic and sacral areas, the lower part of the body.

Wind is located below the navel, and bile is in the center. Phlegm is in the upper body and head. The collaborative action of evaporation and filtration transforms water into nectar essence, which is collected again in the brain and glands. This energetic cycle allows for regeneration.

---

6 G.yu thog yon tan mgon po, 1993, 10.
7 Ibid.

8 Ibid.

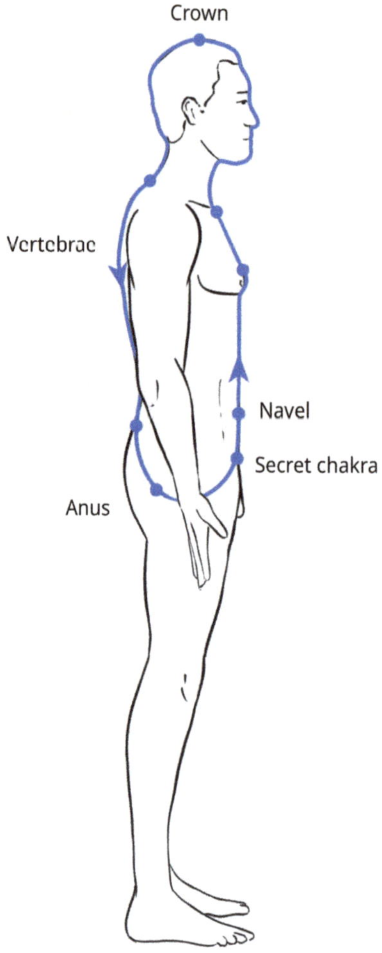

FIGURE 5.5 The humoral energy cycle

Body energy circulation

Wind moves the bile energy, which rises up to the front side of the head and then flows down again from the backside of the body as it cools down, circulating continuously. Bile circulation predominates during the day at the front side, whereas phlegm circulation at the backside is stronger at night. Wind energy circulation predominates principally in the early morning and late evening.

On top of this daily front-to-back humoral circulation, there is also a daily energy cycle from one side to the other. For men, it starts from the left big toe in the morning, continuing to the left thigh, arm, hand, and then reaching the head on midday. It then turns to the right side and reaches the right big toe on midnight. For women, this cycle moves in the opposite direction. The same cycle also takes place on a monthly basis in relation to the lunar calendar, which is the so-called *la* cycle (see Figure 18.1 and Figure 18.2). The difference, however, is that the humoral energies are gross, while *la* is a subtle vital force. Their relationship is like water and nectar, fruit and juice, and rock and diamond. They are connected but nonetheless distinct. The energy circulation front-to-back and sideways takes place along the four directions, keeping the body-mind in balance.

General function of the humors

After having focused on origins and general locations, let's now consider the general humor functions. The *nyépa* regulate the body and mind, sustain health, keep the body systems in order, digest food, transform the nutrients into body constituents, clean the waste products, and give strength. The wind humor governs the whole body by its six qualities or characteristics, while the bile and phlegm humors each have seven qualities. Opposite qualities neutralize the effects of the opposite energy, while complementary energies strengthen each other and sustain the body:

- *Lung* is cold nature, but moves bile heat and freezes phlegm coldness, also giving oxygen to the organs and tissues

- *Tripa* is hot, which melts and vaporizes solid and liquid phlegm, nourishing the body through its metabolic power

- *Béken* is cold and like water, neutralizing the bile heat, stabilizing wind, and sustaining the physical body

By their very nature, these energies struggle with each other to dominate the body-mind. Opposite powers may balance each other out and sustain health, whereas they could also cause disequilibrium and produce disease. The effect of these powers on the body on top of the influence of age produces a complex and delicate situation. When the body is young, the humors are strong and balanced according to the person's constitution. When the body gets older, humoral strength and qualities also degenerate, leading to disorder.

Congenital humoral defects

Serious disharmony of the humors during or soon after conception, or even parental health problems, may not lead to conception or end in abortion. In case conception takes place anyway, a fetus with disorders may develop. This could be termed "hereditary disease" (*lhenkyé né*). Such inborn diseases are also known as co-emergent lesions (*lhenkyé ma*), literally "born with wound." What in modern biomedicine are called genetic and congenital disorders may correspond to these categories, which also include certain tumors (*dré né*). In addition to karmic influences, these are probably related to the parents or unfortunate circumstances during or after conception.

5.3 COLLECTIVE HUMORAL FUNCTIONING (*NYÉPÉ TÜNMONG GI LÉ*)

The collective action and equilibrium of the three humors is the secret of body-mind synchronization. Besides the mind and the fundamental support of life-sustaining wind, the body is coordinated and kept in balance through the functioning of the *nyépa*. Understanding the natural position of the elements within the body will help us to further reveal where the humors dominate and why.

The elements appear inside the body in the following order:

- The space or ether element position is in the head and especially the crown area
- The wind element resides in the throat and chest
- The fire element is in the middle part of the body
- The water element is held in the lower abdomen and thighs
- The earth element is situated in the bottom, especially the legs and feet

The earth gives the base for water, water for fire, and so on. They support each other and thus sustain the balance of the body-mind. This elemental positioning in the body is called *jungtsek*, which refers to their stacked sequence of manifestation from sky to earth.

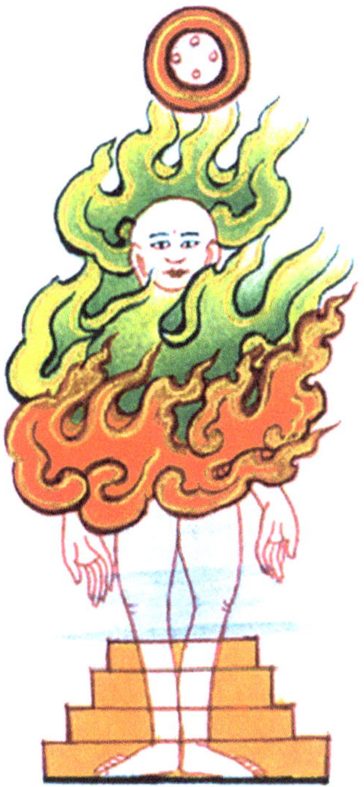

FIGURE 5.6 The sequence of the elements inside the body

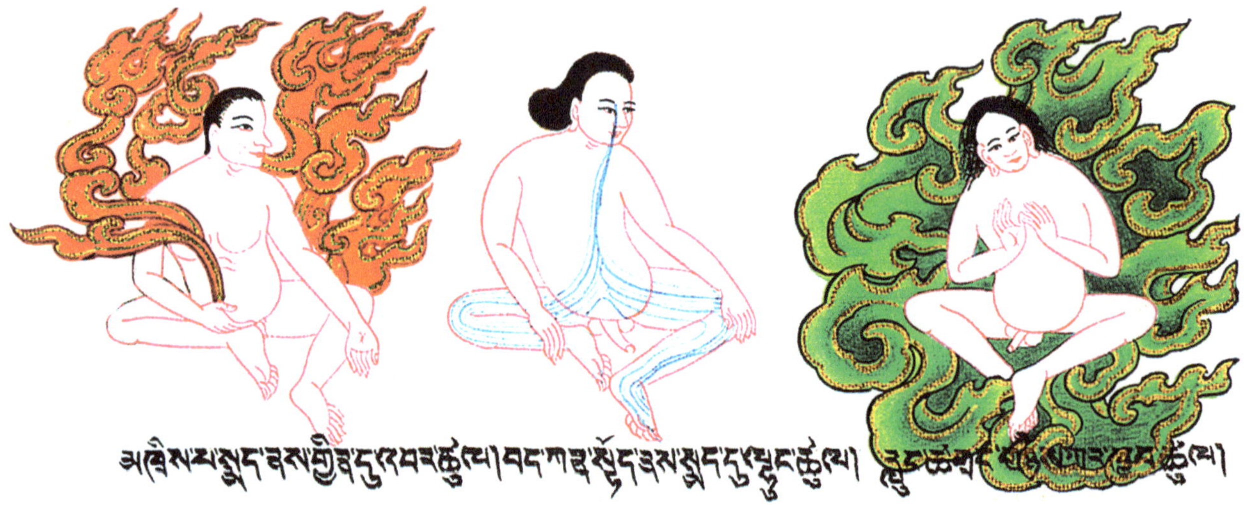

FIGURE 5.7 The humoral forces within the body

Collective elemental and humoral function

The combination and collaboration of the five elements constitutes the three humoral forces. Phlegm is located in the head and flows down like a river. Bile is the fire energy contained in the middle part of the body, of which the heat moves upwards. The wind humor is in the lower area of the body and blows the fire. Wind increases the fire heat, which heats up the phlegm water. This circulating stream of activity is life. This is the process of the collective body energy, balancing the humors just like the changing seasons.

The relationship between the humors

There are many examples which elucidate the positive and negative interactions between the *nyépa sum*. One example (as mentioned in the 15th chapter of the *Oral Instruction Tantra*) goes as follows:[9]

> Wind, bile, and phlegm are like brothers.
> If one faces adversity, the two others also suffer.

The humors, body constituents, and waste products keep each other in check by the body's functioning. However, the humors and emotions must be in balance. Proper nutrition and behavior should be followed, attending to the seasons. This leads to a healthy, balanced body-mind.

On the contrary, imbalanced humors and emotions aggravated by unhealthy food, behavior and going against seasonal law become the cause of body-mind

disorders directly, or to humoral accumulation which may later manifest as disease.

Nevertheless, the body naturally maintains balance. It has the capacity to heal itself. The healing powers are the humors themselves, which can be restored over time. With the help of the seasons, nutrition and behavior, the body waste products are purified automatically, and health is sustained. Therefore, the four or six seasons have major healing potential, naturally supporting the balance of the elements and humors.

In late spring wind increases, activating bile during summer and autumn, after which the body constituents are cooled again in winter and early spring by phlegm. Spring energy gives new life to the body, and in summer flowers blossom, which brings joy. Autumn is the maturation time, and in winter energy is dormant. Spring's waste products are cleaned in summer, and summer's waste products in autumn. Autumn's waste products are processed in winter, and winter's residue during the elemental changes of spring.

Like seasonal changes, the body's biorhythm equally shifts throughout the morning, day and night, clearing waste products every day. This cyclic cleansing and balancing supports health. Summer hydrates (especially monsoon) and winter dehydrates, which is balanced in autumn and spring. The seasons, day and night, and the changing body temperatures are like a cosmic clock. This humoral equilibrium naturally rises and falls to sustain the body, health, mind, and emotions.

---

9 Ibid., 203.

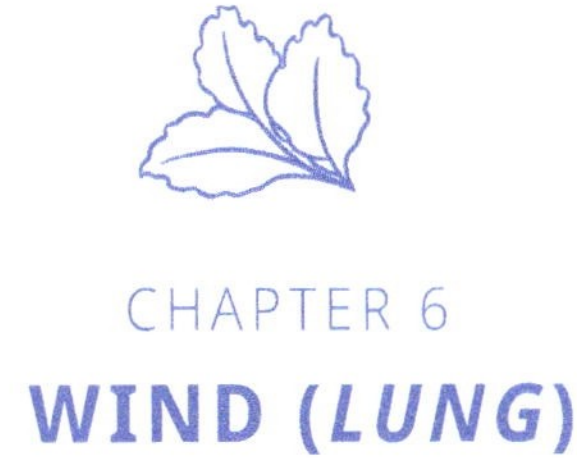

CHAPTER 6

WIND (*LUNG*)

Focusing on the physiology of each humor in turn, *lung* takes first place in Tibetan medical literature because life starts with and is sustained by wind, disease is initiated by wind, and life ends with wind.

6.1 GENERAL WIND (*LUNG CHI*)

Lung is a life force, the breath of the body-mind. It is pervasive and circulates in and outside of the body. It manifests from the mind and cosmic subtle wind energy (*lung trawa*), and is the foundation of the body's respiration, mobility, and strength. *Lung* sustains and governs the function of the mind and the wind humor system. During fetus development, subtle wind forms the central channel (*tsa uma*), which goes upward straight to the head from the umbilical cord (navel chakra), passing by the other chakras. This channel also goes down to the perineum from the umbilical cord, forming the root of the central wind channel which supports the body like a pillar. This is the wind humor trunk, a tree that has countless big and small branches. It is like the piston of a wheel or the handle of an umbrella. The nodes of the central channel are called chakras (*khorlo*). There are five main and 12 minor chakras (the 12 joints). Countless smaller branches of wind ramify like the veins of a leaf, covering the entire body. The fourth chapter of the *Explanatory Tantra* states:[10]

> A channel penetrates downward from the
> navel, forming the secret organ.
> Attachment resides in the male and female
> genitals.
> From there, wind arises, so it is located
> below.

The *lung* branches form a network that also includes the seven body constituents and three waste products. The wind channels distribute nutrition to all bodily organs and tissues. They all live by breathing; this energy is the wind humor. Respiration helps transform nutrients and thus nourishes the body. It eliminates the waste products and thus keeps the body clean. Wind and its channels are like a tree, with fruits maturing at the tips of its branches. The main root of the wind system is life-sustaining wind (*sokdzin gyi lung*), which is located principally in the brain.

Wind is concentrated in the central channel, where the subtle mental consciousness (*künzhi yi kyi namshé*) resides, and where the life fuel energy (*tsé yi lung*) is stored. This is the root and trunk of the Wind humor, and the chakras are the nodes of the tree. The vital and sensory organs are its fruits and flowers. The fifth chapter of the *Explanatory Tantra* says:[11]

> The function of wind is breathing in and out,
> movement, actions, giving force, circulating
> the constituents and waste products,
> clearing the sense organs and sustaining
> the body.

The wind humor has five principal roots (*tsawé lung nga*) and five minor branches (*yenlak gi lung nga*), together comprising the 10 vital wind energies. Besides these, there are 24,000 tiny subdivisions constantly flowing throughout the body, sustaining life, and manifesting emotions arising from attachment, desire, and lust.

The wind humor shares the same nature and characteristics with general wind or air, and neutrally functions alongside bile and phlegm.

There are three main sources for the wind humor:

1. Subtle wind energy coming from the past life along with the bardo consciousness

---

10 G.yu thog yon tan mgon po, 1993, 22.

11 Ibid., 28.

2. Wind elements from the parents during fetus development (especially from the mother)

3. *Lung* absorbed throughout life from food and air (breathing)

Location

The wind humor is found in every part of the body, but it is particularly active in the heart, lungs, colon, small intestine, skin, ears, bones, (hip) joints, and lumbar-sacral area. Its base is in the lumbar and pelvic area, lower abdomen, colon, and in the nervous system.

The five principal winds are mainly located in the head, throat, chest, abdomen, and lower abdomen. These five locations correspond to the five chakras in tantra: the crown chakra, throat chakra, heart chakra, navel chakra, and secret chakra. In short, these winds sustain and manifest the five emotions of closed-mindedness, desire, hatred, pride, and jealousy.

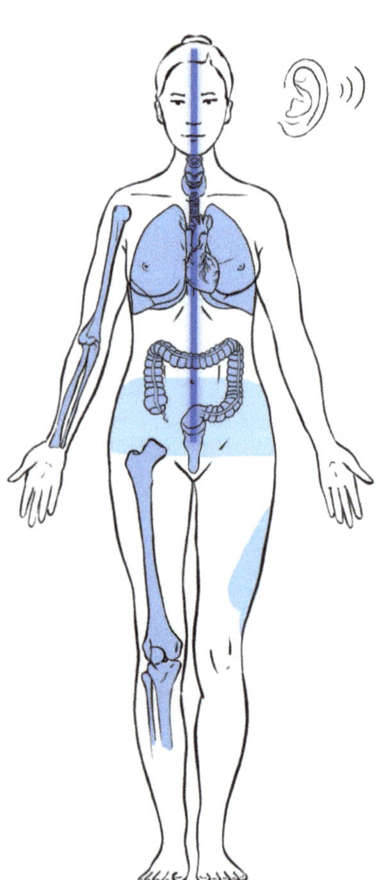

FIGURE 6.1 The main locations of general wind

Function

Wind functions as vehicle of the mind and enables the mind to perceive and to think. It allows for awareness. *Lung* regulates respiration and mobility, and sustains life through breathing; it enables movement, and makes blood, lymph and subtle energy circulate. Wind helps absorb nutrition, transform tissues, clear the sensory organs, and sustain their functions. It controls the senses, as well as the functions of the vital and hollow organs. It transfers memories of the gross mind to the subtle mind. In short, all physical and mental functions depend on the wind humor. *Lung* gives life to the body as well as to the body's microorganisms.

Crippled general wind

When the general wind is severely damaged during fetus development, this may cause congenital diseases such as physical and mental handicaps, neurological disorders, and missing organs.

Six characteristics

Lung has six characteristics (*lung gi tsen nyi druk*): (1) rough (*tsupa*), (2) light (*yangwa*), (3) cold (*drangwa*), (4) subtle (*trawa*), (5) hard (*sawa*), and (6) mobile (*yowa*). These qualities maintain the body by balancing the two other *nyépa*.

Imbalance signs

Wind imbalance implies the increase of its characteristics through wrong diet and behavior. *Lung* itself is first disturbed, and then begins to attack the other two humors, overpowering them and thus creating disorder. This is first reflected in mild wind-increasing symptoms in line with the six characteristics:

TABLE 6.1 The six characteristics of wind

	Wind characteristic	Neutralized qualities of other *nyépa*	*Nyépa* reduced	*Nyépa* increased
1.	Rough/dry	Oily and sticky (mucus)	- Bile - Phlegm	
2.	Light	Heavy	- Phlegm	+ Bile
3.	Cold	Hot	- Bile	+ Phlegm
4.	Subtle	Oily	- Bile	
5.	Hard	Oily	- Bile	+ Phlegm
6.	Mobile	Stable	- Phlegm	+ Bile

1. The body becomes dry
2. Becoming and feeling lighter
3. Sensitivity to cold and wind
4. The mind becomes more fragile, sensitive, and subtle
5. The body becomes hard
6. The body-mind becomes more mobile, causing instability and restlessness

6.2 THE FIVE PRINCIPAL WINDS (*TSAWÉ LUNG NGA*)

The five principal winds branch from the main wind tree. They manifest from the life-sustaining wind of the central channel during fetus development, like light radiating from the sun. If we compare these with tantric sources, we can understand the link with the five chakras.

1. Life-sustaining wind (*sokdzin gyi lung*)

Life-sustaining wind is the first branch to develop from the main wind trunk (*lung uma*), during the first month of embryonal development.[1] At this time, a channel branches off to become the central axis of the body-mind. However, its main place of activity is in the head (brain), like the canopy of an umbrella of which the shaft is the central channel. It is the most vital energy of life. It governs the head and rules the whole body-mind system.[2] It is also called life-span wind (*soklung*) or longevity wind (*tsé yi lung*), which is stored in the central channel like fuel and released throughout life through the nostrils during respiration.

Function

Sokdzin lung is sustained by breaths from the central channel, which contain a small amount of the lifespan wind energy that flows upwards. Each lifespan breath consists of two parts. One part goes to the crown chakra (brain) and is consumed there, becoming body-mind energy which sustains the six consciousnesses and the continuation of *sokdzin lung* functioning. The second part of the breath comes out from the mouth and nostrils with exhalation. Each breath therefore consumes life energy. The quantity of the life energy in the central channel is the basic lifespan of the person and their body-mind force (see Section 4.3). Life-sustaining wind functions in the brain, sensory organs, mouth, nostrils, and esophagus. It regulates the nervous system, brain memory, and supports analytical power and attention. It determines the sense of I, and thus controls the entire body. It helps swallow food, breathe, sneeze, spit, vomit, belch, etc. It clears the mind and the sensory organs, and sustains life. It regulates the central pillar of the body and the respiratory system. It keeps

---

1   The branch winds' manifestation months described here follow Nāropā's Six Yogas.

2   Buddhist tantra states that *sokdzin lung* resides in the heart. One should be aware of this distinction.

TABLE 6.2 The five principal winds

	Principal wind	Chakra (body part)	Emotion
1.	Life-sustaining wind (*sokdzin lung*)	Crown chakra (head)	Ignorance
2.	Ascending wind (*gyengyü lung*)	Throat chakra (upper body)	Attachment
3.	Pervasive wind (*khyapjé lung*)	Heart chakra (chest)	Anger
4.	Fire-like wind (*ményam lung*)	Navel chakra (abdomen)	Pride, greed
5.	Descending wind (*tursel lung*)	Secret chakra (lower abdomen)	Fear, jealousy

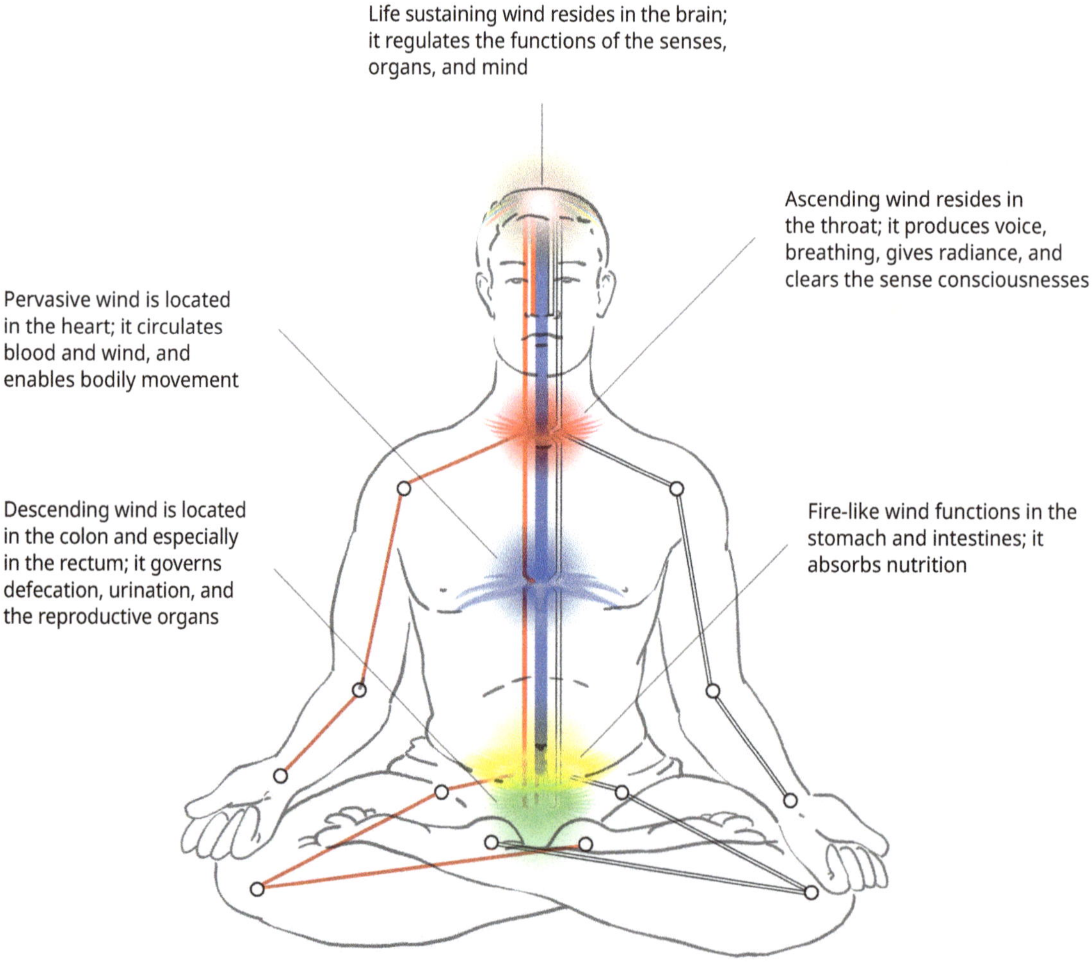

FIGURE 6.2 The five principal winds and the five chakras

the body-mind in balance and holds and sustains the mind and its mental functions.

Psychologically, life-sustaining wind manifests from closed-mindedness (*timuk*), which is why the brain is the seat of ignorance and the main source of our thoughts. The fifth chapter of the *Explanatory Tantra* describes:[3]

> Life-sustaining wind resides in the crown.
> It functions in the throat, the middle of the chest, and when swallowing,
> in respiration, spitting, sneezing, and belching,
> clearing the intellect and sense organs, thus sustaining the mind.

Life-sustaining wind and the brain

The *Explanatory Tantra*'s channel and sense organ development chapter explains that the head is an ocean of channels and the seat of closed-mindedness, which develops the phlegm humor. All three major channels (nerves, blood, and lymph) and especially the endocrine glands and lymphatic water bank (cerebrospinal fluid) are to be found in the brain. Through cerebrospinal channels, fluid flows down like Himalayan rivers flowing downhill, nourishing all body parts. The brain's grey matter and liquid represent the earth and water elements respectively that produce the heavy quality of the brain.

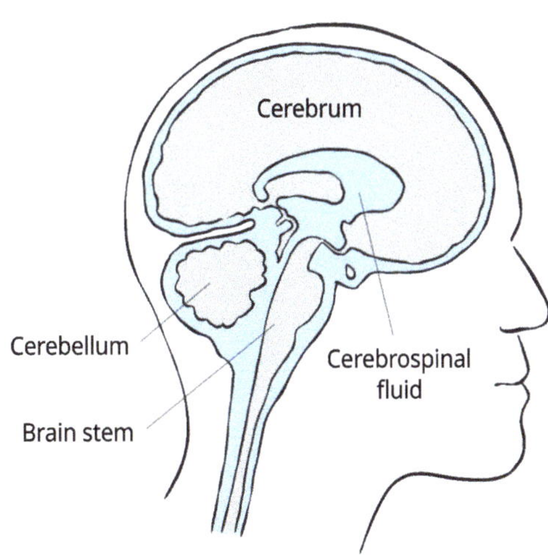

FIGURE 6.3 The ocean of phlegm and its rivers

The qualities of heaviness and coldness manifest *timuk*, the closed-minded gross mind of the brain. More detail is provided in Dési Sangyé Gyatso's *Blue Beryl* commentary on the *Explanatory Tantra*. During life, the middle part (central channel) is the seat of *künzhi* consciousness, which is filled by life-sustaining wind. It appears empty and sky-like. In relation to this, the Kālachakra Tantra states that the middle channel's tip is the seat of (planet) Rāhula (Sgra gcan) while the opposite end represents Kālāgni ("Fire Time").[4] This helps to understand the dual nature of the middle channel: the top is associated with the darkness of an eclipse (which is the source of *béken* and *timuk*), whereas the bottom is fiery in nature. In brief, all brain-based channels and humoral development arises through the action of life-sustaining wind.

Life sustaining wind and the five sense organs (*wangpo nga*)

The five sensory organs function by means of the five sense consciousnesses, which are minor wind branches of life-sustaining wind (see also Section 6.3). The perceptions of the five sense consciousnesses are supported by the brain's five sense faculty nerve channels (as well as blood and lymph). When the eye perceives an image, for instance, wind functions like an electric current which allows the consciousness to recognize the object. These nerve channels are called the 12 sources or bases of perception (*kyéché chunyi*), consisting of six outer or external objects such as form and color, and six inner sense bases. They are fundamental for sensory and mental perception.

From each of the three main channels, eight subchannels branch out, forming 24 sensory channels that envelop the five sense organs from which 500 minor perception channels derive. These 500 channels are divided as follows: 200 branch off from the eight branches of the main blood channel (*trak tsa*), 200 from the water channel (*chu tsa*), and 100 from wind (*lung tsa*). These minor perception channels support the sense organs to see, hear, smell, taste and feel by guiding the sense consciousnesses. The collective function of the five or six (including the mental faculty) consciousness functions in the brain is what is called gross mind (*sem rakpa*).

Gross memory

Each sense consciousness perceives its own object and imputes information into its memory faculty. All senses together produce the common memory of the

---

3   G.yu thog yon tan mgon po, 1993, 28.

4   Sde srid sangs rgyas rgya mtsho, 1994, 85.

brain, which is referred to here as general or gross memory (*drenpa*). The collective experience of the sense consciousnesses is stored in the coiled channel (*khyilwé tsa*) nerves of the brain. Metaphorically, this plexus operates like a computer's hard drive. However, there might not be one single place for gross memory; rather, five or six separate records of memory are "saved"—one from each of the sense consciousnesses. Each of these five or six storages have a significant influence over the mind. Essential memories are transferred to the heart, where the *künzhi* is located. This storage of collective karma collects experiences in the subtle mind. But before transferring memories to the heart, the brain's memory-clearing channels filter each experience. Memories encompassing strong emotions and sensations are transferred, whereas minor feelings are dismissed, a process that takes place mainly during sleep. This explains why things are forgotten.

Malfunction of life-sustaining wind

If the life-sustaining wind function is disturbed by wrong factors, one may lose consciousness and balance, get vertigo, lose control, have wrong perceptions, confusion, sounds in the head and ears, experience feelings of having an empty head, and hallucinate. It may also cause shortness of breath, difficulty breathing in, and difficulty swallowing.

Crippled Life-sustaining wind

A serious defect or disharmony during conception or fetus development may provoke congenital disorders such as handicaps, brain and neurological genetic disorders. *Sokdzin lung* disturbed after birth may become the cause of mental instability and even insanity.

2. Ascending wind (*gyengyü lung*)

Gyengyü lung is the second principal wind that branches from the wind humor tree. It manifests during the third month of fetus development. It resides in the chest, lungs, throat, larynx, mouth and nasal cavity, and especially in the vocal cords and thyroid.

Function

It underlies the ability to speak and the voice, maintains the strength of the body, increases radiance, clears the complexion, generates interest and skills in art and crafts, and clears memory and awareness. It moves upwards to the throat and makes breathing through the lungs, trachea, and nostrils possible. It activates the thyroid and throat chakra during sleep and dreams. *Gyengyü lung* is the main force driving the elimination of minor excretions like sputum and mucus from the mouth, nose, and other sensory organs, as well as the throat, lungs, heart, and chest. In short, it rules the throat and neck areas and produces sound. This wind energy flowing up to the head through the throat is a vital function for the balance of the body-mind. The fifth chapter of the *Explanatory Tantra* states:[5]

> Ascending wind resides in the chest.
> It circulates in nose, tongue, and throat, and produces sound,
> giving strength, radiance, color, effort, and clearing the memory.

Psychologically, ascending wind manifests attachment, desire, and lust. It also provokes anger and nervousness.

Malfunction

Malfunction of this wind could be the cause of many disorders of the upper body: thyroid and lung disorders, insomnia and having many dreams, hysteria, sore throat, loss of voice, breathing difficulties, as well as neck and should pain, and headaches. It may also produce pressure in the sensory organs and head, speech defects, loss of strength, facial paralysis, and loss of consciousness. Hyperfunction of the ascending wind induces frequent dreams and emotions, as well as hyperactive behaviors.

Crippled ascending wind

Disharmony of this wind during fetus development could manifest in various vertebral disorders, such as spondylitis, scoliosis, chicken chest, as well as back, neck and chest deformation. The mother experiencing psychological problems could also influence this wind in the child, leading to fetal malformation, cervical and thyroid disorders.

---

5   G.yu thog yon tan mgon po, 1993, 28.

3. Pervasive wind (*khyapjé lung*)

Pervasive wind or *khyapjé lung* is the third principal wind, which branches off from the wind humor trunk in the fourth month of fetus development. It resides in the heart, chest and shoulders, arms and hands, but also pervades the entire body.

Function

Pervasive wind facilitates movements such as lifting the arms up and down, stretching, bending, and walking. It regulates the body organs and cavities by keeping one's body in balance and allowing a straight posture. It sustains the heart function, makes the blood and wind circulate and thus nourishes the body. In short, it rules all bodily actions, especially in the chest. The *Explanatory Tantra*'s fifth chapter states:[6]

> Pervasive wind resides in the heart.
> It flows across the whole body, lifting the limbs up and down and enabling walking, stretching, bending, contraction, and expansion.
> Most actions such as these depend on this wind.

Psychologically, this wind produces anger, hatred, and related emotions. Therefore, *Gyüzhi* says that desirous or accomplishing bile and anger reside in the heart.[7]

Malfunction

Pervasive wind malfunction manifests as loss of balance, hypertension, chest tension, fear, panic attacks (cf. heart-wind disorder), fainting, loss of speech, cardiac disorders, talkativeness, desire to roam, pains in the joints, shoulders and back, blood circulation difficulties, heart palpitations and rhythm disturbances, in complaining and unfriendly speech which worsens the situation, and so on.

Crippled pervasive wind

A pervasive wind defect or disharmony during conception or fetus development could manifest as congenital cardiac diseases such as mitral valve disorders, arrhythmia, and other heart defects.

4. Fire-like or fire-accompanying wind (*ményam lung*)

Ményam lung is the fourth principal wind, which branches off from the wind humor trunk in the fifth month of fetus development. It resides in the stomach and intestines. It is the wind fan which increases bile's fire, so it is called *ményam*, stabilizing fire-like heat.

Function

It is the firepower which helps the digestive bile to process food, functioning in all digestive organs. It aids the absorption and assimilation of food, maturing the nutrients and transporting the food essences to the liver and body while separating the waste products. In short, it regulates the abdominal area below the diaphragm and above the navel. The fifth chapter of the *Explanatory Tantra* says:[8]

> Fire-like wind resides in the stomach, circulates in the internal organs, digests food, separates food essence from waste products, and matures the constituents and waste products.

Psychologically, this wind manifests hunger for food as well as authority, egotism, pride, and greed.

Malfunction

Malfunction of this wind causes a cold stomach, poor appetite, vomiting, and disturbed blood circulation of the stomach. It also contributes to all acute and chronic digestive disorders, especially in the lower abdomen, including gas formation, hiatal hernia, tension in the heart, back and chest pains, intestinal cramps, constipation, low metabolism, upset intestinal flora, malabsorption, etc.

Crippled fire-like wind

A fire-like wind defect or disharmony during conception or fetus development could manifest congenital abnormalities such as cascade stomach, intestinal and pancreas-based digestive malfunction as well as malabsorption disorders.

---

6   Ibid., 28.

7   Buddhist tantra states that *khyapjé lung* resides in the head.

8   Ibid.

5. Descending wind (*tursel lung*)

Tursel lung is the fifth principal wind, which branches off from the root of the wind trunk in the second month of the fetus development. It resides in the colon, bladder, reproductive organs, thighs, and especially in the sigmoid colon and rectum (*nyéma*). As it operates downwards, it is called the descending wind.

Function

It regulates bowel movement, controls the evacuation of feces and urine, sexual activities, as well as semen and menstruation discharge. It rules conception, fetus development and labor, and thus ensures procreation. The fifth chapter of the *Explanatory Tantra* says:[9]

> Descending wind resides in the sigmoid colon and rectum.
> It functions in the colon, bladder, genitals, and thighs,
> regulating semen and menses, feces and urine, and childbirth.

Psychologically, this wind manifests jealousy, fear, and worries.

Malfunction

Disturbance of this wind manifests in the joints with a boiling pain, and as excessively loose or rigid joints. It also produces lower abdominal disorders such as back pain, constipation, infertility, bladder, urination and ejaculation disorders, menstrual disorders, hemorrhoids, intestinal hernia, and blood circulation disorders. In short, it becomes the cause of all lower body disorders.

Crippled descending wind

A descending wind defect or disharmony during conception or fetus development could manifest congenital colon and reproductive organ defects as well as urinal tract impairments and fistulae.

6.3 THE FIVE MINOR WINDS (*YENLAK GI LUNG NGA*)

The five minor winds are not directly described in the *Gyüzhi;* they are therefore not that well-known in medicine even though they are listed in the commentarial and tantric literature. Nevertheless, they are crucial to grasp the functioning of the brain and sense organs as well as for the field of pathology.

These minor winds all branch off from the life-sustaining wind,[10] and mainly function in the brain. In Tibetan medicine, explanations on brain function are underdeveloped compared to other aspects of anatomy and physiology; this is undeniable. Buddhist philosophy and tantra generally do not pay much attention to brain function either. The physiology of

---

9   Ibid. 25.

10   Different tantras explain different times and causes for its development.

TABLE 6.3 The senses and the five minor winds

	Sense faculty	Sense object	Minor wind	Minor wind element	Sense organ and consciousness	Nerve channel
1.	Vision	Form	*Lu*	Earth	Eye	Optic
2.	Audition	Sound	*Rübel*	Space	Ear	Auditory
3.	Olfaction	Smell	*Tsangpa*	Water	Nose	Olfactory
4.	Gustation	Taste	*Lhajin*	Fire	Tongue	Gustatory
5.	Somato-sensation	Touch	*Norlhagyel*	Wind	Skin	Tactile

these channels has remained unclear for centuries. Knowledge on the *yenlak gi lung nga* therefore must be advanced further. Comparing the tantric five minor winds with the *Explanatory Tantra*'s five hundred sense organ channels could be the basis for further research. These winds seem to largely correspond to the functions of the seven cranial nerves in biomedicine. However, in Tibetan tantra and medicine, *lung* terminology is applied. As is clearly laid out in the Six Yogas of Nāropā, the sense consciousnesses operate through the five minor winds.[11] Such connections and comparisons may fill the gap between Tibetan medicine and modern brain anatomy, and lead to a deeper study of the mind.

Development

The minor winds are secondary wind branches of *tsa uma*, as described in Nāropā's Six Yogas:

- In the sixth month, *lü lung* and the earth element develop the eyes

- In the seventh month, *rübel gyi lung* and the space element develop the ears and all hollow organs, channels, and external orifices

- In the eighth month, *tsangpé lung* and the water element develop and open the nostrils

- In the ninth month, *lhajin gyi lung* and the fire element develop the tongue

- In the 10th month, *norlhagyel lung* and the wind element develop the body's tactile sense and physical wind system

Sakyapa Gyeltsen Pelzang has described a different classification of the five minor winds, in which not all branch from life-sustaining wind.[12] From a medical perspective, however, it seems more logical to accept that the minor winds develop from the life-sustaining wind of the brain, as asserted by Dési Sangyé Gyatso.[13]

---

11 Dpal 'byor don grub, 1995, 76–83.

12 Sa skya pa rgyal mtshan dpal bzang, 1991, 51–54. Different names and origins may be found in the literature, with each tradition having its own reasoning.

13 Sde srid sangs rgyas rgya mtsho, 1994, 130.

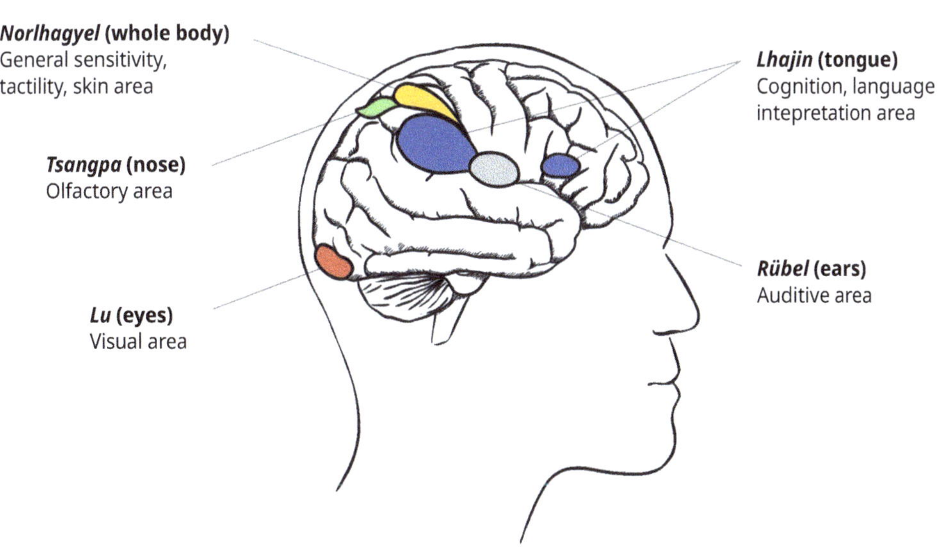

FIGURE 6.4 The activity of the five minor winds in the brain correlates with the five primary sensory areas of modern neuroscience

General function

The minor winds govern the sense organs and are vehicles of the sense consciousnesses and their related emotions. Together, these winds and sense organs perceive images, sounds, etc., and transmit these to the sense consciousnesses. The sense consciousnesses (*shépa*) recognize, process, and analyze this information before storing it in the brain memory bank. This is then later transmitted to the mental consciousness of the *künzhi* in the heart. The minor winds are the primary cause of sensory perception and skills.

1. *Lu* wind

Lu (which means "naga") is a minor eye wind of the earth element.[14] The root of this wind resides in the small intestine, like a coiled snake. It provides the conditions to develop the eyes during the sixth month of fetal development, later operating in the eye organ and brain. *Lu* perceives colors and forms, while also fostering creativity and skill (as in dance and drama). Therefore, it may also be called the artistic wind.

The eye consciousness (*mik shé*) is carried by *lu* wind through the eye and optic nerve to make contact with images. Where the mind wishes to look, there the eyes turn to, and eye consciousness activates.

- The eye organ develops from the fire element and liver

- *Lu* itself is earth element and arises from the small intestine

- Both produce the eye consciousness, which reaches out to external objects

Crippled *Lu* wind

Lu wind defects or disharmony during fetus development could manifest congenital eye disorders such as blindness from birth, perception and other eye defects.

2. *Rübel* wind

Rübel wind (literally "turtle wind") is the ear minor wind. It functions in the ear organs to perceive sound. *Rübel*'s root is in the liver, developing during the seventh month of fetal development. It rules hand, leg, and head movements and can also be called emotional expression wind, articulating hand and body gestures during speaking or work.

- The ear organ develops from the kidneys and space element

- *Rübel* wind itself is space element and arises from the liver

- Both produce the ear consciousness, which reaches out to external objects

Crippled *rübel* wind

A *rübel* wind defect or disharmony during fetus development could manifest congenital diseases of the ear, deafness from birth, missing limbs, and impaired body flexibility.

3. *Tsangpa* wind

The nose minor wind is of the water element and its root develops from the lungs during the eighth month of fetal development. This wind governs the smell faculty, perceives odors, and is involved in sneezing and other nasal functions. It also provokes anger, irritation, nervousness, and other emotions through sensorial contact. Therefore, this wind may be called the nervous wind.

- The nose organ develops from the lungs and earth element

- *Tsangpa* wind itself is of the water element and arises from the lungs

- Both produce the nose consciousness, which reaches out to external objects

Crippled *tsangpa* wind

A *tsangpa* wind defect or disharmony during fetus development could manifest congenital diseases such as nasal organ defects, an angry nature, and fragile nasal cavities.

---

14 The minor wind elements given below follow Sa skya pa rgyal mtshan dpal bzang, 1991, 53.

4. *Lhajin* wind

The tongue minor wind has a fire element nature and its root develops from the heart. The tongue develops during the ninth month of fetus development, experiences taste, and enables yawning. This wind may therefore be called the sleepy wind.

- The tongue organ develops from the water element and heart

- *Lhajin* wind itself is of the fire element and arises from the heart

- Both produce the tongue consciousness, which reaches out to external objects

Crippled *lhajin* wind

A *lhajin* wind defect or disharmony during fetus development could manifest congenital diseases such as sleeping disorders, speech disorders such as stammering, and impairments of eating and swallowing food.

5. *Norlhagyel* or *zhulégyel* wind

Norlhagyel wind is the body minor wind. Its root develops from the kidneys during the 10th month of fetus development. It is bow-shaped and activates the bodily tactile sense, supporting the function of body consciousness. *Norlhagyel* perceives temperature, smooth and gentle or rough and coarse, hot and cold, and feelings of enjoyment or dislike, etc. It is particularly involved in rhythmic movement patterns which can be trained. It may therefore be called the body coordination wind. This wind remains even after death, until the body's complete destruction.[15]

- The body's tactile organ develops from the wind element and spleen

- *Norlhagyel* wind itself is wind element and arises from the kidneys

- Both produce the body consciousness, which reaches out to external objects

Crippled *norlhagyel* wind

A disharmony of this wind during fetus development may manifest congenital diseases such as insensibility and other tactile disorders, as well as impaired growth.

6.4 SOME IMPORTANT SUPPLEMENTARY NOTES ON *LUNG*

Tibetan medical practitioners customarily study the five principal winds and the wind pathology chapters. But they ought to learn more about the wind humor and its branches. A large area of study on wind-nerve function, mind, and emotions is yet to be fully explored. To this end, some extra information on the functioning of *lung* which is generally not elaborated much is added in this section.

Depending on *lung*'s nature, temperature and location, different names have been given to different winds by ancient tantric masters. Without question, body constitution and breathing involve different qualities of wind. Peljor Döndrup states that there are three natural wind genders in his *Secret Explanation of the Vajra Body*. The relative strength of these different types of winds during conception may well contribute to gender, body constitution and personality, which is a fascinating hypothesis for further study.

- Masculine wind (*po lung*) manifests as shorter, rough breaths

- Feminine wind (*mo lung*) manifests as longer, gentle breaths

- Neutral or hermaphrodite wind (*ma ning lung*) manifests as intermediate, smooth breaths

Wind and ageing according to Sakyapa Gyeltsen Pelzang

Life is wind, and wind is life. When life begins, the body absorbs more air (oxygen) until the age of 24, using it to build up the body. In the middle period between 25 and 45, inhalation and absorption of air and exhalation are intermediate and sustain the body. After 45, absorption of air reduces, and exhalation increases. This loss of *lung* from the body leads to ageing and degeneration, and soon the first signs of old age and loss of strength manifest as a result.

---

15 Studying more on the relationship between *norlhagyel, la, tsé,* and the liberation after death ceremony from different Tibetan Buddhist traditions may help to better understand this matter.

Gyeltsen Pelzang also describes that the body has two opposite wind natures, like sky and earth. The sky wind, which corresponds to the upper body, is cooling. It cools down the bile and *médrö* heat which rise upwards. The lower body wind on the other hand is warming in nature and sustains the *médrö*, warming up the phlegm fluids which flow down from the head. These two winds balance the body temperature and regulate the energy flow from the head to the feet and back. This wind circulation endures throughout life. The two opposite winds are called hot and cold wind, or alternatively the upper and lower winds. They are the body's two major wind systems, which include all other specific winds. Upper cold wind (*tölung silwa*) arises from the crown chakra's 32 petals and flows down to the throat, chest, and until the navel chakra. It has a cooling quality, flowing down like a river, pacifying bile. Lower hot wind (*mélung tsawa*) rises from the channels of the navel to warm up the chest, throat, and forehead chakras. It increases bile heat and pacifies phlegm and cold.

Tantric *lung* descriptions are extensive. There are for example 84,000 emotions that arise from 84,000 channels and winds. The *Jewel Mound Sutra* (*Mdo dkon mchog brtsegs pa*) and the *Sutra on Entering the Womb* (*Dga' bo mngal 'jug gi mdo*) also explain in detail 78 groups of winds located in different parts of the body and 80,000 tiny beings (*sinbu*) which are born, live inside and sustain the body, but which may also become the cause of disease and body-mind disharmony. These texts are of great value to study human biology and to advance our knowledge of body-mind interdependence.

21,600 breaths within 24 hours

In general, respiration is carried out by the lungs. However, each breath is a collective undertaking. Breathing is a vital flow of energy. Each inhalation contains earth-water wind (*sa chü lung*) or oxygenated air, while the exhalation contains fire-wind wind (*mélung gyi lung*) with carbon dioxide. Both are essential to sustain life. Inhaled air is distributed to all body organs, tissues, and microorganisms. Exhaled air is a collective product of the vital and hollow organs, blood, nerves, and lymph systems, and body microorganism. In total, a healthy adult takes about 21,600 breaths within 24 hours. From these 21,600 breaths, 675 vital wind energy breaths come from *lung uma*, which contains the life fuel that is consumed every day (see Section 4.3). The remaining 20,925 breaths are physical body wind breaths, products of air and food. There is major breathing, but also minor or subtle breathing of the body's microorganisms and

cells which are countless in number. We should gain more knowledge on the channels and winds and their functions from Buddhist tantra and yogic practices. The body can be seen as a woven basket, a network of major, minor, and subtle channels through which breathing takes place. Wind circulates not only through the nose and mouth, but also through all other orifices such as the eyes, ears, skin pores, and even through hairs.

Lung dzinpa

On a microscopic level, wind and its channels develop from the cosmic subtle wind energy called *lung dzinpa*, which has the inherent potential to attract other elemental particles like a magnet attracting pieces of iron. This life-retaining wind gathers particles from three sources: the quintessence of cosmic air, from the parents' wind energy, and from the subtle wind that carries the bardo consciousness. Being attracted to each other, they unite during conception like water mingling with water. This is the beginning of life-sustaining wind (*sokdzin lung*), the root of the wind humor and the vehicle of mind. More research on the nature and function of *lung dzinpa* could be helpful to better understand the very beginnings of a new human body. Minute subtle wind particles (*trawé lung gi dültren*) are drawn together by *lung dzinpa*, around which the other elemental particles also circle with rainbow-like colors. One could say that *lung dzinpa* has a kind of pseudo-consciousness or intelligence, providing a precondition for the mind to dwell. From this attraction of microscopic particles, the power of the mind and the elements grows, eventually maturing into the body-mind system. As we have seen, wind is the central figure of mind and life, which is why it has been covered so extensively in the tantras. Where there is subtle wind, there is a basis for a consciousness to dwell and for conception to take place if other conditions are fulfilled. It is intriguing to note here some analogies with Western scientific concepts of nuclei. In relation to cell biology, the cell nucleus is the center of fusion at the beginning of new life which also carries information that will influence the future of the organism, while in physics the atomic nucleus attracts other particles and acts as a foundational building block for materials.

In short, consciousness together with *lung dzinpa* may be the first foundation for further body-mind development, especially of the wind humor and channels. Wind and mind are two sides of the same coin, as Peljor Döndrup says:[16]

---

16 Dpal 'byor don grub, 1995, 87.

Like both wind and awareness,
One nature with two aspects.
The self-knower remembers and is clear,
Wind is material, producing illusions.

The body is like a hot air balloon

If we look at the body from a yogic point of view, the body is like a wind bag as stated by Marpa Lotsawa.[17] The body balloon consists of several bigger and smaller wind bags. These bags provide the pressure to stand and move, just like a hot air balloon. Each of the millions of microbes and blood cells are "inflated" by wind in this way. The root of these winds is life-sustaining wind, located in the middle channel. The central channel is like a trunk, the five principal winds are its main branches, and the five minor winds are flowering minor branches. The channels are passages of wind, blood, and nutrition. Healthy channels give good health, whereas impure and blocked channels manifest disease and negative emotions. The winds are fundamental to health.

----

17 Mar pa lo tsa ba, 1995, 2.

CHAPTER 7

BILE (*TRIPA*)

7.1 GENERAL BILE (*TRIPA CHI*)

The bile humor is called *tripa* in Tibetan. *Tripa* means "burning." This refers to *médrö*, the metabolic heat that is able to digest food, transform nutrition to body constituents, and which produces body temperature. *Tripa* is produced by the liver and especially gallbladder, and functions mainly in the middle part of the body and in the digestive tract. The term *tripa* is derived from *nötri*, the gallbladder, which literally means "bile container." Its content acts as the principal source of bile energy and *chuser* (blood plasma and interstitial fluid). Just like the other *nyépa*, *tripa* also has a psychic origin: It is derived from the fire of hatred and anger.[1] The liver produces heat and blood, and the liver's waste products transform to bile juice in the gallbladder. The liver is like burning wood that gives off heat. Wood acts as fuel for the fire, leaving ashes which correspond to the bile juice collected in the gallbladder. This picture perfectly portrays how liver and gallbladder both produce *tripa*. Bile is acidic, oily, and bitter, playing an important role in the digestion of food and the transformation of body constituents. This bile fire protects the body from the coldness and humidity of wind and phlegm. Bile heat dominates the right side of the body, its fire energy being rooted in the right channel (*tsa roma*). This is described in the fourth chapter of the *Explanatory Tantra*:[2]

> A channel from the navel penetrates the center,
> where hatred resides in the blood,
> forming the life channel.
> From it, bile develops in the middle part of the body.

The bile humor has three main sources:

1. Subtle hatred coming from the past life with the bardo consciousness

2. The bile energy received and developed from the fire element of the parents' two reproductive fluids, and especially from the contribution of the mother's nature and menstrual blood

3. After birth, fire energy received from nutrition throughout life

Location

General bile operates mainly in the middle part of the body, where it actively functions in the stomach, small intestine and especially the duodenum, pancreas, liver, and gallbladder.

Function

The fifth chapter of the *Explanatory Tantra* reveals:[3]

> Bile rules hunger, thirst, appetite, and digests food.
> It gives body temperature, clears the *dang*, generates bravery, and intelligence.

Healthy bile gives a balanced temperature to the body. Bile absorbs nutrition, transforms and matures it into body constituents, sustains the organs, and clears the sense organs and skin. *Tripa* also stimulates intelligence, clear memory, pride and ambition, a

---

1 The psychic cause of *tripa* is not explicitly mentioned in the *Explanatory* and *Oral Instruction Tantras*.

2 G.yu thog yon tan mgon po, 1993, 22.

3 Ibid., 28.

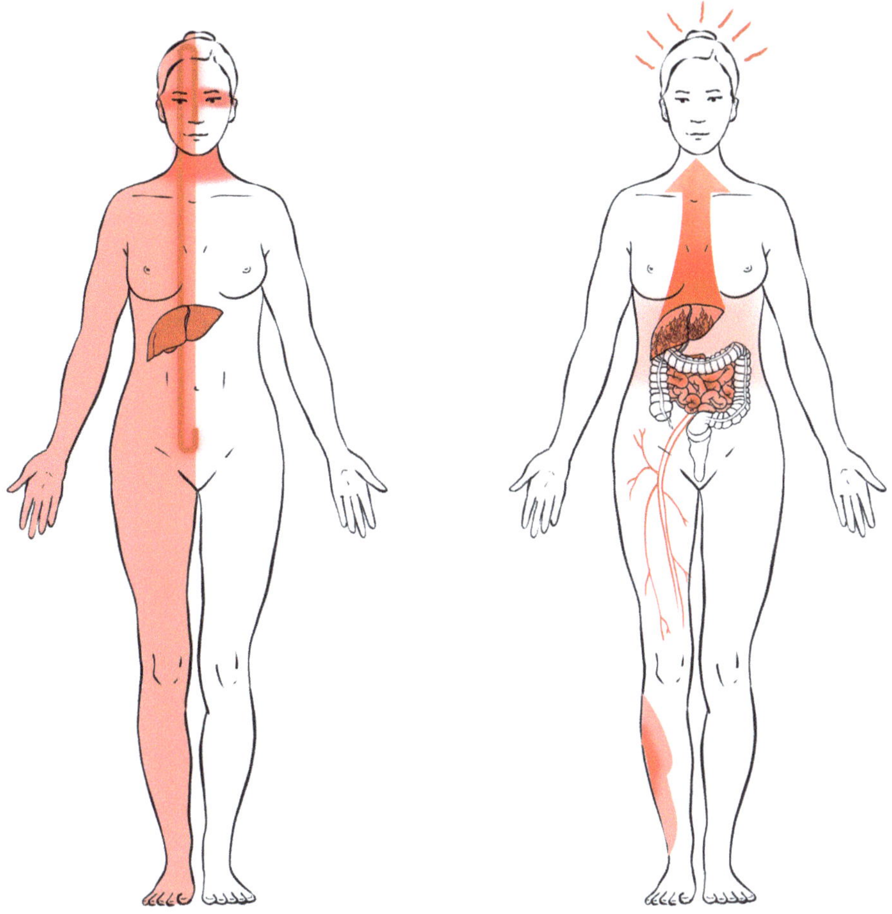

FIGURE 7.1 The main locations of general bile

sense of perfection, willpower, and an egotistic mind. Bile produces blood, serum, perspiration, the skin, the eyes, and of course bile juice and salts. It regulates intestinal functioning and eliminates the waste products from the body.

Crippled general bile

A severe bile humor defect during conception or fetus development may cause hereditary and congenital diseases that involve disorders of the blood and of organs such as liver, spleen, heart, gallbladder, small intestine, and skin, as well as abnormal body temperature and impaired digestion.

Seven characteristics

Tripa has seven characteristics (*tripé tsenyi dün*): (1) oily (*numpa*), (2) sharp (*nowa*), (3) hot (*tsawa*), (4) light (*yangwa*), (5) malodorous (*drinam*), (6) purgative (*truwa*), and (7) moist (*sherwa*). Bile's properties keep the other two humors in equilibrium by reducing phlegm's humidity and neutralizing the coldness and dryness of wind.

Imbalance signs

When *tripa* is disturbed by wrong diet, behavior, the seasons, old age, and mental factors, it shows an increase in the seven bile characteristics, leading to the following signs and symptoms, amongst others:

TABLE 7.1 The seven characteristics of bile

	Bile characteristic	Qualities neutralized	*Nyépa* reduced	*Nyépa* increased
1.	Oily	Rough/dry	- Wind	+ Phlegm
2.	Sharp	Sticky	- Phlegm	
3.	Hot	Cold and cooling	- Phlegm + Wind	
4.	Light	Heavy	- Phlegm	+ Wind
5.	Malodorous	Wet/thinness	- Phlegm	
6.	Purgative	Rough/dry		
7.	Moist	Rough/dry		

1. Oily blood, organs, skin, face, hair, or body
2. Sharp disease symptoms that are acute and aggressive
3. Hot body temperature manifesting as fevers and infections
4. A light disease nature, with fast-changing symptoms
5. Malodorous sweat and foul urine
6. The body expels bile through purgative diarrhea
7. Bile patients sweat profusely; they become moist and dehydrated

7.2 THE FIVE PRINCIPAL BILE BRANCHES (*TSAWÉ TRIPA NGA*)

Five principal bile branches are included under the general bile humor, which govern general and specific body functions:

1. Digestive bile (*tripa jujé*)
2. Color-transforming bile (*tripa dangyur*)
3. Accomplishing bile (*tripa drupjé*)
4. Seeing bile (*tripa tongjé*)
5. Complexion-clearing bile (*tripa doksel*)

1. Digestive bile (*tripa jujé*)

Tripa jujé is the body's main digestive fire or metabolic power, also called *médrö* or "fire heat." This fire is derived from the liver and gallbladder, and produces the heat and acidity necessary to digest food. It operates in the stomach, duodenum and pancreas, small intestine, and colon, aiding the transformation of food into the body constituents.

Function

Digestive bile digests food, directs hunger and thirst, and assimilates food essence (*dangma*) from the stomach and intestines. It absorbs and assimilates nutrients, matures and transforms these into constituents, and thus sustains body heat. The *Explanatory Tantra's* fifth chapter states:[4]

Digestive bile resides between where digestion has and has not taken place.
It digests food, separates nutrients from waste products, increases body heat,
and sustains and strengthens the four other branches of bile.

---

4   Ibid.

Malfunction

Impaired digestive bile decreases *médrö* and manifests indigestion, poor absorption, gastric, abdominal, and chronic peptic disorders, and potentially esophageal and laryngeal inflammations. In particular, the tongue turns yellow, and appetite is poor.

Crippled digestive bile

A defect during fetus development may cause congenital diseases such as chronic colon, liver, gallbladder, duodenal and pancreatic disorders.

2. Color-transforming bile (*tripa dangyur*)

Tripa dangyur resides in the liver. This bile transforms nutrition into blood and gives (especially reddish) color to the body constituents. That is why it is called color-transforming.

Function

It transforms *dangma* received in the liver from the digestive system into red blood and other tissues, giving them color: blood becomes red, bile yellow, bone and fat white, etc. The *Explanatory Tantra*'s fifth chapter says:[5]

> Color-transforming bile resides in the liver.
> It transforms food essence into the colors of
> all body constituents

Malfunction

Malfunction of this bile manifests as liver weakness, poor digestion, and may produce yellow urine, stomach swelling and heavy abdomen, loss of strength, anemia, edema, eyesight disorders, tiredness, and sleeping disturbances.

Crippled color-transforming bile

A serious defect during fetus development may cause congenital diseases such as liver angioma and liver malfunction, different types of inherited anemia, eyesight weakness, and gallbladder malformation.

―――――――
5   Ibid.

3. Accomplishing bile (*tripa drupjé*)

Tripa drupjé resides in the heart. It is also called desirous bile because it grants interest, wishes and enthusiasm to the mind.

Function

It gives strength to the heart, produces pride, braveness, intelligence, awareness, self-perception, and gives the willpower and determination to fulfill one's desires and wishes. The *Explanatory Tantra*'s fifth chapter says:[6]

> Accomplishing bile resides in the heart.
> It gives courage, pride, intellect, and
> interest to fulfil one's wishes.

Malfunction

Malfunction of this bile provokes heart palpitations, strong breathing, abnormal thirst, poor appetite, trembling, pain in the chest, and sensations of heat in the heart and lungs. Psychologically, it manifests lack of desire, fear, lack of will and interest, depression, pessimism, and self-criticism or narcissism.

Crippled accomplishing bile

A defect during fetus development may cause congenital diseases such as heart problems (mitral and aortic mitral heart disorders, arrhythmicity), and a tendency towards depressive complaints. This could manifest cardiac-mental imbalances such as anxiety, fear, panic attacks and paranoia, amongst others.

4. Seeing bile (*tripa tongjé*)

Tripa tongjé grants eyesight and the ability to perceive objects. It resides in the eyes.

Function

It is the light of the body that perceives the world through the eye organs and consciousness, including colors, shapes, forms, and distances. The *Explanatory Tantra*'s fifth chapter says:[7]

> Seeing bile resides in the eyes and
> perceives forms.

―――――――
6   Ibid.
7   Ibid.

Malfunction

Malfunction of this bile manifests headache and pain after drinking alcohol. The eyes become yellow, may develop myopia or perceive close objects but not distant ones, wrongly perceiving colors and forms, cataract, various other eye disorders such as night and color blindness, and even complete blindness.

Crippled seeing bile

A defect during fetus development may cause congenital diseases such as eye organ malformation, or the development of myopia, blindness, and perception impairments.

5. Complexion-clearing bile (*tripa doksel*)

Tripa doksel resides in the skin. It gives color to and sustains the skin, so it is also called skin-coloring bile.

Function

It functions in the skin by clearing its color and complexion. *Tripa doksel* maintains the skin and its temperature, acting as a fire barrier that encircles the body and protects it from negative influences. The *Explanatory Tantra*'s fifth chapter states:[8]

> Complexion-clearing bile resides in the skin and clears the complexion.

Malfunction

Malfunction of this bile results in increased skin temperature, and the skin becoming dark-blue and rough. It produces a poor complexion and poor radiance, which contributes to various dermatological disorders.

Crippled complexion-clearing bile

A defect during fetus development may manifest congenital diseases such as abnormal skin color, skin disorders, poor hair growth, and dermatological allergies.

---

8   Ibid.

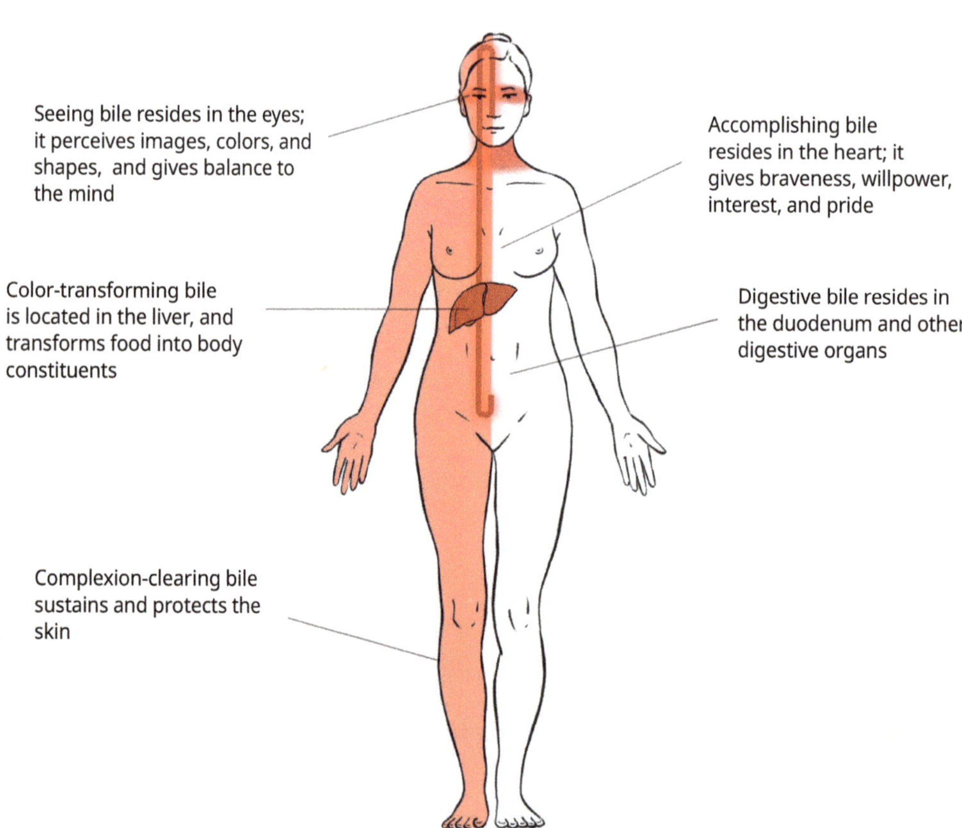

FIGURE 7.2 The five principal bile branches

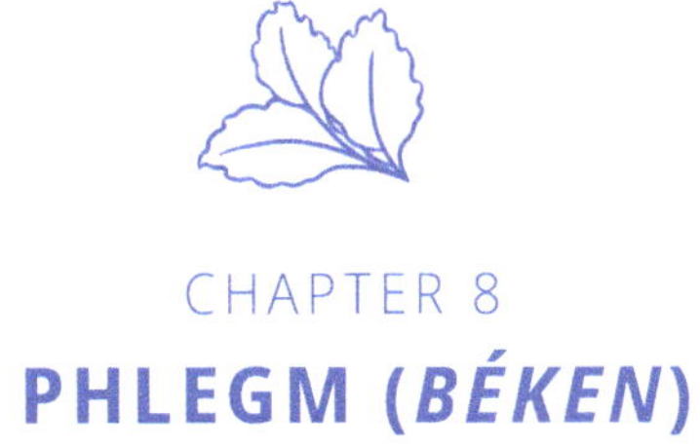

CHAPTER 8

PHLEGM (*BÉKEN*)

8.1 GENERAL PHLEGM (*BÉKEN CHI*)

The phlegm humor is called *béken*. *Bé* refers to earth, and *ken* to water; *béken* is the combination of these two elements. It is an archaic Tibetan loanword for "mucus." Earth provides the qualities of solidity, heaviness, and form to the body, and water gives moisture, coldness, and the cohesion that holds different parts together. The phlegm humor gives the body form and binds the body particles together into tissues and organs.

Psychologically, the phlegm humor is derived from *timuk* or closed-mindedness, hence its heavy and dull quality. The brain is described as an ocean of phlegm, and as such represents the major source of body water. From the brain, channels branch down through the spinal column to the organs and body tissues. *Béken* gives elasticity to the body as well as stability, tranquility, and a phlegmatic appearance. It is a masculine lunar energy that dominates the left side of the body. Phlegm sustains the physique and regulates endocrinal and lymph fluid secretion in the brain and elsewhere. Phlegm humor energy is water-dominated and cooling, which refreshes the body and balances *tripa*. The *Explanatory Tantra*'s fourth chapter says:[1]

> A channel goes up from the navel
> and develops the brain,
> from where closed-mindedness
> generates *béken*.
> Therefore, it is in the upper part
> of the body.

There are three main sources of *béken*:

1. The subtle closed-mindedness continuum of the bardo consciousness

2. The physical earth and water elements from the parents, and especially from the father's sperm

3. Phlegm energy received from nutrition throughout life

Location

The phlegm humor is mainly located in the head, chest and above the diaphragm, and especially in the brain and lungs.

Function

Béken directs the body fluids, and is active in the chest, throat, lungs, brain, food essence, muscles, fat, bone marrow, reproductive fluids, feces, and urine. It also functions in the nose, tongue and especially in the spleen, stomach, kidneys, and bladder. Phlegm dominates the esophageal tract from mouth to stomach, and thus aids digestion. It induces sleep and patience, connects the joints, and lubricates the body and its tissues. It keeps the organs and skin smooth and produces the body fats and oils. It allows for physical growth, and especially sustains whitish tissues such as the brain, glands, and ligaments. *Béken* rules the endocrinal glands and the lymphatic system, fluid circulation, and provides firmness and stability to the body-mind. The cool and wet nature of the phlegm humor opposes the heat of bile, while its qualities of heaviness and

---

1 G.yu thog yon tan mgon po, 1993, 22.

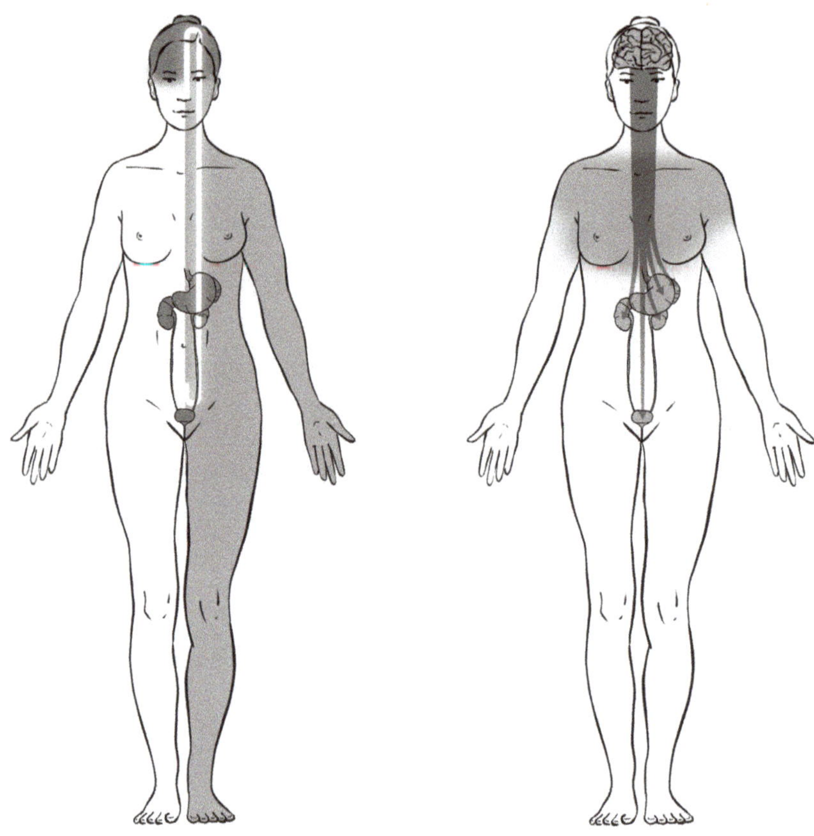

FIGURE 8.1 The main locations of general phlegm

gentleness (smoothness) balance the roughness of wind. The *Explanatory Tantra*'s fifth chapter says:[2]

> *Béken* keeps the body-mind stable and induces sleep.
> It keeps the joints fixed, gives rise to patience, and smoothens and oils the skin.

Crippled general phlegm

A serious defect could manifest in phlegm humor function during or after conception, or fetus development. Theoretically, hereditary phlegm disorders come from problems with the father's contribution. This could lead to congenital diseases such as brain malformation, defects of the glands, spleen, bones, spine and bone marrow, nervous system, endocrine, lymphatic and urinal systems, reproductive organs, and other physical constituent imbalances.

Seven characteristics

The phlegm humor has seven characteristics (*béken gyi tsenyi dün*): (1) oily (*numpa*), (2) cool (*silwa*), (3) heavy (*chiwa*), (4) blunt (*tülwa*), (5) smooth (*jampa*), (6) stable (*tenpa*), and (7) sticky or slimy (*jarbak*). These qualities sustain phlegm, and nourish the body and organs. They counterbalance the bile and wind qualities, bringing harmony and health.

Imbalance signs

An excess of *béken* will dominate the other two humors, and will show the following symptoms:

1. Obesity caused by excess production of fat because of its oily quality
2. The body cools down, weakening the digestive fire and metabolism

---

2 Ibid., 28.

TABLE 8.1 The seven characteristics of phlegm

	Phlegm characteristic	Qualities neutralized	*Nyépa* reduced	*Nyépa* increased
1.	Oily	Rough/dry	- Wind	+ Bile
2.	Cool	Hot	- Bile	+ Wind
3.	Heavy	Light	- Wind - Bile	
4.	Blunt	Sharp	- Bile	
5.	Gentle	Rough/hard	- Wind	
6.	Stable	Light	- Wind - Bile	
7.	Sticky	Dry/coarse	- Wind	

3. The body-mind becomes heavy, feelings of heaviness
4. Body-mind actions become slow, feelings of sluggishness
5. The skin becomes smooth, slippery and soft
6. Body, mind, and disease tend to stagnate
7. Increase of mucus and saliva due to the sticky nature of phlegm.

8.2 THE FIVE PRINCIPAL PHLEGM BRANCHES (*TSAWÉ BÉKEN NGA*)

The phlegm humor is divided into five branches that carry out specific functions. These are the principal phlegm branches:

1. Supportive phlegm (*béken tenjé*)
2. Decomposing phlegm (*béken nyakjé*)
3. Experiencing phlegm (*béken nyongjé*)
4. Satisfying phlegm (*béken tsimjé*)
5. Joining phlegm (*béken jorjé*)

1. Supportive phlegm (*béken tenjé*)

Béken tenjé is the principal phlegm branch, sustaining the functions of the four other phlegm branches. It resides in the chest, lungs, and throat.

Function

Supportive phlegm sustains the body water system: the cerebral, endocrine, lymphatic and urinary/renal systems. *Béken tenjé* distributes the fluids in and towards the blood and body tissues, and rules thirst and salivation. It collects fluids from the body through the lymph channels to the chest, and then sends them to the brain through throat channels. The brain transforms and distributes the liquids back to the body. The *Explanatory Tantra*'s fifth chapter says:[3]

> Supportive phlegm resides in the chest.
> It is the base that supplies the rest of the
> phlegm branches and water functions.

Malfunction

Malfunction of this phlegm could manifest as loss of appetite, tension in the shoulders, pain in the back and front of the chest, acidity, and vomiting of sour liquids.

Crippled supportive phlegm

In case this phlegm is crippled by severe early-life causes, it may lead to malformation of the thymus gland and chest, and lymphatic impairments may occur.

---

3 Ibid., 28–29.

2. Decomposing phlegm (*béken nyakjé*)

Béken nyakjé mainly resides in the upper part of the stomach, but also functions in the mouth, esophagus, and other parts.

Function

It is active in the mouth, esophagus, stomach, small intestine, colon, and especially in the stomach, where food is mixed and processed. It functions like water when cooking food, breaking down and decomposing nutrition during digestion. *Béken nyakjé* helps absorb and assimilate nutrients and liquid, sending these to the liver. The *Explanatory Tantra*'s fifth chapter says:[4]
> Decomposing phlegm resides in the area where digestion has not taken place.
> It decomposes food and liquids, making them soluble.

Malfunction

Malfunction could manifest all types of digestion difficulties, stomach disorders, malabsorption, as well as feelings of a hard or tense stomach. In short, it becomes the cause of chronic phlegm indigestion disorders called *mazhuwa*.

Crippled decomposing phlegm

Serious defects may produce congenital malformation of the stomach, and poor metabolic power (*médrö*), becoming the source of chronic stomach disorders.

3. Experiencing phlegm (*béken nyongjé*)

Béken nyongjé resides in the tongue and other body organs.

Function

It allows for the perception of flavor (the six tastes: *ro druk*) principally, as well as perceptions of "good" or "bad" related to the other sense organs such as the eyes, ears, nose, and skin. *Béken nyongjé* also produces bliss during sexual orgasm by means of the *samséu* channel, which is connected to the brain.

The *Explanatory Tantra*'s fifth chapter says:[5]
> Experiencing phlegm resides in the tongue and perceives taste.

Malfunction

Malfunction of this phlegm leads to loss of taste and appetite, lack of thirst, the feeling of having a cold tongue, pain in the lips, and hoarseness.

Crippled experiencing phlegm

Such a defect may produce congenital malformation of the sense faculty of the tongue and the associated brain area, which may lead to impaired speech, stammering and other tongue congenital diseases.

4. Satisfying phlegm (*béken tsimjé*)

Béken tsimjé is located in the head, including the brain (*lépa*).

Function

Satisfying phlegm governs the feeling of satisfaction of the mind and heart coming from the consciousnesses of the eye, ear, nose, tongue, and body. This phlegm gives a sense of like or dislike for music, for example. It is also active in the throat, stomach, sex organs, and the body's tactile sense, giving sensation and satisfaction. The *Explanatory Tantra*'s fifth chapter says:[6]
> Satisfying phlegm resides in the head and satisfies the senses.

Is serotonin a function of satisfying phlegm?

Not much detail has been provided in the *Gyüzhi* or other traditional medical literature on satisfying phlegm. The few lines that are available are paraphrased below under the heading "malfunction." In the author's understanding, the sense organs are a source of contentment and satisfaction for the body-mind, and so is digestion and the distribution of *dangma* in the body. A lack of satisfaction due to sadness, stress or hormonal changes also influences the stomach and intestines, and can thus disturb

---

4   Ibid., 29.

5   Ibid.

6   Ibid.

the absorption of *dangma* and its distribution. Both a reduction in nutrition (gross, physical *dangma*) and of the subtle *tiklé* involved in energetic circulation could manifest in decreased brain power and clarity of mind, and depressive mental states. Like a flashlight with low battery, the whole brain (and its memory) becomes dark, cloudy, and confused by the heavy quality of phlegm. Satisfying phlegm, digestion, and serotonin are therefore likely important factors in depression. One could interpret serotonin as a product of satisfying phlegm of the stomach and intestines, which nourishes the brain and mind. Serotonin interacts with *béken tsimjé* in the brain (in particular via the pituitary gland in the hypothalamus, which links the nervous system to the endocrine system). It is clear that food gives a positive reaction in the mind, giving satisfaction when the stomach is filled. In this case, we see serotonin is active in the stomach and intestines, whereas depressed patients often have a bad relationship with food. Detailed research on each humor would be helpful to better understand Sowa Rigpa and human body functions. Many factors may lead to depression, but malfunction of life-sustaining wind, accomplishing bile, and fire-like wind are likely involved. In biomedicine, the exact physiological pathways of depression are still unconfirmed, but low serotonin levels in the stomach, intestines and central nervous system have been indicated.

Malfunction

It manifests vertigo, lost control over the eyes (drunken eye), hearing disturbances, sneezing, an excess of nasal mucus, catching frequent colds, and a heavy feeling in the fontanel area. This phlegm disturbance could also cause extreme or exaggerated thoughts, a fixated mind, or loss of interest and depression, anorexia, and bulimia.

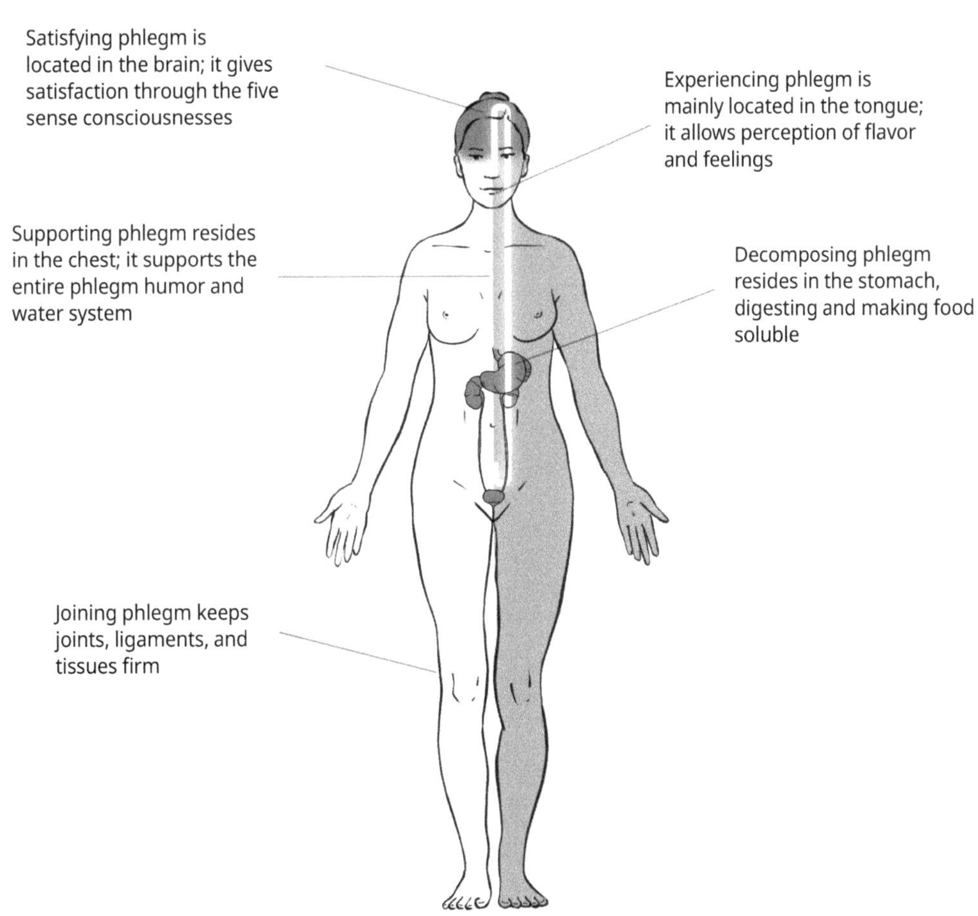

FIGURE 8.2 The five principal phlegm branches

Crippled satisfying phlegm

A serious defect may produce congenital malformation of the sense organs as well as pernicious mental irregularities that could lead to eating disorders.

5. Joining phlegm (*béken jorjé*)

Béken jorjé resides in the joints.

Function

Joining phlegm lubricates the joints and strengthens cartilage, tendons, ligaments and related structures, keeping them firm. *Béken jorjé* controls movements of the limbs. The *Explanatory Tantra*'s fifth chapter says:[7]

> Joining phlegm resides in all joints.
> It connects the joints, and controls
> contraction and retraction.

Malfunction

Rigidity or pain of the hands, feet, and joints, and swollen joints could manifest. This can develop further into osteoarthritis, arthritis, rheumatism, and various joint and ligament disorders.

Crippled joining phlegm

Such a severe defect may produce congenital malformation of joints, articulations, and dry connective tissue.

---

7   Ibid.

CHAPTER 9

BODY CONSTITUTION

The term used to denote a person's general constitution or body type is *rangzhin*, which also means "inherent nature" or "essence." As a result of the particular assemblage of the five elements engineered by one's karma, people have a certain physiognomy from birth. The details of this process are described in embryology (cf. Chapter 13). Vāgbhaṭa gave a similar example in his *Ashtāngahridayasaṃhitā*:[1]

> Beings are born in various bodies, like
> melted copper poured in different molds.

The elements are represented by the ore; the mold is the mother's womb, and the blacksmith represents karma. The womb shapes the elemental combination of the child in accordance with its karmic tendencies, leading to its physiognomy. Constitution can also be called a mudra or symbol, a sign of the natural state of the body. If you know the correct *rangzhin*, it is easier to apply the right remedy to restore health. Each person has their own characteristics that derive from different contributions. Some constitutions show particularly strong influences in physical features, while others do not. Some physical shapes and forms may change due to wrong diet, bad behavior, or disease and medication. However, the deep nature and subtle personality in general do not change, but it does develop more clearly with age, just like a blossoming flower.

9.1 BODY CLASSIFICATION (*LÜ KYI YÉWA*)

In general, the body can be classified according to gender, age, and body constitution.

The classification of gender consists of three groups: male, female, and intersex. The cause of the gender or sex is related to basic psychic differences as well as the parents' energetic contributions. There are also three age categories: childhood, adulthood, and old age:

- From birth to 16 years old is the development stage, which is considered childhood. During this period, the body is ruled by *béken*.

- From 17 to 50 is adulthood. It is the mature stage. During this period, life is more stable and governed by *tripa*.

- From 50 to 100 is considered of old age. It belongs to the wind element. Body strength decreases as the energy of the elements declines.

Notwithstanding the age or gender classification, each individual has their own specific body constitution.

9.2 INTRODUCTION TO BODY CONSTITUTION AND ITS CAUSES

Tibetan medicine recognizes seven body constitutions (*rangzhin dün*), which characterize the inherent nature of a person. There is actually considerable variation in body types, but this can be generalized into seven main groups. It appears that constitution and personality are furthermore strongly related to ethnicity (clan, family) and especially one's parents, geographical influences, as well as nutrition and way of life. All influence the elements. Body constitution has three main causes:

1. A distant cause, which is karma
2. An indirect cause, namely the five elements
3. Direct conditions: the parents' humoral energies

---

1 Pha khol, 1989, vol. 1, 255.

Body constitution determines the physiognomy and personality of each person, yet physical characteristics usually take precedence in constitutional diagnosis. Both derive from the combination of the elements (with a concept similar to genetic recombination) and humors of the parents. The mother's psychology and lifestyle certainly contribute to the child's constitution. For example, parents who are ruled by the wind humor and element will likely have a child with these same characteristics.

There are three single, three double, and one combined constitution, which makes seven general body types in total. Generally speaking, body constitutions do not change. However, in some cases they may be altered through biomedical hormone therapy.

A collective constitution (*düdé rangzhin*) is also seen in larger groups of people, for example in a family, in clans, different ethnicities, and in people who live at high versus low altitudes. Further differences are found between peoples from different countries and regions, showing variation in color of skin, hair, and eyes, for example. There is no personal choice in getting a particular constitution, but special astrological techniques attempt to influence the probability of obtaining a child of a desired gender and *rangzhin*. Despite these collective tendencies, coincidental factors could lead to any one of the constitutions.

Different constitutions have a different *médrö or* digestive fire:

- Wind-constitutional people have an unstable digestion

- Bile-constitutional people have a strong and fast digestion

- Phlegm-constitutional people have a slow digestion

Different constitutions also have different intestinal functioning:

- Wind constitution people have hard stomachs. They are prone to having a hard stool or to being constipated.

- Bile constitution people tend to have sensitive intestines, and to suffer from diarrhea.

- Phlegm constitution people have an intermediate intestinal function, which is considered "normal."

9.3 THE SEVEN BODY CONSTITUTIONS

In this section, we will cover the seven specific body constitutions one by one. The constitution or typology of a person is dominated by various humors. This gives rise to the natural physiognomy of each individual, a person's appearance, distinguishing features, and temperament. The seven *rangzhin* are:

1. Wind constitution (*lung gi rangzhin*)
2. Bile constitution (*tripé rangzhin*)
3. Phlegm constitution (*béken rangzhin*)
4. Wind-bile constitution (*lungtri rangzhin*)
5. Phlegm-bile constitution (*bétri rangzhin*)
6. Phlegm-wind constitution (*bélung rangzhin*)
7. The combined constitution (*düpé rangzhin*)

The first three are called single constitutions. In the second three, two humors predominate together. In the final constitution, all three humors are equally represented.

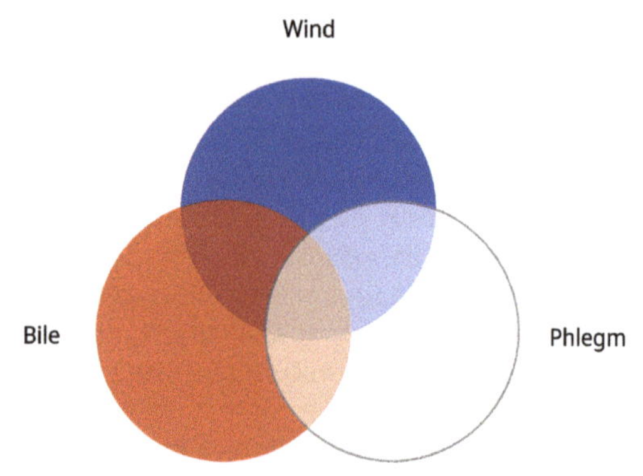

FIGURE 9.1 Seven body constitutions arise from the three humors

Three single constitutions

A single constitution is strongly governed by one humor. For example, if wind is dominant over bile and phlegm, this is called wind constitution. Bile and phlegm then act as secondary *nyépa*. The dominant single humor shows its nature and characteristics more clearly.

1. Wind constitution (*lung gi rangzhin*)

Wind element or humor people's nature is like the wind. Such people are thinkers and emotionally sensitive. They naturally have thin bodies, can be short or very tall, and have difficulty gaining weight. They have a light-bluish or darkish complexion, rough and dry skin, small and sharp eyes with dark irises, and their sensory organs and extremities, including their fingers, are either short or long, and dry. Their thorax and bones (and cervix for women) tend to curve inward when they get older. Some strong wind constitutional bodies develop a chicken chest or a mildly deformed back with kyphosis.[2] Their joints and veins are clearly visible. They have dry hair, prominent body pores, and fragile nails. They also have cold bodies and little muscle tissue. Wind types are sensitive, and thus cannot tolerate cold, wind, high temperatures, or abrupt sounds. They are nervous and may suffer from hyperactivity. Their bodies easily produce sounds. They are extrovert and creative, with lots of ideas, but they have difficulty bringing projects to completion. They are unstable by nature and can change their activities and ideas at any time. *Lung* persons are talkative, walk noisily, and they often have chest and intestinal complaints. They have a quavering voice, speak often, and tend to talk in incomplete sentences, and their volume of voice is either weak or loud. Many of them do not have a sweet singing voice. Nevertheless, they like to sing songs, dance, play or listen to music. They like sports and particularly archery, and love to argue and laugh. They are light sleepers and have many dreams. Wind types become drier with age. Women enter menopause earlier than in other constitutions, and may have a fragile, unstable mind.

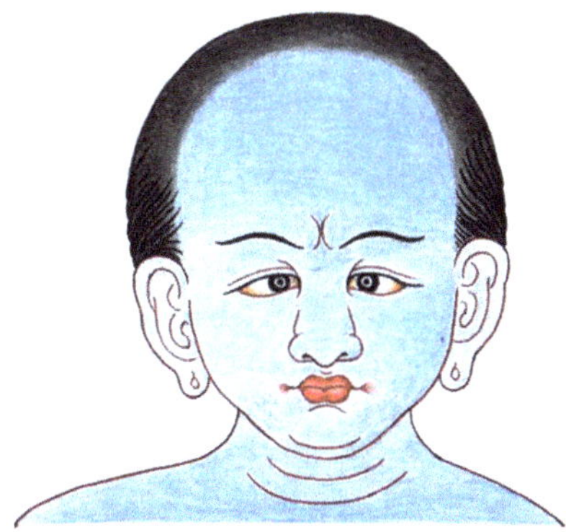

FIGURE 9.2 The wind constitution head: elongated at the top, with a flesh-like brain

Their taste preferences for food are sweet, sour, bitter and hot. They have difficulty tolerating coffee, (green) bell peppers, and sometimes carbohydrates. Fasting can easily make them sick. Their body nature is like an arid soil where crops hardly grow. This means that they do not put on weight even when they have a good appetite. They have open pores through which their body constantly loses energy. Their life span is shorter than that of other constitutions, and they generally do not have stability of wealth in their lives. They have a tendency to suffer from wind disorders and psychological instability.

The character of wind constitution people is similar to the vulture, crow, and fox.

2. Bile constitution (*tripé rangzhin*)

People dominated by the fire element and bile humor have a rational, sharp mind, and a medium-sized body. Their minds are more stable than that of wind types. They have red-yellowish or brownish irises, and oily and red, yellow, or coffee-colored hair. Their skin has a yellowish or reddish hue. *Tripa* types have a broad chest and broad shoulders with a thick neck and an oily face. They have a quick and strong digestion, quickly getting thirsty. They are able to digest raw vegetables and salad and generally assimilate food without difficulty. They naturally have a higher body temperature, a stronger body odor, and tend to sweat a great deal. They have good memory, are intelligent, and have a strong ego, although they may suffer from mental insecurities. They easily get headaches due to hyperfunction of liver and gallbladder, and suffer from acidity and small intestine problems. They are prone to allergies, infection and inflammation, hypertension, shoulder aches, cataract, bad blood circulation, gastritis, colitis, skin rash, hemorrhoids, and high cholesterol. Women of this constitution often suffer from cervical pain as well as premenstrual syndrome. In short, bile types tend to suffer from disorders originated from liver and gallbladder malfunction. They are short-tempered and impatient.

Their favorite food and drinks have sweet, bitter, astringent, and cooling qualities. They cannot digest milk and related animal products well, and do not tolerate too much garlic, wine, and fatty foods. These items tend to make them feel angry or ill. Their lifespan and wealth are moderate.

The character of bile constitution people is similar to the tiger, monkey, and harmful spirit (*nöjin*).[3]

---

2 Severe deformations such as Marfan syndrome and "bamboo spine" (ankylosing spondylitis) also belong to extreme wind constitutional disorders.

3 *Nöjin* means "harmful spirit," but they are in fact powerful heavenly beings and Mount Méru guardians. They are gods of wealth, and generally peaceful. However, they easily turn wrathful and aggressive, being offended by anyone acting against the Dharma.

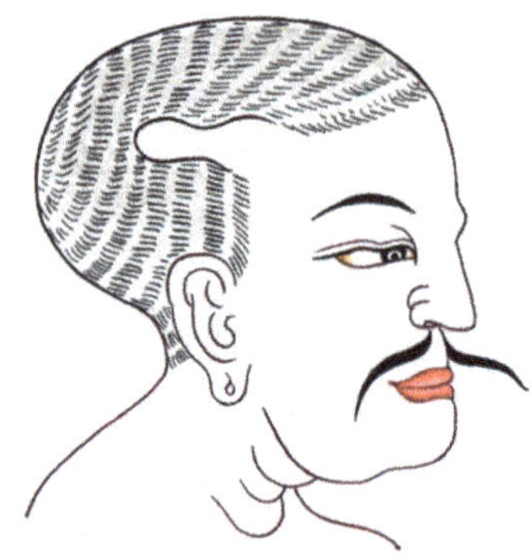

FIGURE 9.3 The bile constitution head:
with a protuberant occiput, and a butter-like brain

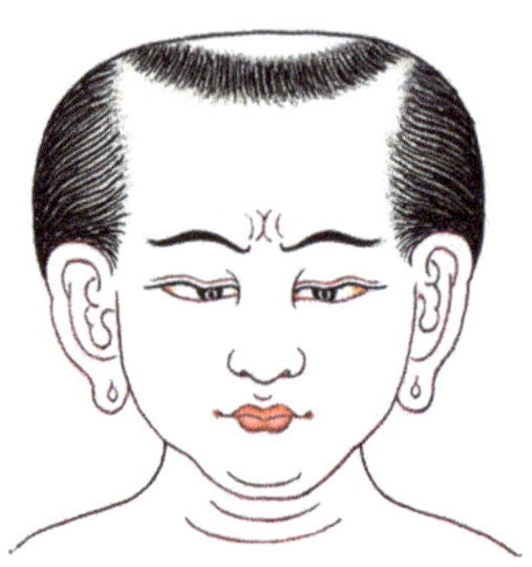

FIGURE 9.4 The phlegm constitution head:
triangular, with a beehive-like brain

Bile constitution has two subdivisions: hot bile and cold bile (*drangtri rangzhin*). The latter has inherent poor gallbladder function, which cools down and weakens digestive bile. It manifests metabolic disorders such as cold bile disorder, yellow bile, or brown phlegm. In this case, the influence of the phlegm and wind humors can be seen clearly in the reduction of digestive bile function.

3. Phlegm constitution (*béken rangzhin*)

Earth and water element or phlegm-dominated constitutions have a stable, down-to-earth mind. They are slow and profound thinkers. Phlegm constitutional people naturally have larger-sized bodies, white, dampish, smooth and soft skin, and a tendency to curve backwards when they get older. They have big greenish or grey-blue eyes with pronounced white sclera, and a low body temperature. People with this constitution easily put on weight. Their face, hands, and fingers have a smooth, beautiful shape and color to them. Their hair is often black, strong and straight. They have a slow digestion, are not particularly hungry or thirsty, and demonstrate great patience when facing problems. Their sleep is heavy, and they tend to be sluggish. They talk little and often have complaints related to the kidneys, bladder, stomach, and spleen. They show a tendency towards obesity, water retention, poor or slow digestion, diabetes, and the need to urinate frequently. With time their body shape tends to become pear-like; the lower abdomen and hips become larger while the upper part of the body reduces. They have a good heart and are tolerant, but are prone to melancholy and sadness.

A *béken* type's favorite food can be described as hot, sour, and astringent, with a liking for roughage. They have digestive difficulties and may be intolerant to an excess of carbohydrates (strong phlegm constitution), cucumber, salad, raw food, and sugar. Excessive eating, insufficient physical movement, and staying in cold and damp places will make them ill easily. Women of this constitution enter menopause later and most of them do not suffer from premenstrual syndrome. They enjoy a long life, prosperity, and wealth.

Their personality and character are similar to the lion, elephant, and buffalo.

Three double constitutions

If two *nyépa* are combined in equal or similar strength in the body, this is called *denpé rangzhin*. There are three types of constitutions dominated by two humors. Generally speaking, you may find these three groups are most common in society. They are: (1) wind-bile, (2) bile-phlegm, and (3) phlegm-wind.[4]

4. Wind-bile constitution (*lungtri rangzhin*)

This is perhaps the most common constitution. Wind-bile constitution people have a fast, sharp mind and are frequently anxious. They are thin, with bile-type skin and hair color, and easily suffer from digestive complaints, headaches, tinnitus, poor liver or gallbladder function, cystitis, eye weaknesses, allergies,

---

4 The three double-combined constitutions each have two variants depending on which humor is mentioned first. The first-mentioned humor is stronger, but still close to the second one.

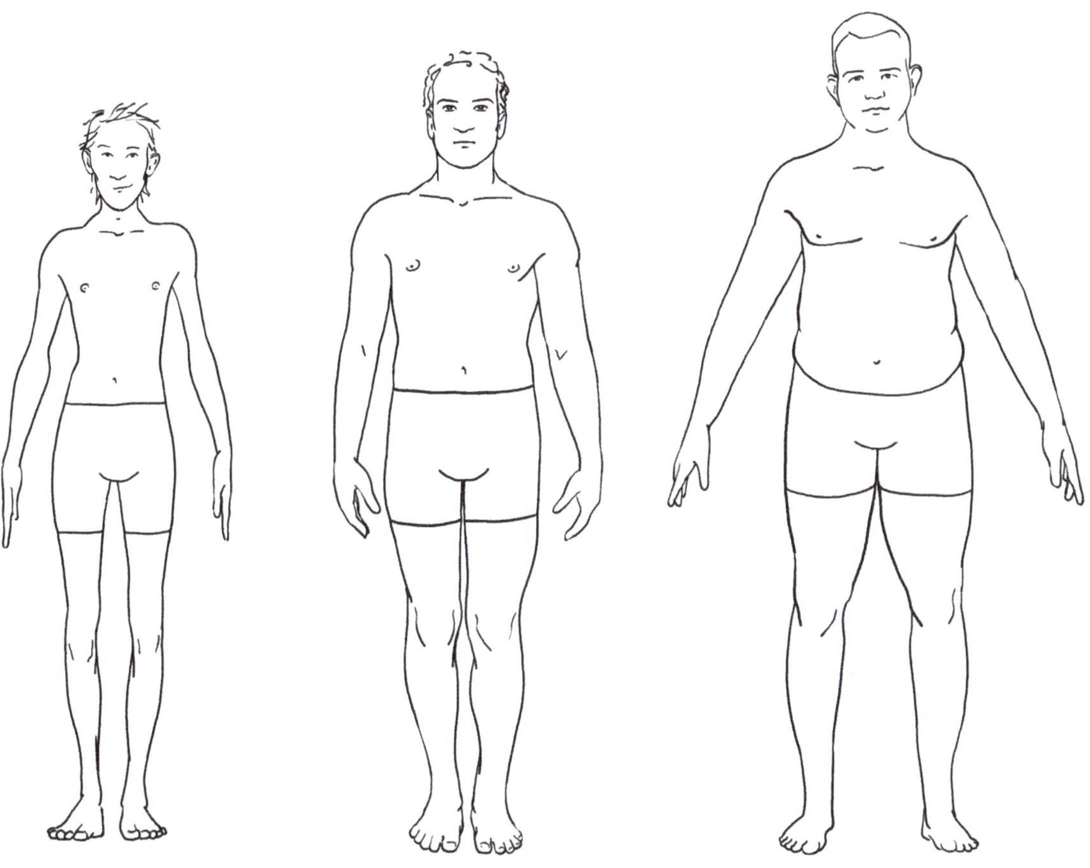

FIGURE 9.5 Wind, bile, and phlegm body types

acidity, and dry skin. They may have difficulties digesting bell pepper, milk, and alcohol, and tend to develop a nickel allergy. They easily get afraid, suffer from anxiety, and may develop hypersensitivity.

This combined constitution has two sub-types: (1) general or hot wind-bile, and (2) cold wind-bile.

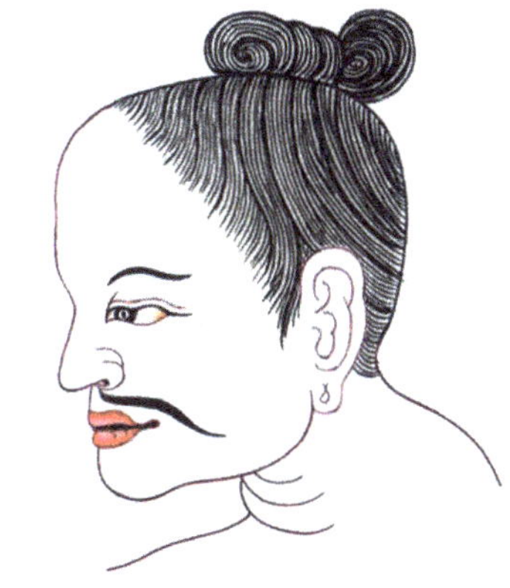

FIGURE 9.6 The wind-bile constitution head: square, with a buttermilk-like brain

If the wind combined with bile nature is hot, the patient will have a hot body and warm hands and feet. The bile and wind heat goes to the head, face, neck and hair, and produces an oily skin, with pimples and greasy hair. They are prone to migraines and headaches as well as colitis and tinnitus. They have difficulties tolerating white wine, champagne, fizzy water, bell peppers, coffee, milk, and fatty foods. They tend to get cold and easily get throat infections when exposed to windy places.

Cold wind-bile occurs if the wind is combined with the cold bile type (due to constitutional gallbladder weakness). They manifest cold hands, nose and feet, frequent headaches, neck and shoulder aches, and digestive problems. They are physically thin but with a tendency to get high blood pressure. Women suffer more from menstrual pain. Generally, these people, especially women, develop migraine and headaches. Food intolerances are the same as those of wind and bile constitutions. They are psychologically "in conflict" and have problems making decisions, which is similar to the bile-phlegm constitution.

5. Phlegm-bile constitution (*bétri rangzhin*)

These people have straight bodies and stable personalities, yet are prone to psychological conflict.

This combined constitution has two sub-types: (1) general or hot bile-phlegm, and (2) cold bile-phlegm.

Hot bile-phlegm types are caught between the two opposite elements of fire and water. In size they are between the bile and phlegm constitutions, but usually more substantial and stable in nature. They tend towards mental conflict, but they are not dependent on others. Instead, they live with their conflict alone. They also physically suffer from conflictive humors (hot as well as cold disorders) that manifest disharmony such as high blood pressure, and glandular, colic, liver, gallbladder and digestive complaints, headaches, bad blood circulation, plus a tendency for gallstones. With age, they feel their body is divided into two parts: feeling hot in the upper and cold in the lower half.

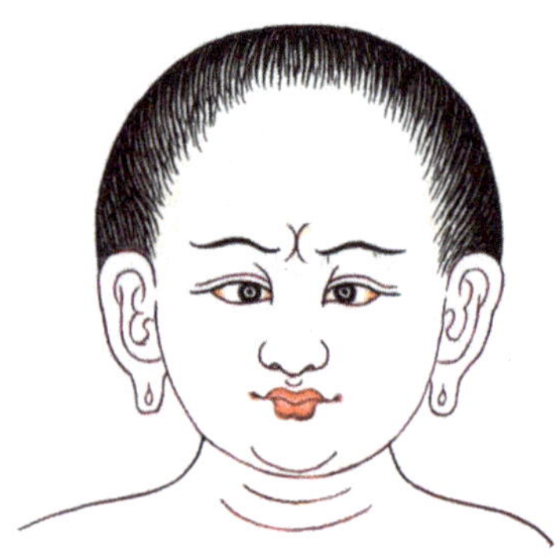

FIGURE 9.7 The bile-phlegm head: rounded, with a curd-like brain

Cold bile-phlegm individuals are generally more skinny, with a cold body and a propensity to sweating. This proneness to being thin and the lack of physical substance tends to be more prevalent in women. It manifests cold feet, hands, and nose. These symptoms are also found in the cold wind-bile type, but cold bile-phlegm types are characterized by the presence of more mucus, fat and thickness, demonstrating more phlegm signs. Externally, they suffer from poor blood circulation and internally they have high blood pressure. Their nature is like boiled hot water. Many people of this type, and especially young women, get headaches and suffer from premenstrual pain. This constitution also manifests high cholesterol, gallbladder malfunction, and gallstones can develop in the later part of life. Men may suffer from high cholesterol and heart complaints.

6. Phlegm-wind constitution (*bélung rangzhin*)

People having this constitution have a large, beautiful, clean and clear appearance. However, they have a tendency to mental confusion, having a cloudy mind. They like to consult others to confirm their ideas. They do not trust themselves, which can make them dependent on others. Generally, the mind is slow and easily suffers from melancholy and depression. Their body produces cold sweat, and they put on weight easily. Gas formation, hypertension, heart disorders, diabetes and cold kidney disorders are quite common in this constitution.

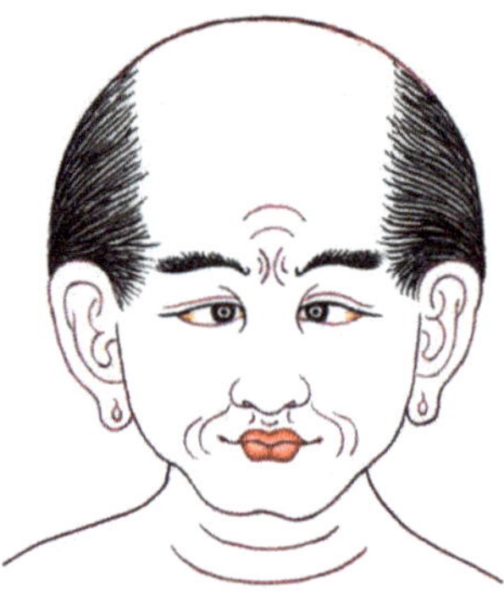

FIGURE 9.8 The phlegm-wind head: wide, with a milk-like brain

One triple constitution (*düpé rangzhin*)

The combined constitution

When all three humors contribute equally, the resulting constitution is called *düpé rangzhin*, the "[totally] composite nature." This type possesses characteristics from all three humors.

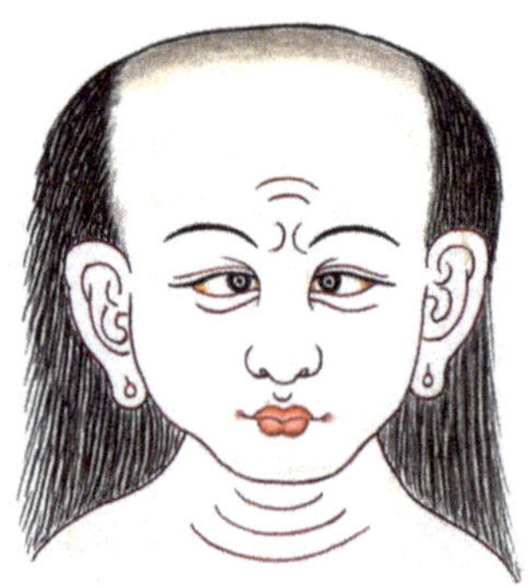

FIGURE 9.9 The triple combined constitution head: flattened, with a water-like brain

The three single constitutions are considered to be the lowest or most inferior quality of the body, while the double combined constitution is intermediate. The totally combined constitution is superior: the most balanced of all body types. It is the standard body in Sowa Rigpa. Such an ideal body constitution is rare.

9.4 *RANGZHIN* AND BLOOD GROUPS

It is interesting to try to compare the *rangzhin dün* with the four major blood groups of modern biomedicine (the ABO system) and the Rh system (positive or negative). A, B, and O might correlate with double humor constitutions, and AB with the triple combined one:

- Blood group A: phlegm constitution
- Blood group B: bile constitution
- Blood group O: wind constitution
- Blood group AB: triple combined constitution

This is a tentative proposition, and there might be many exceptions. More research is needed to uncover the relationship between blood and body constitution. These four blood groups could also relate to the four humors theory in Tibetan medicine (and in the ancient Galenic tradition), carrying the subtle nature of a person's constitution. Such ideas could be a secret key to reveal the body constitution as well as personality of patients on a deeper level, and may give new possibilities in preventing disease and finding right treatments. Yutok Yönten Gönpo described a concept akin to "four humor bloods" (*duwa nam zhi*) as well as "seven body constitution blood types" (*trak rik dün*) in the venesection chapter of the *Subsequent Tantra*. So far, such concepts have not been elaborated or compared to biomedicine. There are more possibilities in our modern times for Tibetan medicine to take one step further in understanding anatomy and physiology, building on the *Gyüzhi*.

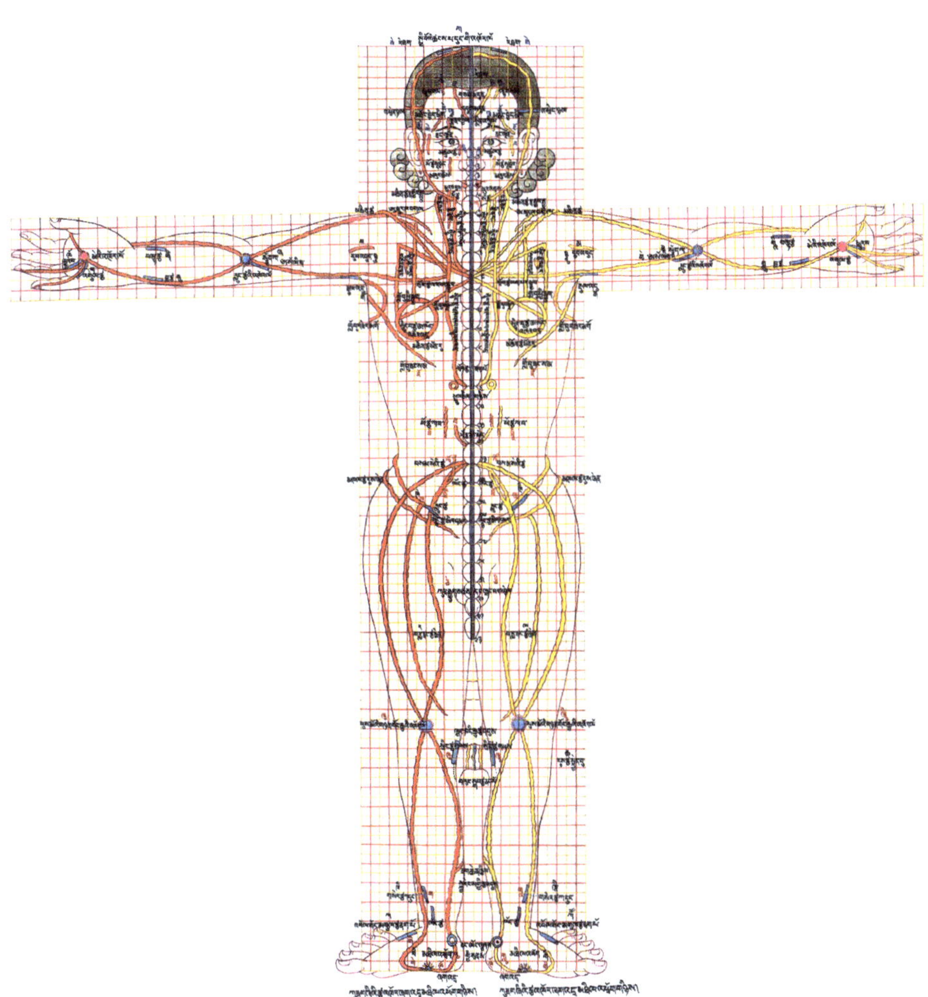

FIGURE 9.10 The standard body proportions as depicted in the Tibetan medical paintings

Summary

Knowing the constitution can help to better understand the body-mind, including the natural behavior and personality of individuals. It also acts as a guide to a healthy daily life by paying specific attention to, nutrition, behavior, seasonality, and psychology. Constitution is an important key that reveals the origin of disease, and unlocks the door of proper diagnosis and treatment.

PART 3

DIGESTION AND THE CONSTITUENTS

ཟས་འཇུ་ཆུལ་དང་ལུས་ཟུངས།

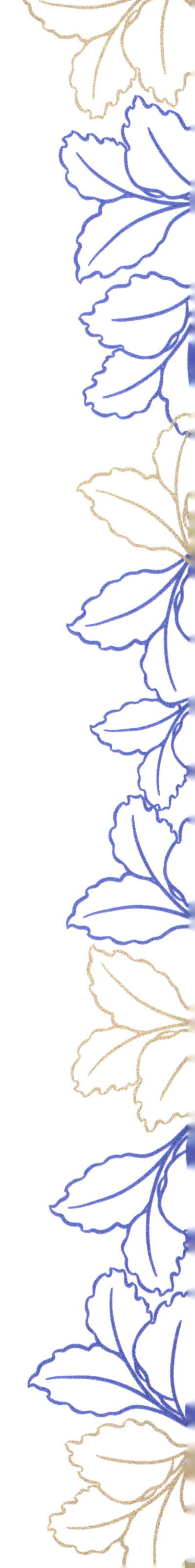

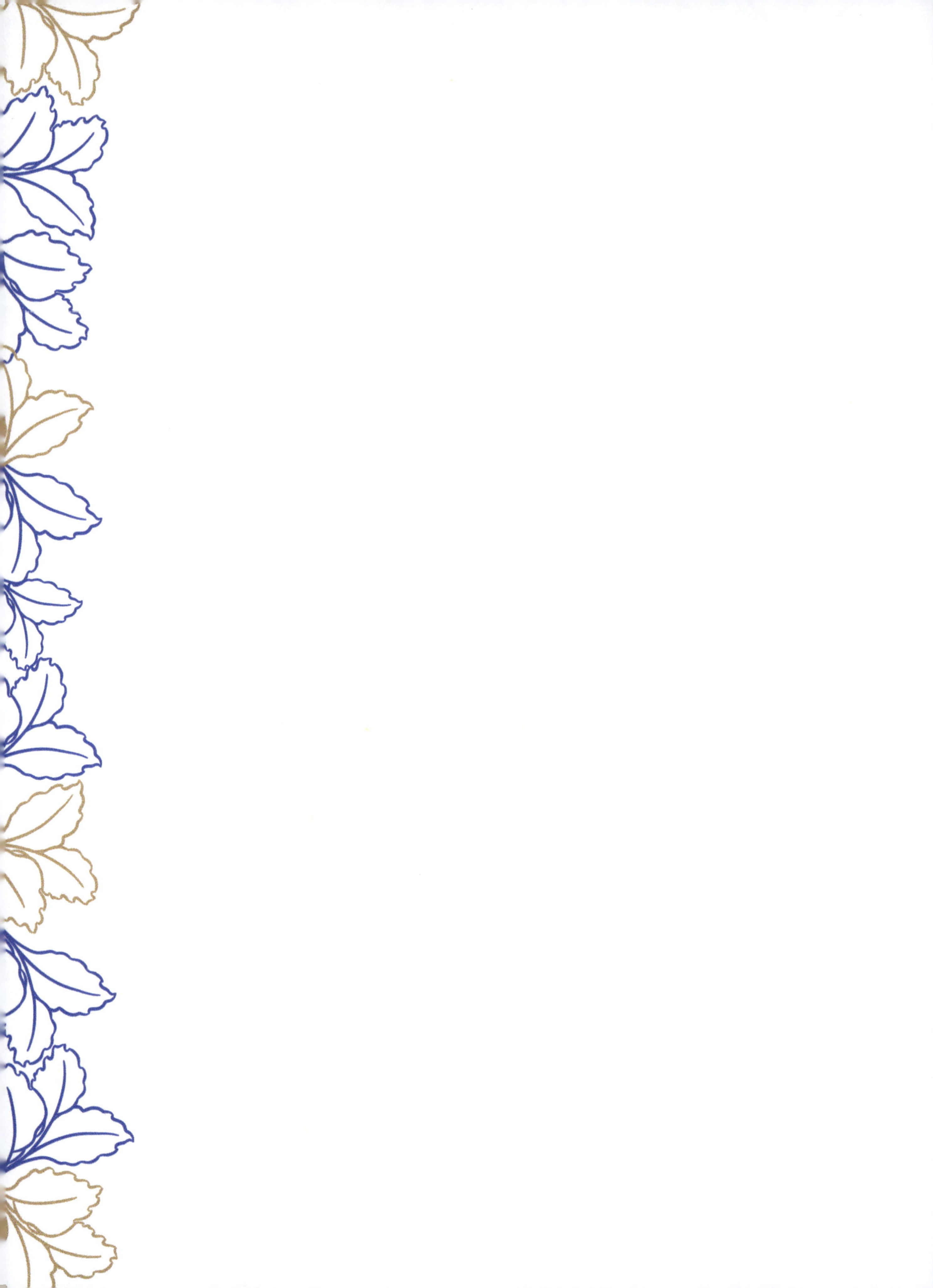

CHAPTER 10

THE DIGESTIVE SYSTEM

The digestive system or process (*zé jutsül*) operates automatically within the body by means of *médrö*, the power of the digestive fire. Digestion functions through the cooperation of the three humors and the digestive organs. This system starts to develop before birth, and starts to work with the intake of mother's milk. The first stage takes place in the stomach, followed by the small intestine and colon. Digestive bile acts like a kitchen fire, decomposing phlegm like water in a cooking pot, and fire-like wind functions like gas. Together, these three energies help "cook" the food as it proceeds through the digestive tract. In Tibetan this is called *zé juwa*, the digestion of food. Food essence or nutrition (*dangma*) is absorbed and sent to the liver. There, it transforms into blood that sustains the body-mind, flowing like the mighty river Ganges that nourishes the earth and supports vegetation. *Dangma* contains the energies that sustain all three humors as well as the seven body constituents. In other words, it contains the necessary carbohydrates, proteins, fats, minerals, and vitamins. In this sense, *dangma* is the most essential substance for sustaining life. The digestive organs are the essential machinery for *dangma* processing and extraction. A healthy stomach is like a fertile land where abundant crops can grow. The *Explanatory Tantra*'s 28th chapter states:[1]

> The stomach is like a field.
> *Médrö* must be sustained.
> Whoever knows this,
> is a skilled physician.

The three main organs of the digestive tract are the stomach, small intestine, and colon, where decomposing phlegm, digestive bile, and fire-like wind predominate respectively.[2] Other organs have supporting functions. The liver, for example, is like wood that conducts fire. The gallbladder ignites the fire in the duodenum, while the spleen and kidneys regulate the liquid in which food dissolves. The heart, lungs, and colon provide wind (movement) and desire for food, whereas the tongue and stomach give satisfaction.

The digestive process can be divided into general and specific digestion. The first refers to the general processes taking place in the stomach, small intestine, and colon. The specific digestion is a more subtle transformation of the nutrients. *Dangma* is absorbed from the digestive organs and sent to the liver through the portal veins, called the nine absorbing channels (*dangma lenpé tsa gu*). The number nine in this case is symbolic. We should understand that there are many nutritional absorption channels connecting to the liver, corresponding to the portal vein system in biomedicine. Absorption takes place through the seven bodily constituents (*lüzung dün*): *dangma*, blood, flesh, fat, bone, bone marrow, and the reproductive fluids. Along this process, waste products (*drima*) such as urine, feces, and sweat are eliminated. This is an important form of natural cleansing. The strength of the body constituents and the humoral energies increases or decreases depending on the efficiency of general and specific digestion. A healthy digestion gives positive health and long life, while poor digestion impairs health and shortens life, as we are taught in the *Explanatory Tantra*.

General digestion

General digestion starts in the mouth. Food is swallowed through the activity of life-sustaining wind. As soon as the foodstuffs reach the stomach, digestion is regulated by the three energies of decomposing phlegm, digestive bile, and fire-like wind, which respectively act like water, fire, and wind (gas) in cooking.

---

1 G.yu thog yon tan mgon po, 1993, 91.

2 In general statements "stomach" includes the small and large intestines.

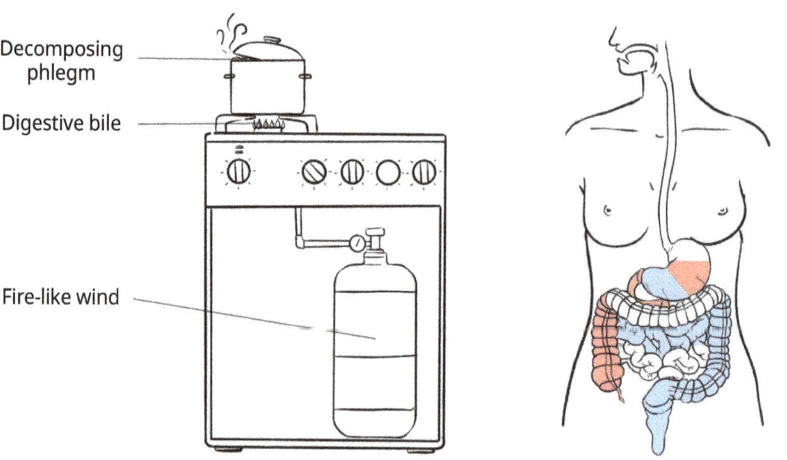

FIGURE 10.1 General digestion is like cooking food

The first digestive stage starts in the mouth but principally takes place in the (upper) stomach, where *béken nyakjé* acts like cooking food with water. *Tripa jujé* dictates digestion in the stomach, and is especially active in the duodenum and small intestine. This second stage is like filtering, sending the digested essence to the liver. The digested food reaches the large intestine, where the third process takes place under the action of *lung ményam*, just like gas sustains fire. It separates, absorbs, and transports *dangma* to the liver through the portal veins and other channels.

The stomach mainly digests foods based on the earth and water elements, which have a sweet (and salty) taste, such as milk and wheat products. The resulting frothy liquid (*dangma*) or "food essence" takes on a phlegm-like quality, and is absorbed and sent to the liver. There, it becomes blood and increases the phlegm constituents such as flesh and fat. This equally increases the cooling power of *béken*, which has heavy and oily qualities.

The second stage takes place in the duodenum and small intestine. Here the fire element, including foods with sour and hot tastes such as spices, alcohol, and greasy animal fat, is absorbed and transformed into a sour liquid (another type of *dangma*) with a bile quality. This then goes to the liver and becomes bile, blood, sweat, and other bile constituents. This increases the bile humor, which has hot, sharp, and oily qualities.

The water and air food elements are processed in the colon. These have bitter and astringent tastes, such as lettuce, fibers, and coffee. The resulting *dangma* is sent to the liver, where it becomes blood and produces wind constituents like bones, nerves, tendons, and skin. It also increases the wind humor's lightness and instable character.

Specific digestion

After the general digestion process is complete and the different types of nutrients have been transported to the liver, specific digestion begins. The nutrients are transformed into subtler constituents in seven stages.

1. *Dangma*
   Immediately after the processing of the nutrients by the three digestive functions, the first resulting constituent is food essence, which was separated from the food in the digestive organs. It is basically colorless, but the color of food can influence it. It generally has a sweet taste and goes to the liver via the portal vein system.

2. Blood (*trak*)
   When *dangma* reaches the liver, it transforms into blood within a day. The blood becomes the main contributor of life along with the other body constituents.

3. Muscles (*sha*)
   Blood transforms into flesh (muscles) within a day, which protects and gives strength to the body.

4. Fat (*tsil*)
   Then, it becomes fat on the third day. This lubricates the body and protects it from dryness and cold.

5. Bone (*rüpa*)
   On the fourth day, the essence of fat becomes bone, which keeps the body firm.

6. Bone marrow (*kang*)
   On the fifth day, the bone essence becomes bone marrow, a resource and reservoir of bodily power.

7. Reproductive fluid (*khuwa, tiklé*)
   During the sixth day, the essence of bone marrow transforms into reproductive fluids, which are a highly refined material essence that ensures future generations.

The final product: radiance (*dang*)

Dang is the most refined food essence. It is a quintessential subtle liquid, a substance of light. It is the essence of the reproductive fluids, which is sent to the heart. Radiating from the heart, it brightens the whole body and especially the face. It is like sunlight reflecting on a flower, like spices added to food, moisture in the soil, and air to life. A strong *dang* sustains life, protects health, and gives courage. Poor or weak *dang* leads to loss of physical and mental strength. *Dang* is physical yet subtle, and therefore does not count as one of the seven body constituents. This liquid nectar light is related to the modern concept of hormones.

In short, the five elements in the food essence chain nourish and increase the five elements of the body in the form of seven constituents. The duration of the whole process, from *dangma* to reproductive fluids, takes six days of transformation. There are exceptions, however, such as in the case of some aphrodisiac medicines.

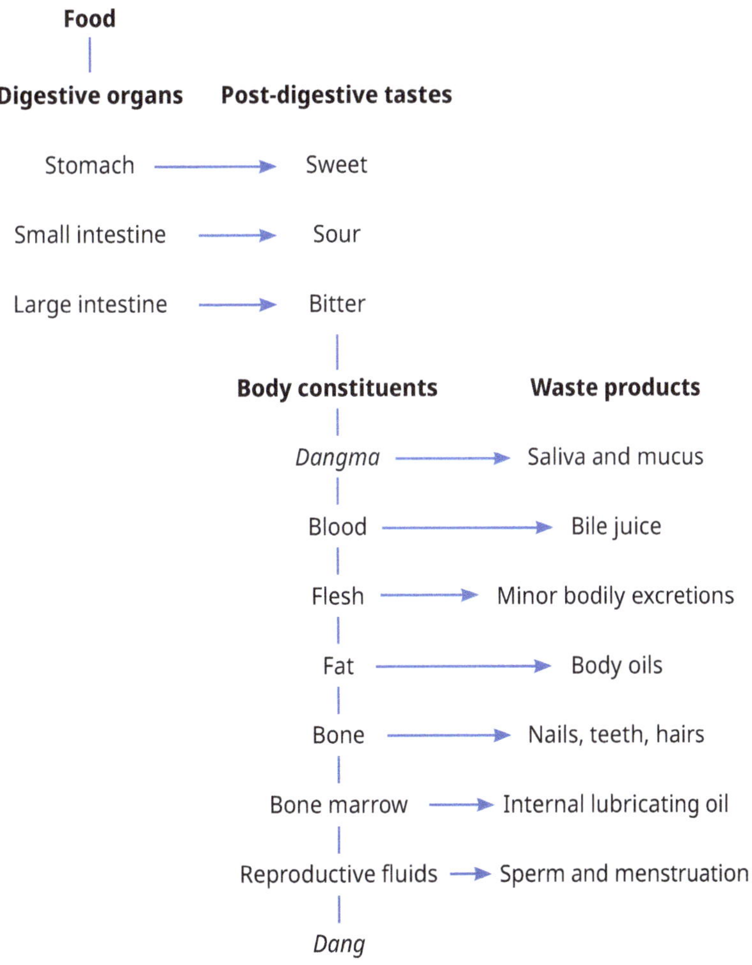

FIGURE 10.2 The specific digestion process

CHAPTER 11

THE CONSTITUENTS AND WASTE PRODUCTS

11.1 THE SEVEN BODY CONSTITUENTS (*LÜZUNG DÜN*)

Seven constituents, which are products of food, make up the physical body. In Tibetan these are called *lüzung dün*, "the seven bodily sustainers." They give form, shape, and power to the body-mind and protect the organs. They are like soil for crops or the building blocks of a house, as we are told in the *Explanatory Tantra.*

Dangma

Dangma means "food essence," and roughly corresponds to chyle. *Dangma* is absorbed by the liver in three stages of digestion, where it becomes blood: from the stomach, small intestine, and large intestine. It comprises the nutritional energy that is needed for body maintenance and development. *Dangma* is an important building block of *béken* activity.

The *dangma* waste products become saliva and mucus in the stomach and intestines, and other organs.

Blood

Blood is the first substance to be refined from *dangma* as it is transformed into blood and colored red by color-transforming bile in the liver "blood bank." It is of the nature of fire and is the principal transporter of all the energies in the body. Blood carries bile heat, nutrients, fluids, and the vital energy of the organs, tissues, and cells. The amount of required blood for a healthy person is traditionally measured as seven cupped hands. Generally, there are seven different types of blood (see Section 9.4). The liver transforms *dangma* into blood within 24 hours, which is then distributed through blood vessels. There are two groups of blood channels: *traktsa marpo*, the red blood channels or arterial system, and *traktsa nakpo*, the dark blood vessels or veins.

The blood waste product is bile, which is stored in the gallbladder. This bile is itself subdivided further into two parts. The pure part is *chuser* ("yellow fluid"), which mixes with the blood, becomes plasma, and which acts as the blood's vital energy that also protects the skin (in the form of interstitial fluid). The second bile part is the waste product called *trikhu*, bile juice. It is released into the duodenum, where it powers the digestive fire, digests food, and regulates the intestines.

Chuser, the yellow fluid

The term *chuser* is mentioned in each of the *Four Tantras*, but more so in the *nyamyik* literature of collected medical experience. Many physicians are convinced that *chuser* influences numerous disorders, including infections and chronic inflammatory conditions involving hidden fever (*gaptsé*), arthritis, rheumatism, skin diseases with necrosis (*tiksak*) and pus formation, as well as organ malfunction, blood and lymph vessel inflammation. Besides these major ailments, the appearance of external wounds and blisters, fractures, and hair loss may also be caused by unhealthy *chuser*. As it appears to be a significant factor of both infectious and noninfectious diseases, we can assume that this yellow fluid also plays a vital role in health maintenance.

As introduced above, *chuser* is a blood residue or byproduct that is produced by the liver and gallbladder. There, refined bile juice (bile *dangma*) transforms into *chuser* that is secreted into the bloodstream. From a biomedical perspective, we can recognize it as plasma, a yellowish liquid making up about 55% of the total blood volume (and that is closely related with the interstitial fluid between cells). Although red blood (cells) and *chuser* are distinct entities, both are interdependent in their functioning and sustainment of the bile humor. The waste products of bile juice refinement enter the intestines, aiding the breakdown of foodstuffs. These bile residues are finally excreted, giving urine its yellow color and odor.

The *Gyüzhi* does not give details on *chuser* function, yet the *Explanatory Tantra*'s chapter on body similes expounds that the gallbladder is like a bag of nutrients or spices hanging in one's kitchen. The content of the bag in this analogy refers to bile juice, but especially to the high-quality refined bile that sustains and protects the red blood and bile humor by means of its hot nature, strengthening the *médrö* to digest food, contributing to body heat, and defeating pathogens. *Chuser* invigorates the blood just like nutritious ingredients make food more nourishing. Although the 59th chapter of the *Oral Instruction Tantra* and the *Subsequent Tantra*'s urine analysis chapter both state that it is a waste product of the blood (and thus also connected to bilirubin), *chuser* is in fact the main bile energy that flows through the body like a river, carrying the red blood while also acting as a defense system. *Chuser* and blood flow together through the arteries and veins, but the former has traditionally been deemed less important. The reddish tinge of plasma indicates its derivation from blood, whereas its yellow color points to its identity as bile's refined liquid (*trikhu*).

Chuser is active mainly between the flesh (muscles) and skin, contributing to its radiance (*dang*), as well as in the joints. The necessary amount in the body is measured as four double handfuls. Besides guarding and circulating the blood, it therefore also acts to protect the skin and lubricate the joints. It seems that *chuser* is closely involved in wound healing, and that it constitutes a powerful protective force against foreign agents such as bacteria, parasites, and viruses, playing a significant part in our immune system.

Flesh

Flesh or muscle tissue is a refined substance of blood. It belongs to the earth element and is a basic physical component. It covers the body, forms the organs, moves the articulations, and maintains the body's strength. The waste products of flesh are minor products such as tears, earwax, dandruff, and sweat.

The *Blue Beryl* lists 45 vital muscles (*sha né*), alongside 14 tendons (*gyüpa*) and nerves.[3] There are 190 blood channels that could be life-threatening if injured. Here is a general list of the quantities of the important components of a standard body:

- The quantity of fleshy tissue (*sha*) of the body should be 500 fist-sizes for a man and 520 for a woman (20 extra fist-sizes for the breasts and hips)

- 45 vital muscles, of which five in the head, four in the neck, 18 in the abdomen, and 18 in the extremities; all these have an essential life-protecting role

- Five sensory organs (*wangpo go nga*)

- Five extremities (*yenlak nga*): arms, legs, and head.

- Five solid organs (*dön nga*): heart, lungs, liver, spleen, and kidneys

- Six hollow organs (*nö druk*): stomach, small intestine, large intestine, gallbladder, urinary bladder, and reproductive organs (including breasts)

- Nine orifices (*gogü buga*)

- 20 fingers (*dzupmo*), five on each hand and foot

- Head (*go*) and brain (*lépa*); the size of the brain is two cupped hands

- 900 tendons (*gyüpa*)

- 19 ligaments (*chuwa chugu*)

- Three principal channels (*tsa sum*)

Fat

Fat is the refined part of flesh. It maintains the body's oil system that lubricates and nourishes the skin, organs, and tissues. It belongs to the water and earth elements, being cold and phlegmatic in nature. For a healthy person, the prescribed amount of fat (solid) and oil (liquid) in the body is two cupped hands. Fat maintains the glands and lymphatic system, and guards the body heat. The fatty tissues include eight vital lymph nodes (see Section 17.5). The waste product of fat becomes the body oils, which keep the skin young and nourished.

---

3 Sde srid sangs rgyas rgya mtsho, 1994, 114.

Bone

Bone is a refined product of fat. Its pure essence produces bone marrow, the spinal cord (white and grey matter), and brain. Bones support the structure of the body. It belongs to the earth element and is a house for wind. The skeleton is comprised of approximately 360 pieces of bones and tendons. There are 32 vital bones to which damage could be life-threatening. There are many different shapes and sizes of bone tissue:

- 23 general bone shapes

- 20 main vertebrae

- Five cervical vertebrae

- Three coccyx (tailbone) segments

- 24 ribs (12 on each side)

- 20 fingers and toes

- 12 big joints (six in the arms and six in the legs)

- 210 minor joints

- 360 pieces of bones in total, including cartilage and some tendons

The bone waste products become hair, teeth, nails, and other minor products:

- 20 finger and toenails

- 32 teeth (eight front teeth, four eye-teeth, 16 chewing teeth, four corner or wisdom teeth)

- 21,600 hairs on the scalp[4]

- 3,500,000 body hairs

Bone marrow

Bone marrow is a refined product of the bone constituent, and is an important substance that nourishes all the organs, tissues, nerves, blood, and lymph. It vitalizes the body-mind, sustaining bodily strength and the power of eyesight. It belongs to the earth and water elements and has a heavy quality, which supports

béken. The waste product of bone marrow provides lubricant for the body, feces, urine, and body pores.

Reproductive fluids

The reproductive fluids are digestion's final refinement of nutrition, being directly derived from bone marrow as well as the reproductive organs. The reproductive fluid, include sperm and (pre-)seminal fluid for men, and ovum and normal vaginal discharge for women. Sperm and egg are the products of many body parts which finally come together like a fruit absorbing water. We cannot perceive this elemental transformation directly, but we can see the result. Because they are the final nutritional product, they are called the "storehouse of treasures" (*nor gyi bangdzö*) in the *Gyüzhi.* Semen is a phlegm-dominated constituent, whereas menses are derived from bile energy. Millions of *khuwé bu* (spermatozoa) are produced in the testicles. A large quantity of *khuwa* manifests in men who naturally have more physical strength, desire, and sexual attraction. The reproductive fluids are collectively called *khuwa kar mar,* meaning "white and red fluids," in medicine. In tantric literature, *kham kar mar,* "white and red essential natures," is used.[5] Both refer to semen and menstruation (including ovum). *Tiklé* (drops) is also applied in common and tantric language, especially when referring to semen, while the term *khu chu* is used for seminal fluid. Tibetan medicine recognizes sperm as alive, as reflected in the name *khuwé bu* or "sperm being".

A woman's menstruation is called *datsen,* the "monthly sign" of the hormonal cycle. Its nature is fire, hence its red color. *Datsen* is related with the moon phases; the menstrual cycle is the female body's biological clock, which also indicates when it is possible to conceive a child. *Datsen* is light and warming in quality, which makes women more active, sensitive, creative, and susceptible to subtler feelings than men. Detailed description of the follicles and ovum are lacking in Sowa Rigpa, but the menstrual cycle is recognized (see also Chapter 12). A strong, healthy and regular follicle development and menstrual flow gives physical strength, desire, and sexual attraction.

Both reproductive fluids contain vital energy, nourishing the body tissues and organs. They manifest sexual interest, pleasure, romantic emotions, lust, neuroticism, courage, and aggressiveness. The *khuwa kar mar* also grant vigor to the body, keeping it youthful. It maintains the heredity and stimulates male and female characteristics. The refined essence of the reproductive fluids is *dang*: the radiant light of the body.

---

4   This symbolic number of hairs corresponds to the average number of breaths in a day.

5   Another tantric term used is *jangsem kar mar,* white and red *bodhicitta.*

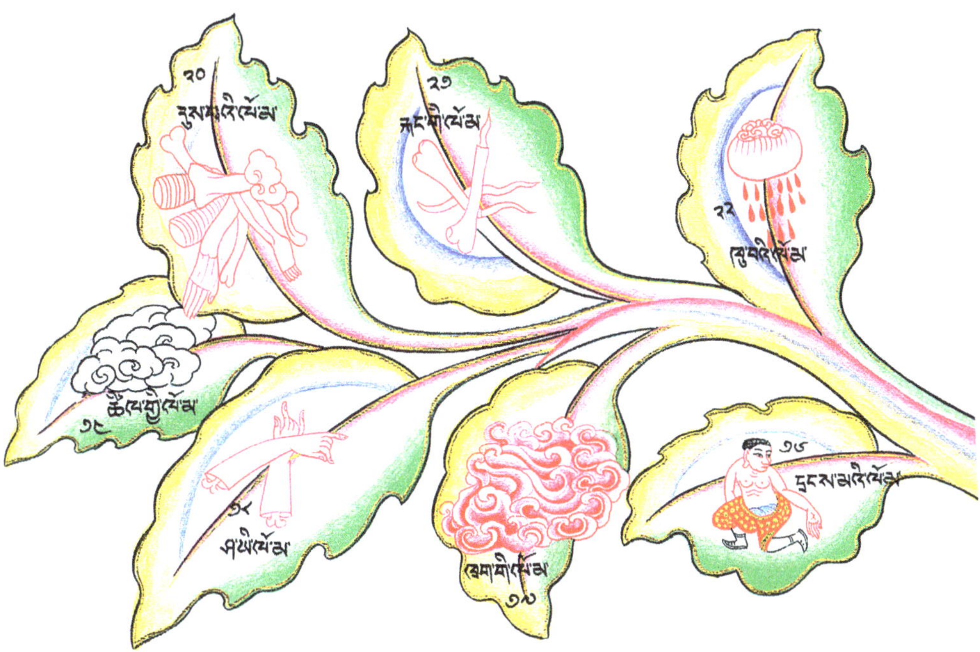

FIGURE 11.1 The seven body constituents and their minor residual products

The reproductive fluids are considered waste products because they are released through the reproductive organ after *dang* is absorbed and sent to the heart. Men produce semen, which accumulates in the testicles and is ejaculated upon sexual orgasm. Women produce follicles which become the ovum, and accumulate blood and tissue on the inner lining of the uterus. With time, the latter is released and flows down, becoming the monthly menstruation if fertilization does not occur. The male and female fluids are both residues of high refinement and value, being essential in keeping good health, high spirits, and in the production of offspring.

Dang

Dang is the final refinement of the food essence energy, which is generated from the reproductive fluids of the testicles and ovaries. It does not count as one of the seven body constituents as it does not lead to more refined substances. *Dang* is a subtle liquid that produces the body's radiance and complexion. It is a luminous energy that is concentrated in the heart, but is also pervasive. It gives vital energy to the blood, organs, and tissues, and its effect is especially visible in the face and on the forehead, chest, and skin. This radiance is expressed as an encircling halo of light (aura) that reinforces the body and sustains mental stability and consciousness. It grants intelligence, self-awareness, pride, courage, and ambition. A strong and large aura is a sign of good health and long life, and *vice versa*. The *Explanatory Tantra*'s chapter five states:[6]

> The reproductive fluids, the constituents'
> final product, is supreme *dang*.
> It resides in the heart yet pervades the
> whole body.
> It sustains life, generates radiance, and
> brightness.

This sublime light is distributed from the heart to the brain and other organs and tissues, then radiating through the skin. The function of *dang* is the same for women and men. *Dang* is abundant during youth, when the body is healthy like a fresh flower. Abundant *dang* production reflects good health and a strong mind, whereas poor *dang* is a sign of weakness that could lead to decreased disease resistance. Psychologically, poor *dang* is accompanied by feelings of weakness, fragility, anxiety, and fear. As you can see in Figure 11.2, *dang* not only radiates from the skin as body complexion but also from the five main chakras. Each chakra contains subtle *tiklé* that sustain mind and life, and which manifest the five mental poisons: closed-mindedness, attachment, hatred, pride and jealousy respectively, from head to toe. In each

6 Ibid., 27.

of these energy centers, a white and red moon can be seen opposite to each other. These represent the *tiklé* obtained from the parents; they are the root source of physical development and the material condition for the mind and emotions. They also correspond to the quintessence of the five elements (*jungwa ngé dangma*), which may be somewhat related to the concept of hereditary material (DNA). These *tiklé* carry information on body constitution, health, capacities, etc., in relation to the parents. In the middle of the two half-moon signs, there is a dark-colored *nāda*, a sign for smoke that symbolizes the neutrality of consciousness. All this is sustained in the body by *dangma*.

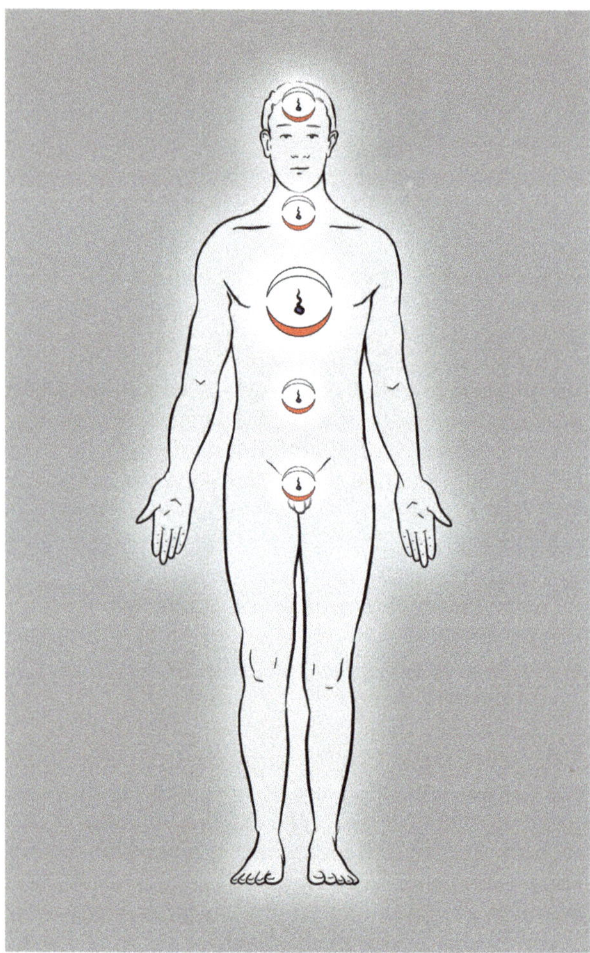

FIGURE 11.2 Radiance and the *tiklé*

Dang actually has five colors that represent the quintessence of the five elements, which together create radiance, complexion, and life energy, regenerating the body organs, tissues, and even the waste products. In short, *dang* is the essential power of the body-mind, giving rise to emotions. Each organism constantly produces *dang*, which simultaneously flows out of the body like candlelight. *Dang* is causally connected to the *la* body, the energetic second body that usually goes together with each person like a shadow (see Section 18.1).

11.2 HORMONES (*KHAM KYI DANGMA*)

Dang gives physical strength and maintains youthfulness. When *dang* decreases, the person appears older as the skin shrivels, and weak like a plant lacking water and minerals. *Dang* therefore acts like a generic hormone to some degree, even influencing the person's mood. The cause of decreasing *dang* is described in the *Explanatory Tantra*, chapter 11:[7]

> *Dang* decreases by mental sufferings,
> resulting in fright, emaciation, weakness,
> unhappiness, and loss of radiance.
> Having milk and meat broth acts as healing
> medicine.

In Sowa Rigpa, there is no unique term that can adequately cover all different aspects of hormones as they are defined in biomedicine. Yet, the author has coined *kham kyi dangma* as a general term to interpret hormones, creating a bridge with biomedicine. This refers to "natural essences" of the body that are distributed to the organs and constituents, developing different genders and other characteristics. *Kham kyi dangma* can be interpreted as the ultimate product of the reproductive fluids in the form of a liquid quintessential substance. Gathering in and being distributed from the heart like the distillation of essential oil, it reaches everywhere like sunrise. *Kham kyi dangma* is indeed the essence of the reproductive fluids or *tiklé*, but not *dang* itself. It is more gross than *dang*. *Kham kyi dangma* are produced in the process in-between the reproductive fluids and *dang*, although there is an undeniable relationship with bone marrow as well. According to biomedicine, many important hormones are secreted by the pituitary gland of the hypothalamus in the brain, from where they reach other organs such as the thyroid and reproductive system. Many types of hormones are defined, and it is important to know their physiology in detail. Under the following two headings, we will briefly cover hormone function based on *Gyüzhi* medicine and tantric sources.

Hormone-related concepts in Sowa Rigpa

In addition to *dang*, which has been introduced above, three relevant terms are discussed here: *tsap*, *potsi*, and *motsi*.

---

7   G.yu thog yon tan mgon po, 1993, 40.

Tsap

The *Gyüzhi*'s gynecology chapters indirectly refer to female hormonal imbalance when covering the group of gynecological diseases called *tsap né*. *Tsap*[8] can be said to refer to hormones here, and *né* stands for disease. The nature of hormones is not clearly described, however, two types of *tsap né* are discussed which correspond well with biomedical etiology: *traktsap* (premenopausal stage diseases) and *lungtsap* (menopausal disorders). *Tsap* is a specific term used to refer to female hormonal imbalance (see also Chapter 12), which does not cover *kham kyi dangma* in general.

Potsi **and** motsi

These Tibetan terms, literally meaning "male" and "female essence," were invented by Dr. Samten to refer to the male and female hormones in the nineties, as described in his groundbreaking book.[9] They are produced in the testicles and ovaries, are suitable names, but do not cover all types of hormones. *Potsi* likely corresponds to testosterone, *motsi* to estrogen, progesterone and prolactine.

Tantric interpretation of *tiklé*

Tantra is referred to as *sang ngak*, which literally means "secret mantra," that which protects the mind from suffering. It is esoteric and generally restricted from public exposure. However, on this particular subject and on a medical level, tantra offers profound explanations that allow for deeper insight into human physiology and the psyche. Tantra uses different sets of terms for the gross and subtle forms of semen, menstruation, and *dang*. The two reproductive fluids are frequently called *kham kar mar*, meaning the two natures (and their colors) of men and women.

Tantric sources rely on the term *tiklé* (meaning "essence drop") when explaining the subtle physiology of the *vajra* body, in this context mainly referring to the man's semen or white *tiklé*. Menstruation, including the ovum, are generally not considered *tiklé* but are referred to as *kham mar*, the red nature substance. A metaphorical term is applied to the inner subtle *tiklé*: *jangchup kyi sem gyégyur gyi rikchen* or "evolving relative *bodhicitta*." This is discussed as a

luminous nectar that flows in the body, changing in alignment with the moon phases and thus naturally increasing and decreasing like ocean tides. For our purposes here, we can understand this as hormones or *kham kyi dangma*.

Tantra gives much attention to these natural essences, treating both the gross and subtle reproductive fluids as important. The gross *tiklé* or essence drops (semen and menses) which produce *dang*, are the quintessence of all body-mind power. They are involved in the manifestation of sexual pleasure and ecstasy. Through the application of advanced tantric techniques, the intensity of this moment can light the *tumo* fire and melt the central *tiklé* of the brain, which is tiny, pear-shaped, and hanging downwards. This *tumo* heat then stimulates the subtle *tiklé* to flow downwards into the bloodstream like rain drops from clouds, like butter churned from milk, or juice pressed from fruits. This process, which might also be interpreted as the generation of a unique bioelectric impulse, is stimulated by gross *tiklé* movement. When both *tiklé* reach the genitals, they create extraordinary bliss that arises within a state of meditative absorption. The gross *tiklé* may ejaculate, but the subtle *tiklé* are not lost. In this manner, sexual union can present a great opportunity to unite compassion and wisdom, but for ordinary people it often has the opposite effect: the gross *tiklé* are lost without any spiritual benefit. It is quite safe to say that the pear-shaped *tiklé* in the brain, hanging upside down, is a metaphor for the pea-sized pituitary gland. From a medical point of view, the subtle *tiklé* released in the blood stream are *kham kyi dangma*. Tantric practitioners strive to retain the *tiklé* and to distribute them throughout the body, thus experiencing a deeper state. Therefore, men should not loose semen unnecessarily.

The *tiklé* always exist in the body, yet change in amount every day in relation to the waxing and waning moon. The inner *tiklé* cycle is referred to as *jangchup kyi sem gyégyur gyi rikchen*. The flow of this cycle is in opposite directions in men and women (see Section 18.1). In men, it starts from the left foot's first joints of the toes at new moon, and in women on the other side, from the right foot. Evolving relative *bodhicitta* has five components: *tsa* (channels), *lung* (wind), *drö* (heat), *tiklé* (essence drops) and *nampar shépa* (consciousness). The subtle channels are like a house, *lung* circulates like a horse, *drö* gives energy, *tiklé* are like a treasure, and *nampar shépa* is the house owner. These five aspects are like a space shuttle traveling inside the body sky, aiming to land on the moon surface of Buddhahood. This is called the *vajra* body, each part being described in detail in tantric physiology and metaphysics. To study this in depth requires opening the door to tantric mysticism. The utmost subtle *tiklé* is located in the heart center,

---

8 Dictionaries and other medical literature keep silent on the interpretation of this term, some saying it is an ancient term in Zhangzhung language. In common language, *tsap* refers to "serious" or "risky:" *tsapchen*, for instance, means "danger."

9 Bsam gtan, 1997, 21.

where it holds the assembly of the five element colors. This is the light of the *künzhi*. It can be interpreted as the seat of the five mental poisons, the base of the Five Buddhas, or the seed of the future body-mind. Much could be explained, but one can discover it only through realization in practice. In summary, it is the most subtle essence of the body-mind, yet not enlightened and still material. In tantra, many *tiklé* terms are used, and these should be interpreted in light of their specific contexts.

11.3 THE THREE WASTE PRODUCTS (*DRIMA SUM*)

The substances that remain after the digestion, refinement, and absorption of *dangma* are *drima*, which means "dirt" or "impurity." These are referred to as gross waste products since they did not themselves become part of the body constituents. They are considered less essential, but are not completely useless. In fact, the *drima sum* play a significant role in health maintenance. Efficient elimination cleans the body system of residues that could otherwise contribute to minor as well as major diseases. The three main waste products are (1) feces, (2) urine, and (3) perspiration.

1. Feces (*shangwa*)

Feces is the major excrement (*dri chen*), which is gradually separated from solid food during the digestive processes in the stomach and intestines intestines. *Shangwa* is of phlegm nature, and a phlegm waste product. It serves as the solid basis for the other waste products as well as for the body constituents.

2. Urine (*chin*)

Urine is the liquid waste product of food. It is filtered out from the stomach, small intestine and (especially) the large intestine, transported to the kidneys, and then stored in the urinal bladder. Blood (derived from *dangma*) is also filtered in the kidneys, of which the residue equally becomes part of urine, which then acquires a particular color, sediment, odor, etc. Urine has a phlegm nature and provides a base for the body liquids in the bladder. *Chin* eliminates wastewater, especially when water is in excess in the body.

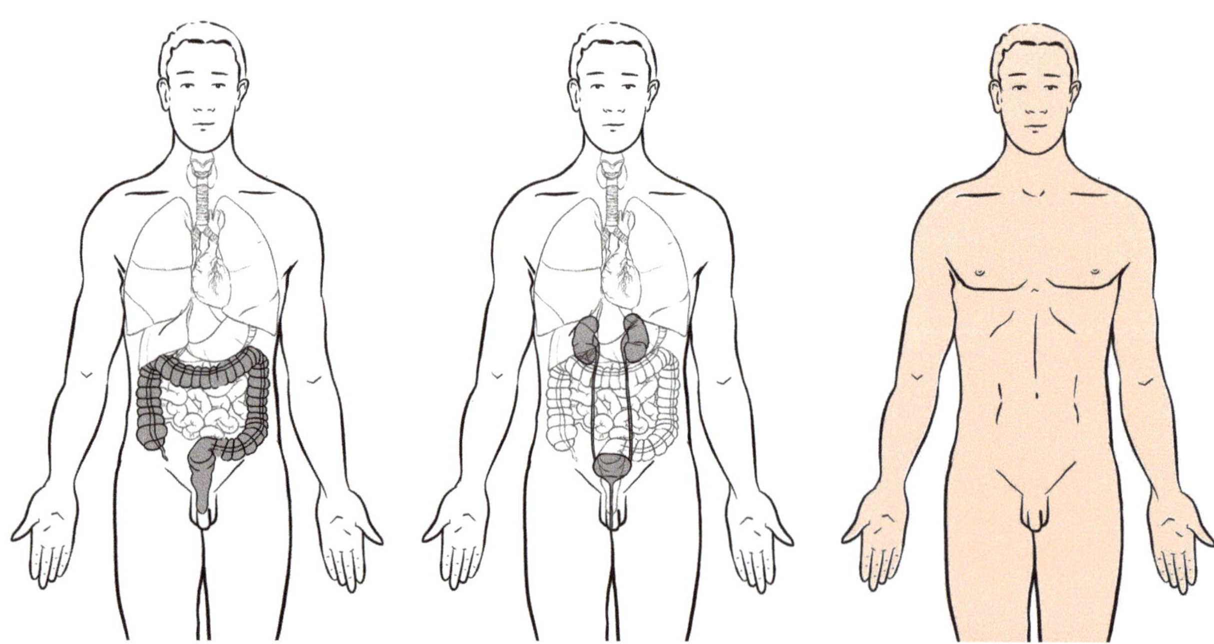

FIGURE 11.3 The elimination of feces, urine, and perspiration

3. Perspiration (*ngül*)

Perspiration has a subtler quality than the first two excrements. *Ngül* is a collective term for the minor waste products, and is generally of bile nature. It carries bile heat through the sweat glands, which is eliminated through the body pores as sweat. There are numerous other minor waste products: tears, nasal mucus, earwax, hair, nails, and so on. Each minor waste product (they have different natures) has responsibilities in purifying the body and sensory organs. When these are blocked in their places, imbalance may arise. For example, the skin might become inflamed if sweat is blocked in the body pores, and if tears are blocked an eye infection may result.

The humors are sustained and supported by the seven body constituents, which are in turn sustained by the three waste products. The body constituents and waste products are interdependent. They maintain the body-mind system by balancing each other.

11.4 *SINBU*

Sinbu is a general term for "tiny beings" in general, but here we will focus on those living in and on the human body. *Sinbu* can be visible or invisible to the naked eye, and include intestinal worms and parasites, insects, fungi, bacteria, viruses, as well as so-called "blood parasites" (*traksin*). Recent scientific studies have revealed that there are more bacterial cells than human cells in our bodies (and many times more viruses), which are all part of the human microbiome. This finding is surprisingly reminiscent to what the Buddha declared more than two millennia ago, namely that "the body is composed of a mass of *sinbu*."

There are at least two distinctive conceptions of *sinbu*. In Tibetan medical texts, these tiny beings are approached mostly as disease-causing agents, whilst Buddhist sutras emphasize their function as components contributing to body-mind formation and sustainment. Nevertheless, both sources accept that they exist in the body and could lead to illbeing when disturbed by wrong diet and behavior. It thus appears they are both a fundamental precondition for good health as well as potentially major factors in pathogenesis.

Sinbu in the sutras

One of the most detailed descriptions of *sinbu* is found in *The Sutra on Entering the Womb Expounded*

to Ānanda (*Dga' bo mngal 'jug gi mdo*), which is part of the important Mahāyāna *Jewel Mound Sutra* (*Mdo sde dkon mchog brtsegs pa*) collection. Dési Sangyé Gyatso's *Blue Beryl* quotes this text together with the *Kālacakratantra* and related sources on embryology. What follows is based on these works, and on Karma Trinlé's extensive survey of the Tibetan Buddhist canon on *sinbu*.[10]

The Sutra on Entering the Womb shows us the lives of *sinbu* as perceived through the meditative eye of the Buddha looking at his own body, from head to toe. Through this teaching, we can understand that *sinbu* live in communities across the human landscape, similar to what one can see when looking down upon areas with vegetation, villages, cities, and countries while flying through the sky. The sutra systematically covers 80 groups of *sinbu*. Each group has 1,000 subtypes, making 80,000 *sinbu* in total. Each of these further consists of subfamilies, leading to countless numbers. Therefore, the body actually consists of masses of microorganisms. They live in and on us just like humans and animals inhabit the world. Consequently, our bodies do not just belong to ourselves but house many living beings. The channels are said to house *sinbu*. However, they are also categorized according to different body locations, which seems contradictory. The *Blue Beryl* provides the following quote:[11]

> In the four directions of the body,
> five channels with 10 branches each.
> Each branch has 100 minor branches.
> Overall, 80,000 channels exist.
> This is the abode of 80,000 *sinbu*:
> the body is filled with impurities.

In *The Sutra on Entering the Womb*, it is said that *sinbu* first appear seven days after childbirth, when they begin to multiply and form communities in specific places: the scalp, the root of hairs, sense organs, skin, vital organs (especially liver, spleen, and gallbladder), stomach, intestines, bladder, fat, ligaments and tendons, bones and bone marrow, etc. They consume and transform bodily products day and night, which can be interpreted as their contribution to digestion, food essence refinement, and the formation of the constituents. *Sinbu* thus also separate gross and subtle waste products, and support excretion.

Disharmony of each group of 80 *sinbu* has the potential to manifest specific diseases as listed in the sutra. In general, however, we can infer that when *sinbu* are agitated by unwholesome factors, their human hosts will similarly be affected. If they become aggressive, the host will show signs of aggression. If they are depressed or aroused, this eventually impacts the

---

10 Karma 'phrin las, 1988, 66–74 and 75–123.

11 Sde srid sangs rgyas rgya mtsho, 1994, vol. 1, 94.

entire body. From this point of view, the gross mind and its emotions are not solely regulated by the heart and brain. *Sinbu* even codetermine the five sense organs and eight consciousnesses according to Sakyapa Gyeltsen Pelzang.[12] The collective power of *sinbu* is akin to the voice of the people forcing leaders to change the policies of the country. Therefore, when the tiny beings become ill, this manifests physical and mental disorders. This is an intuitive way to grasp the Buddhist teaching of interdependence: there is no single causal factor that generates the mind and its activities. The sutra states there are 101 disorders that manifest from *lung*, 101 disorders from *tripa*, 101 disorders from *béken*, and 101 from their combination, making 404 disorders in total. These are together referred to as "inner sufferings," which implies that the internal balance of the body-mind *sinbu* has been altered.

The sutra expounded to Ānanda further describes that at the end of one's life, 78 different local winds will destroy the 80 *sinbu* collectives one by one in a microscopic apocalypse. When this has been completed, life force is consumed, breathing stops, and the person will die. This means that life itself is a communal energy. Body, mind, and life are composite products of collective activity. As the *Heart Sutra* equally proclaims, truly nothing exists independently.

Sowa Rigpa on *sinbu*

In the *Gyüzhi*, *sinbu* are explained in chapter 50 of the *Oral Instruction Tantra*, which is mostly about parasites. This topic, covering external parasites, intestinal worms, and "blood parasites," is usually not studied extensively in relation to medical practice. As stated in this chapter:[13]

> External *sinbu* are lice and louse eggs.
> Phlegm, wind, bile, and blood have four inner *sinbu*:
> phlegm *sinbu* are found in the stomach;
> wind *sinbu* in the colon; bile *sinbu* on the teeth, eyes, skin, anus, and genitals;
> blood *sinbu* have no legs but are round and red in color, living in the blood and traveling to all parts via the channels.
> These become the prime cause of all *nyen né*[14] and leprosy.
> White and black brain worms also derive from them.

Whereas the externally visible *sinbu* are more easily understood and treated, several internal types are also listed. *Béken* parasites can appear like a ball of yarn (referring to tapeworms), *tripa* parasites look similar to maggots (pinworms), and *lung* parasites are stick- or spoon-shaped (threadworms, *Strongiloides* spp.). The blood *sinbu* are described in more detail in chapter 26 of the *Oral Instruction Tantra*, which lays out seven types:[15]

> Seven toxic blood parasites live in the blood.
> They are reddish like copper, tiny, and invisible.
> Any moment, they can travel from head to toe and to all parts of the body.

Blood *sinbu* may become the cause of leprosy and so-called brain worm infections. The Dési also discusses these as a major cause of *nyen né*, especially the type called *parpata*.[16] This type of blood *sinbu* is the product of the wrath of the eight classes of spirits. When angered, their toxic breath infests the sky like clouds, manifesting *parpata* that resemble tiny tadpoles or lizards. After entering through nose and mouth, they contaminate the body's own blood *sinbu*, leading to severe *nyenrim* infections that can turn into deadly epidemics.

Concluding remarks

Sinbu are the unsung heroes of the body-mind, its powerful working population. They work without interruption, continuously being replaced by others of their kind in all major tissues. They sustain the strength of the humors, regulate digestion, hunger, the body constituents, and waste products. *Sinbu* also promote sleep, influence body temperature, blood and *chuser* activity as well as the functions of the organs, maintain the skin and hairs, play a role in sexual desire and conception, and more. They are the citizens of the body country whose actions represent the nation's power, operating in-between body and mind, linking the humors and constituents. The body-mind is coproduced by these tiny beings.

Due to a lack of technology such as microscopes in Tibet, bodily microorganisms (*lü kyi trasin*) have not been a central focus of study in Sowa Rigpa. Nonetheless, it is clear they are highly important for deepening our knowledge of physiology and pathology, and even psychology.

---

12 Sa skya pa rgyal mtshan dpal bzang, 1991, 72.

13 G.yu thog yon tan mgon po, 1993, 322.

14 Aggressive contagious diseases, including viral infections.

15 Ibid., 265–66.

16 Sde srid sangs rgyas rgya mtsho, 1992, 177.

11.5 HEALTH THROUGH BALANCE (*TA MEL NÉ MÉ*)

When the three humors, body constituents, and waste products are in equilibrium or homeostasis, then the body-mind functions optimally. This is *Gyüzhi*'s concept of positive health, in which the contribution of each component also depends on the individual's body constitution. This state is referred to as *ta mel né mé*. In short, body and mind are in sync and work according to their normal daily, monthly, and yearly rhythms (see also Section 5.3), and in accordance with the person's constitution and environment.

Ta mel né mé has two aspects: maintaining and sustaining. Maintaining implies keeping the body-mind system operational, healthy, and clean through the balance of the humors, body constituents, and waste products. Sustaining refers to the support obtained through digestion, and the transformation and detoxification of *dangma*. The former is a top-down process, the latter works bottom-up.

The maintenance of harmony between the humors, constituents, and waste products can be compared to governing a country, or to a court of law. In the latter case, the wind humor functions like a judge who acts with neutrality (temporarily), whilst bile takes on the role of the prosecutor, who attacks first. Phlegm can be seen as taking up the defensive position. The body constituents are the witnesses and supporting parties, who can cast their vote in favor of one party or the other. The judge keeps the trial procedure in harmony until the prosecutor and defense present their final case. In the end, just as a court judge does, wind allies itself with the most convincing, strongest party, subduing the other humors. This is the start of a disorder. Therefore, the *Oral Instruction Tantra* says:[17]

> Wind is the disturbing cause of all disease:
> inviting, finishing, scattering, and spreading.
> Since its nature is aggressive and rough,
> wind manifests countless disorders.

The *Root Tantra* lists 25 components or factors of health: *nyépa sum* (each consisting of five branches), *lüzung dün*, and *drima sum*. These are the forces and building blocks necessary to construct a house for the mind and its emotions. They are responsible for both positive and negative health. If these 25 vital components are in order, and are supported by suitable food, and a good psychology, environment, and karma, this will bring wellbeing. If negative factors disturb this system, various disorders may manifest.

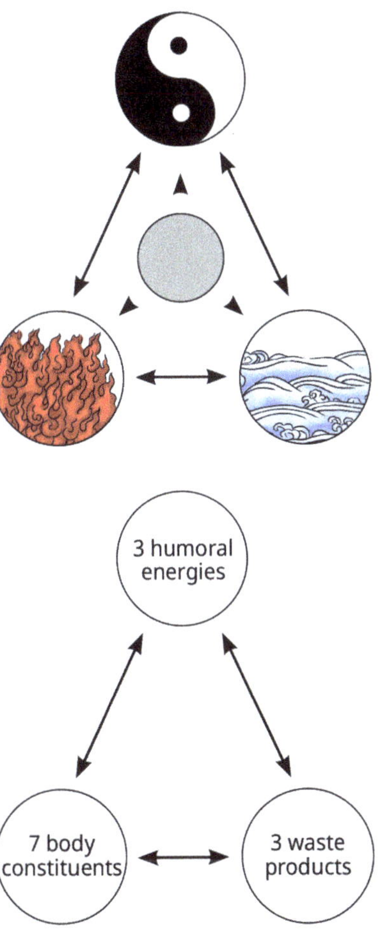

FIGURE 11.4 The medical theory of balance

17 G.yu thog yon tan mgon po, 1993, 105.

BODY DEVELOPMENT

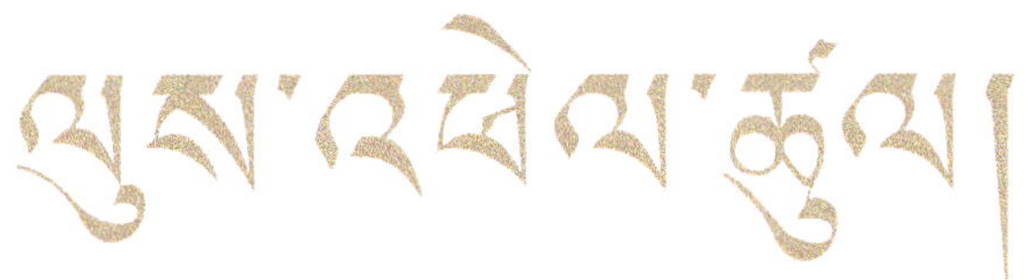

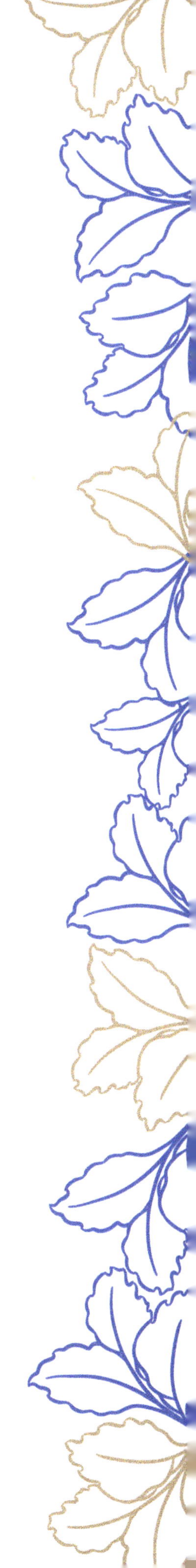

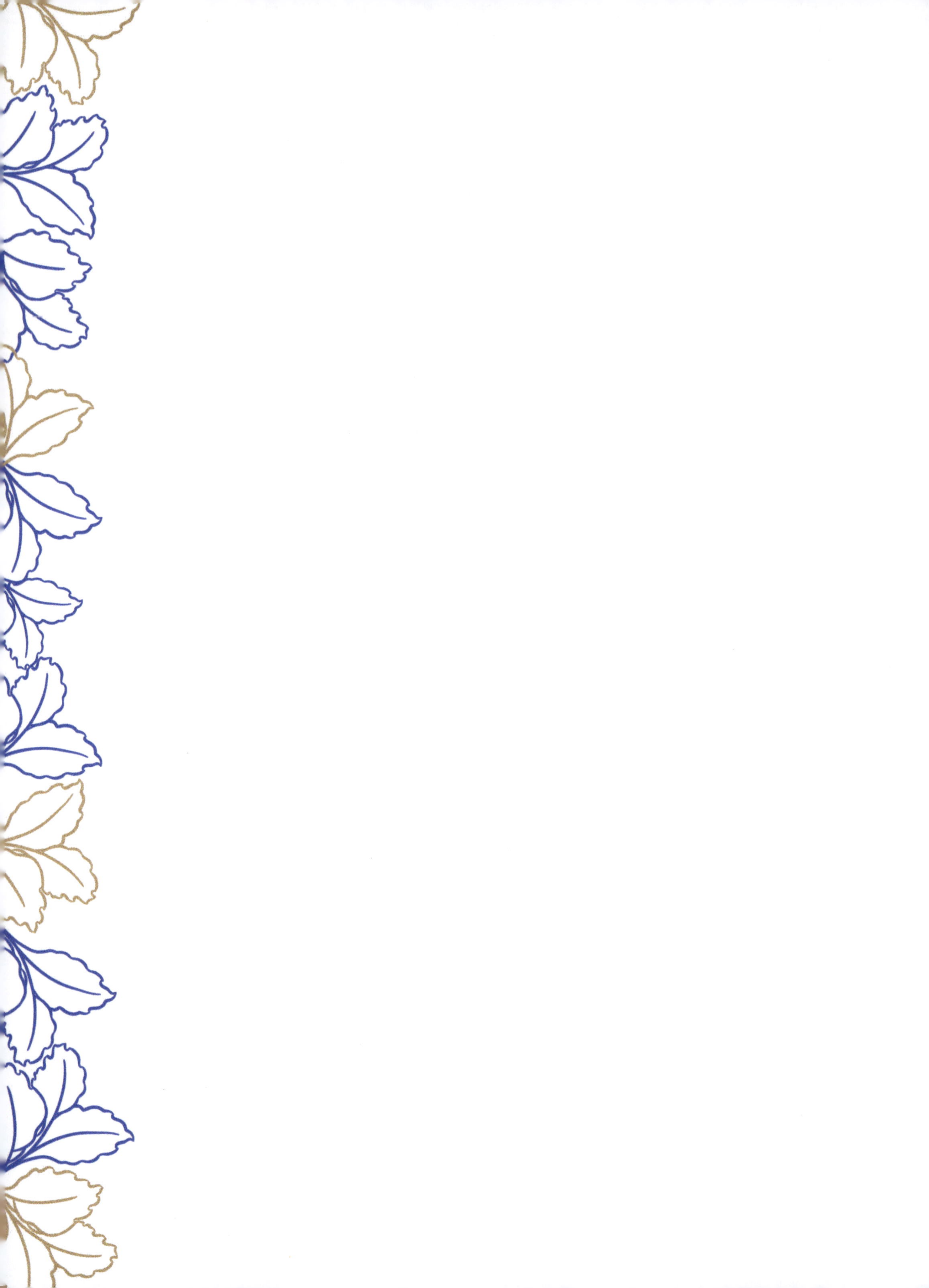

CHAPTER 12

WOMEN'S PHYSIOLOGY

Having described the humors and constituents, Part 4 will cover the development of the physical body (*lü*). All body-mind functions are governed by the humors. Therefore, from a functional point of view the term "humoral physiology" may be used. It comprises *lü*, the humors, and gross mind. Body constitution, for example, determines a person's physique as well as mentality. If the body is a house, the organs are its inhabitants; mind is the owner, and the *nyépa* are workforces. Understanding the *nyépa* is emphasized more than analysis of the physical body in Tibetan medicine. The anatomical explanations found in the *Root* and *Explanatory Tantras* and their commentaries are therefore relatively brief. More detail is found in the chapters relating to wounds from the *Oral Instruction Tantra*. Nevertheless, anatomy and humoral physiology are equally important.

Bodily development (*lü peltsül*) starts prior to birth, during embryogenesis. To comprehend this process more deeply, this chapter first focuses on the female reproductive system as a basis for further discussion on conception, pregnancy, and fetal development.

Women are praised in Buddhist tantras, which furthermore teach that they should be treated with respect and not discriminated against. From a tantric perspective, women are sources of power, wisdom, and the creators of entire worlds. Numerous female buddhas and exceptional practitioners are known. In society, feminine beauty is praised like precious jewels and flowers. Starting from religious, cultural, and philosophical views on the female body in South Asia and Tibet, this chapter discusses aspects of women's psychology and physiology, especially the menstrual cycle and hormones.

Partly due to the complexity and delicate nature of the female body-mind, women have been considered an "inferior rebirth" compared to men. Moreover, they have also been seen as "impure," especially during menstruation, which is generally kept hidden in Tibetan communities. The *Oral Instruction Tantra*'s gynecology chapter introduces women's physiology as follows:[1]

> The body is derived from the three mental poisons and four elements.
> By past life's karma and desire, male or female gender manifests.
> Due to inferior merit, a female body is obtained: breasts, a womb, and menstruation are added.
> The final constituents are the white and red fluids.
> The red menses flows from 12 years old.
> Sperm is held in the womb, generating flesh as well as the body.
> The white fluid goes to the breasts and nourishes.

Nevertheless, the true importance and situation of women in society is aptly described by Gendün Chöpel:[2]

> Women can give pleasure and happiness.
> A female partner is like a gift of karma.
> The heart feels joy seeing this form goddess.
> She is a fertile field that generates excellent progeny,
> a nurse that gives care in case of illness,
> a poet who consoles the saddened mind,
> a helper who does all domestic work,
> a life-long friend who sustains happiness.
> A wife, karmically connected through previous lives,
> possesses these six qualities.
> Women are said to be unreliable and promiscuous,
> This is horribly untrue.

---

1   G.yu thog yon tan mgon po, 1993, 375.

2   Dge 'dun chos 'phel, 1967, 20. These words are honest and truthful, showing the social nature of relationships. Similar points are made in Nāgārjuna's *Letter to a Friend*.

> Committing adultery is not different for
> males and females.
> As a matter of fact, men are even worse.

As quoted above in the *Gyüzhi*'s description on the cause of gender, the bardo consciousness that will obtain a female body is driven by strong desire, leading to attachment for the father (and strong anger towards the mother). This bardo connection could partially explain why male children tend to be closer to their mother while daughters have a special bond with their father. It might also be the case that intense bardo emotions result in a female body with heightened emotional intelligence. Strong anger in particular contributes to the fiery bile nature that is deeply rooted in the female consciousness, which is stimulated further by the more significant elemental contribution from the mother. However, Buddhist sources concur that there is no fundamental difference between the minds of men and women. Differences we observe are related more to bodily conditions. Although women develop specific characteristics, their male side derived from the father continues to be present. Each human being therefore has a dual nature. This is also why self-identification problems of the bardo consciousness at the time of conception could manifest as psychological trauma, hormonal development disorders, and intersex individuals.

When the female newborn's *médrö* starts to function, *dangma* is transported to the liver where the process of body constituent transformation continues up until bone marrow. From puberty onwards, this further results in a red reproductive fluid (*kham marpo*). This generative substance then deeply influences the psyche as well as the activities of the ovum and follicles, like a fortifying elixir. It determines the female biorhythm and organ functions, preparing the body for conception on a monthly basis. This body clock tends to correlate to the lunar phases, with menstruation happening during waxing moon, yet there is significant variation depending amongst others on the date of birth. The residual or gross red essence is called *datsen*, the monthly sign of fertility. Its subtle aspect is the ovum. Taken together, *kham marpo* is a vital feminine force and source of good health as long as the menstrual cycle is regular. It is the body's solar system and origin of new life.

12.1 MENSTRUATION

The menstrual cycle is fundamental for health and wellbeing. Menstruation is a natural form of cleansing by means of the removal of *lung* energy and blood residues. Bile and blood waste products remaining in the body stimulate anger and irritation. The monthly sign usually begins around the age of 12 as stated earlier,[3] its flow being initiated by descending wind (*lung tursel*). Women enter menopause around 50, or more precisely when their body needs to refocus its vital energy on sustainment. Hereditary factors as well as lifestyle and environment lead to individual differences in terms of menstruation, which in turn affects reproductive fluid formation, bone marrow and uterus activity. The cycle is governed by life-sustaining wind (in the brain, where the hypothalamus and anterior pituitary gland secrete hormones) along with pervasive wind (in the heart), which together control *tursel lung*. This natural process generates fertility and prepares the body for pregnancy. In relation to this process and the changing nature of *kham marpo*, we can roughly distinguish the following life stages for women:

- Age 0–11: childhood

- Age 12–16: menarche (first menstruation) and puberty

- Age 17–40: young adulthood (fertile stage)

- Age 41–50: middle age transition (premenopausal stage)

- Age 51–65: menopause

- Age 66–: old age

In women of reproductive age, the absence of periods (amenorrhea) is often interpreted as a gynecological disorder. Emotional trauma, deficient blood, blocked menstrual flow, and *motsi* imbalance could be involved, further creating symptoms such as swollen legs, weight gain, acne, bad sleep, headaches, heart palpitations, indigestion, increased blood pressure, white discharges, and bursts of anger.

The source of menses

Menses are considered a waste product of reproductive fluid and a product of blood, bile, and other vital energies. In young women, menstruation indicates failed conception, implying a "waste" of uterine blood and hormones. When expelled by descending wind on the first day, it is generally a bit darkish in color, flowing for three to five days.

---

3   The Dési mentions the age of 13. Sde srid sangs rgyas rgya mtsho, 1992, 463.

It is remarkable to observe the many physical, mental, and emotional aspects involved in the menstrual cycle. Woman of wind-bile, bile-wind, and bile-phlegm constitutions generally experience these signs and symptoms more. Before the period, the body-mind tends to be sensitive, nervous, angry, tense, and impatient. Afterwards, woman become gentler and more receptive. Each of these feelings arise from various influences, not from a single organ, like the season of spring making flowers blossom. Besides the direct role of the reproductive organs, the liver indirectly contributes to the production of menstrual blood, whereas the gallbladder is implicated in hormone-stimulated sexual heat. General attachment and emotions rise from the heart. The lungs generate anxiety and impatience. The spleen adds to the blood while the kidneys grant sexual power. At the same time, the intestines—and the mesenteric organ in particular—are central figures in heat generation and *motsi* regulation in the lower abdomen. If fire is disturbed, the flames burst in various directions.

Excess heat can injure the intestines and create major gynecological disorders such as endometriosis, myoma, fibroma, as well as cysts, thus becoming a significant cause of menstrual pain, constipation, and irregular periods. Many women suffer from constipation and headaches. Yet, treatment with purgative and headache formulas only works symptomatically and does not resolve the root problem. Based on deeper study and clinical practice, practitioners should investigate *motsi* imbalance as an underlying cause for these and other diseases such as certain allergies and skin disorders, digestive system malfunction and anxiety, and depression. On the other hand, one should proceed with great caution when aiming to medically influence these delicate hormonal cycles.

12.2 ESOTERIC PERSPECTIVES ON THE FEMALE BODY

The female body is like Mount Méru, with its red essence *tiklé* flowing through the three main channels like rivers. The subtle mental poisons form the streams of these three channels, yet a woman's body is mostly governed by attachment and anger since the time of conception. Dominated by fire, the right channel (*tsa roma*) gives rise to the bile and blood humors that rule the right side of the body. It is this aggressive mind and fire energy that ultimately produces the gross and subtle *kham marpo*. The female body nature is therefore like a volcano that erupts every month, shaking the body-earth while creating its seasons (marked by two equinoxes and

solstices) as well as day and night. This bodily heat corresponds to the sun, the planet Mars, summer, and the fire element. It is the destructive energy of hatred and anger. Nonetheless, when channeled the opposite qualities of motherly care, loving kindness, and compassion arise, so women are equally powerful creators and protectors of life. A young woman's body and hormones are like a new moon, and women in the middle of their lives shine like the full moon. Menopause is like the waxing moon, as the body light of the *tiklé* starts to decline.

Kāmadeva

Kāmadeva (Garap Wangchuk) is a Hindu god of desire, love, and lust. He is a symbol of affection in both Hindu and Buddhist religion. As a god of love, his domain spans all worldly romantic love, eroticism, and sexuality. He is one of the most powerful devas, controlling entire realms through his blessings of sensual enjoyment. Practically speaking, narcissism, sexual desire, and craving for luxury are all incarnations of Kāmadeva on a personal level.

Kāmadeva appears as an unbelievably handsome and sweet-talking young man dressed in beautiful garments, an excellent singer and dancer. He is extremely attractive, and his consort Rati is a female goddess of unimaginable beauty. They are manifestations of the desirous love of all beings and all delusions spring from their activity as they grant their gifts to the children of the world. Kāmadeva rides a multi-colored parrot or cuckoo, representing the five sensory perceptions of form, sound, odor, taste, and touch in the form of female divinities. He holds a bow made of sugarcane, and his arrows are adorned with honey and fragrant flowers. All beings shot by his arrows enjoy samsaric pleasures. Religious people who attempt to renounce the world are his favorite victims. In this manner, Hindu mythology recounts how Kāmadeva's five arrows woke up Śiva from deep meditative absorption, after which he had sex with Pārvatī. Angered by his reaction, he turned the god of love to ashes using his third eye. Kāmadeva also appeared to Gautama Buddha in the form of Māra, attempting to prevent the Buddha from attaining liberation. The god of love is content as long as worldly beings are ruled by desire and attached to the daily activities of samsara.

On a collective and more symbolic level, Kāmadeva resides in one of the highest godly realms of Mount Méru called "Mastery Over Others' Delusions" (Gzhan 'phrul dbang byed). Yet Kāmadeva has been born in our mind streams as desire and attachment since the very beginning, hiding in our hearts. Since we continuously enjoy ourselves through the blood, *tiklé*, channels and chakras—and especially our brain, heart, sex organs, and other parts (the 36 areas where body hair grows)—it is exceedingly difficult to renounce and get rid off desire. *Potsi* and *motsi* hormones can be interpreted as Kāmadeva's blessings. Without this soul of samsara, life has no taste. At the same time, his blessing is the source of all psycho-physical disorders.

12.3 *TIKLÉ* AND HORMONES

In a Tibetan medical context, red *tiklé* or "essence fluid" is used as a general term for the menstruation (including ovum). Menstruation, also known as *kham marpo*, is actually its waste product (*nyikma*) on a gross outer level.

Subtle red *tiklé* are in fact no longer red in color. It is a white substance that turns into breast milk during and after pregnancy. When not breastfeeding, it sustains bodily energy and stimulates feminine characteristics and beauty. This white essence (*kham karpo*) is coproduced by bone marrow and the reproductive organs, and is also referred to as *nyikma*.

The very subtle *tiklé* produce radiance (*dang*), which is like a flower's nectar. This essence of bone marrow and reproductive fluid rises to the heart, energizing and prolonging life. It rejuvenates the organs, strengthens immunity, and makes our lives colorful by boosting the mind, like the rising sun shining on a mountain. *Dang*, the most refined body product, is mainly generated by inner red essence *tiklé* in women. These *tiklé* represent the vital force of the blood and its root organ, the liver, which also produces bile and is nourished by the gallbladder. Body temperature, *motsi* heat, as well as the digestive fire all derive from the red *tiklé*, which can be visualized as a branching river or tree of fire particles flowing through the channels. During the fertile stage, this blood energy infused by hormones stimulates follicular development, ovulation, and finally menstruation, like a tree producing flowers and fruits each year.

The *la* cycle is a subtle bodily movement of energy that depends on the very subtle *tiklé*. The force of this luminous quintessential liquid rises until full moon, and then falls until new moon (see Section 18.1). This lunar waxing and waning significantly influences the flow of *motsi* in the female body and thus also regulates emotions. If the inner *la* circulation is harmonious, this means the feminine energetic cycle is balanced. *La* is a link between the outer and inner environment, which furthermore corresponds to the

relationship between the activities of the brain (rationality) and heart (emotionality).

Hormones and their function

Although hormones play a major role in the functioning of the female body-mind, these have not been laid out clearly in classical medical sources. In the following few paragraphs, biomedical terms and understandings are therefore integrated with Tibetan medical and tantric concepts.

The term *motsi* was first introduced to Sowa Rigpa by Dr. Samten, in his book *New Dawn*.[4] In biomedicine, this corresponds to the female sex hormones, including estrogens (mainly produced by the ovaries) as well as progesterone (from the adrenal glands and gonads). From a Tibetan medical perspective, these are regulated by *düpé tsa*, the channel connecting the brain and reproductive organs via back vertebra 13 (BV13, corresponding to the 12th thoracic vertebra). This channel regulates fertility in both men and women, and also transmits sexual pleasure from the genitals to the brain (especially during orgasm). Because of the latter function, *düpé tsa* is also called *déwé kham gyuwé tsa*: the "entering the realm of bliss channel." In Tibetan medicine, the kidneys (at the level of BV14 , 1st lumbar vertebra) are generally the organs that govern reproductive functions such as arousal and fluid production. Ultimately, however, hormonal activity is regulated by a complex neuroendocrine system of feedback interactions under the control of the hypothalamus and pituitary gland,[5] which fall under the power of life-sustaining wind. In tantra and in the context of *tumo* practice, a *tiklé* the size of a bean that is located inside the brain at the level between the eyebrows is described hanging down like a drop of milk; the body's essential nectar that has bliss-generating potential. This likely refers to the pituitary gland and its function. Numerous aspects of health and life are determined by hormones released in the blood, which rejuvenate the tissues and stimulate feelings including desire as well as depression.

Estrogens (estradiol most prominently) and progesterone are the two main female sex hormones. Estrogens make women feel powerful, feminine, and attractive, whereas progesterone has a more tranquilizing effect, giving satisfaction. When progesterone levels are high (luteal phase), women may feel melancholic.

---

4 Bsam gtan, 1997, 21.

5 Four major neuroendocrine systems have been identified: (1) the hypothalamic-pituitary-adrenal axis, (2) hypothalamic-pituitary-gonadal axis, (3) hypothalamic-pituitary-thyroid axis, and (4) the hypothalamic-neurohypophyseal system.

High estrogen levels combined with progesterone deficiency can result in irregular menstrual periods.

Follicle-stimulating hormone (FSH) and luteinizing hormone (LH) are involved in sexual maturation as well as in female follicular development and ovulation. Gonadotropin-releasing hormone (GnRH), which is itself released by the anterior pituitary gland, stimulates the secretion of both FSH and LH through low- and high-frequency pulses. This pulsating movement implies *lung* activity, which acts to synchronize the body clock.

Prolactin, which stimulates breastmilk production, is another *motsi* category hormone that is secreted from the pituitary gland. Referred to as *kham karpo* above, it appears that this white regenerative fluid is equally governed by *sokdzin lung*.

The primary sex hormone in males is testosterone. Predominantly synthesized in the testes, it is also produced in small amounts in the adrenals. Excess of this androgen (*potsi*) in women could manifest symptoms such as oily skin and acne, increased body hair growth and other masculine characteristics, as well as infertility and polycystic ovarian syndrome.

The thyroid (*drésher menbu*) produces two hormones: triiodothyronine (T3) and thyroxine (T4). They are mainly responsible for the regulation of metabolism, increasing the basal metabolic rate and supporting bone and nerve growth. Hyper- and hypothyroidism can both negatively affect the menstrual cycle. In Sowa Rigpa, the thyroid is ruled by ascending wind.

Sinbu and gynecology

Gyüzhi's gynecology chapter affirms the existence of two types of uterine microorganisms (*ngel sin*) that are involved in sexual and reproductive activities, but may also become the cause of many disorders. Named *marutsé* and *aso*, they appear to act as agents of the hormones in the vaginal area and womb. As *motsi* affects them, they in turn influence vaginal physiology, acting as vital intermediaries in desire and satisfaction in a way similar to the intestinal bacterial flora. *Ngelsin* are an interesting topic for further study, especially the links between *marutsé* and estrogen, *aso* and progesterone, and with *Lactobacillus* bacteria such as *L. crispatus* and *L. jensenii* respectively.

Hormones, pregnancy, and menopause

When women in their fertile stage do not get pregnant, this may elicit *traktsap* disorders in the long run, including headaches, constipation, high blood pressure, weight gain, oily skin, as well as impatience and anger. Symptoms such as these can be understood as a type of body language. The absence of pregnancy may, however, also vitiate *motsi* activity to the extent that ovarian cysts and other abnormal growths start to appear, as well as hormone-based breast and blood circulation disorders. It seems that pregnancy in fact also has health benefits for women, whereas contraceptive pills might force the body to produce growths such as cysts and fibroids instead of a child. In this regard, the arrows of the God of Desire present opportunities for regaining health. Nonetheless, women who have had several children may equally have to deal with this kind of diseases, even though the level of aggressiveness generally appears to be less. In conclusion, the life of women is akin to that of a fruit tree that matures in order to blossom and produce seed. If this process is thwarted, the organs become discontent and suffer. Without any sexual contact, this suffering could manifest as disease.

Hormones are our lifelong friends, accompanying the body and giving it strength, providing the full spectrum of emotional (dis)satisfaction. In the most fertile stage, body strength peaks and anger emanates from the aggressive *motsi* power. In menopause, *motsi* declines, leading to feelings of nostalgia, fear of abandonment, melancholy, pessimism, anxiety, hysteria, mood swings, and so on. The gross, rational mind cannot understand the changes that take place as hormonal functions decrease. The subconscious mind of the heart, on the other hand, intuitively knows what is happening, but feels lonely and fearful in this transitory period as the wind humor takes over the body-mind.

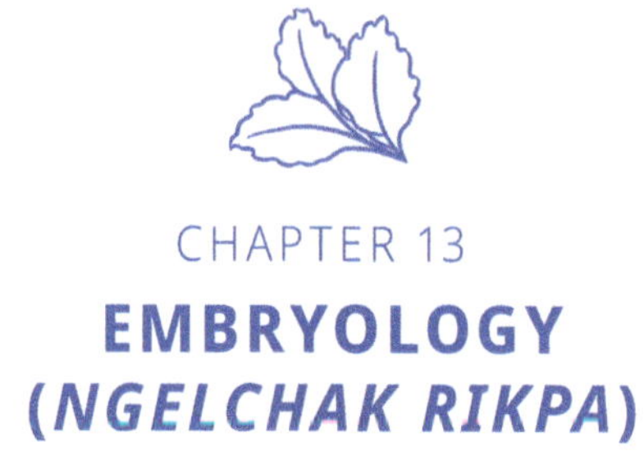

CHAPTER 13

EMBRYOLOGY
(*NGELCHAK RIKPA*)

The body is called *lü*, meaning "base." It is the house for the mind, and is comprised of the humors, organs, tissues, and waste products. The term also refers to "composed" or "assembled," and to the aggregates. *Lü* appears in the Tibetan verb *rak lüpa*, which signifies "to depend on." All positive and negative actions of the body-mind indeed depend on the physical body and its functions, just like a car depends on its parts.

Embryology, also called *chaktsül rikpa*, is described in the second chapter of the *Explanatory Tantra*, which provides a week-by-week and month-by-month description of a child's development. After conception, the growing child's body receives air, blood, and nutrition through the umbilical cord (*tétak, butak*) of the mother, similar to growing crops by means of irrigation. This is called *drupa lü*, which the structural formation of the body. *Gyüzhi* commentators elaborate further on the subject, along with tantric sources. There is also some detail on child conception in the *Sutra on Entering the Womb*.[1] Together, these texts provide many insights that supplement this chapter.

13.1 CAUSES OF THE PHYSICAL BODY

The physical body is produced by three main causes plus life-retaining wind energy (*lung dzinpa*), each of which will be discussed in more detail below.

1. The direct cause: the parents

The direct physical cause refers to one's parents, who give rise to the body's white and red parts. The blood, blood vessels, flesh, organs, and other major tissues develop from the mother's red energy, while skin, bones, bone marrow, nerves, the brain, spinal cord, lymphatic system, fat, reproductive fluid (semen), glands, and ligaments develop from the father's white energy. In the context of the *nyépa sum*, the red parts of the body develop from the bile humor, whereas the white body parts come from phlegm. The nervous system, bones, and skin originate from both the father and the mind's wind element.

2. The indirect cause: the five elements

The elements earth, water, fire, air, and space are concentrated in the father's sperm and the mother's ovum. These five elements work to develop the child's body through the mother, and later by means of food.

3. Bardo consciousness

The third cause of life is the bardo consciousness (*bardö nampar shépa*) of one's past life. This consciousness enters through the father's nostrils and reaches his sperm—which becomes its carrier—to

---

1 There exist two Tibetan translations of this text which differ slightly. The version used here is based on the translation from Sanskrit, which was republished by Kar ma 'phrin las, 1993.

TABLE 13.1 The symbolism of the three primary causal factors of the body

Factors	Correspondences		
Sperm	Moon	Body	Earth and water
Bardo consciousness	*Nāda*	Mind	Wind
Ovum	Sun	Speech (energy)	Fire

enter the mother's womb at conception.[2] Life and physical development thus begin with the union of the three components of sperm, ovum and bardo consciousness. The body develops from the parents' two energies, which arise from the five basic elements, while the mind arises from the *künzhi* and the subtle mind, which develop from the bardo consciousness. Mind produces mind. The subtle mind (*sem trawa*) is carried over from previous lifetimes, and originates neither from the parents nor from other elements. It produces the six sense consciousnesses and gross mind (*sem rakpa*). Contact of the sense consciousnesses with external objects is the condition that leads to emotions, which come to rule the body-mind.

The combined result of the three main factors produces the child's physical body, which is comprised of five vital organs (heart, lungs, liver, spleen, and kidneys) and six hollow organs (stomach, small intestine, large intestine, gallbladder, urinary bladder, and reproductive organ). Five extremities (including the head), five fingers, and five sense organs also form, corresponding with the five elements. The body becomes the base of the three humors and the mind, and wind energy in particular helps to transport these through the channels together with blood, water, and consciousness.

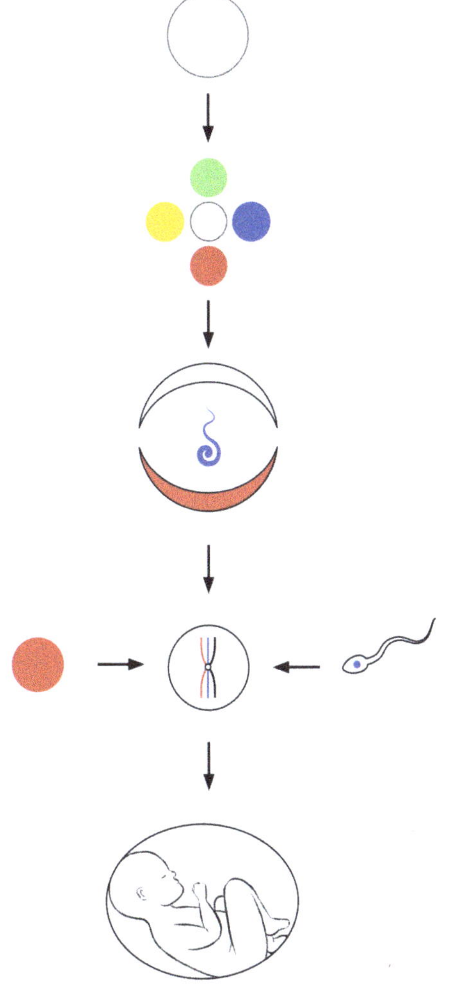

FIGURE 13.1 Conception: the bardo consciousness, five subtle elements, union of male and female *tiklé*, and embryogenesis relying on the five gross elements

---

2 It is interesting to note that modern bioscience holds that spermatozoa fertilize the ovum, which is similar to the Tibetan medical understanding. Biomedicine cannot ascertain the role of the bardo consciousness, however.

4. *Lung dzinpa*

The fourth cause of the body is *lung dzinpa*, life-retaining wind energy. It is wind element's quintessence, which exists as a potential within each of the four elements and attracts other particles like a growing fruit, or a magnet attracting iron. *Lung dzinpa* thus provides a nesting place for consciousness during and after conception (see also Section 6.4). As long as *lung dzinpa* is there, the elements can support life. *Lung dzinpa* is a life-holding, magnetizing energy, which acts as a center for the *bardo* consciousness and sustains the body. Deterioration of *lung dzinpa* results in weakening subtle element energies, becoming the cause of dissociation of the elements and body parts. When there is no *lung dzinpa* in the union of the two energies of the parents, conception will not take place. *Lung dzinpa* disturbance after conception could lead to abortion. All principal and minor *lung* channels develop from its particles, which are sustained through breathing. *Lung dzinpa* gives rise to *soklung*, the lifespan or life fuel wind present in the central channel.

13.2 CONCEPTION FACTORS (*CHAKPÉ GYU*)

The *Gyüzhi* states that life is determined by one's past lives, through the combination of the qualities of the five basic elements and the parents' body constitutions. Karma influences an individual's particular bodily constitution and health. It directs the bardo consciousness to connect with the parents, and additionally matures the elemental energies. The *Explanatory Tantra* illustrates the impact of karma through an analogy: a goldsmith whose molds make different designs. Karma is like the goldsmith; the womb is like the mold, and the elements of the parents' energies are like the materials. Karma unites the consciousness, sperm, and ovum, forming the beginnings of the body and new life. Without consciousness, the two physical energies alone cannot be united in fertilization; there would be no reaction. Irrespective of whether a child is conceived by cloning or insemination, bardo consciousness must be present along with the two reproductive materials. This is a basic tenet of Tibetan medicine and Buddhism.

Body development commences immediately following conception (*ngel dzinpa*) in the mother's womb, where the parental gross and subtle elements begin to be transformed. According to the theory of conception in *Gyüzhi* medicine, the *bardo* consciousness and the two parents' energies are brought together by karma and the emotions of the bardo consciousness, such as attraction toward the parents. This can be compared to a magnet that attracts metal, or the

gravitational relationship between earth and sky. When the bardo consciousness perceives a karmically related couple having sexual contact, it generates attachment according to its own karmic background. If the bardo consciousness is going to have a female body in its next life, it feels attraction for the man and jealousy towards the woman, and if it will be male it will feel attraction towards the woman. At this stage, the bardo consciousness does not realize that the couple will be its future parents. Next, the bardo consciousness enters through one of the father's nostrils and travels with his breath to eventually reach his sperm. If the child is going to be male, the consciousness enters through the father's right nostril, whereas the left nostril is associated with female offspring. The sperm carrying the consciousness then enters the mother's womb and joins with the ovum. At the point of this union of mind and matter, the woman feels a sense of satisfaction and heaviness while the bardo mind goes into a dormant state immediately after conception. But the *lung* associated with the bardo consciousness now begins to grow the body and gross mind. It is called *soklung a*, the fundamental seed that will produce weekly branch winds to develop the fetal body-mind.

From the first week after conception until the 24th week, the bardo consciousness remains dormant as *soklung a* continues to actively shape the growing infant. The child begins to feel comfort and discomfort during the 24th week, and in the 25th week it starts to breathe through its mother. In the 26th week, the dormant consciousness awakens and the child remembers some of its past life and bardo experiences. In accordance with its karma, the bardo consciousness suffers from different hallucinations as is detailed in the *Sutra on Entering the Womb*.

Varying karma and fortune result in different phenomena or illusions during the moment of conception. An important issue to note is that the hallucinations of the bardo consciousness at the point of conception remain a subtle memory within the child that becomes an important influence on their psyche. A Tibetan saying states that a happy child has descended from heaven, and a crying, fearful child from hell. Similarly, some bardo consciousnesses manifest at conception in a state of tranquility and others with negative emotions. Such different bardo emotions can influence the developing child's personality and behavior after birth.

For a new life to come into existence, there are five factors to consider which must be present at conception:

1. The five energies of the elements must be present and in harmony

2. A favorable karmic connection must be established

3. The bardo consciousness must be searching for a new life

4. The parents' two energies must be of good quality

5. The menstrual cycle must be regular, of high quality, and synchronized

If these factors are present, conception can take place. If any of these required factors is absent, even when there is no physical disorder, it could lead to infertility. Each of the five factors will now be laid out in further detail.

1. The elements (*jungwa nga*)

There are two levels of elements: gross and subtle.

The five subtle elements (*trawé jungwa nga*)

The mind's subtle wind contains five subtle elements that are part of its physical elemental energy. They are subtle earth, water, fire, air, and ether or space.

These accompany the mind, taking the form of a *lung* or of tiny particles of the elements themselves. Wind is also called the vehicle of the mind. Practically, wind is the energy of the mind that allows for movement. One could say that subtle *lung* is the power of the mind. It is the dynamic material force behind the development of the body as well as the formation of the whole world. This is what was described above as *lung dzinpa,* which has the power to assemble and multiply the elemental energies. This concept is somewhat related to that of DNA (deoxyribonucleic acid), which transmits heredity and consists of a sequence of the same four nucleotides in every life form on Earth. The nucleotides would then correspond to the four subtle elements, suspended in space. As can be seen in Figure 13.2, four subtle elements surround the central space element. In other words, they are dancing in space according to their own rhythms. This figure also contains the corresponding astrological symbols, further demonstrating their sequence of manifestation and dissolution.

The third part of this illustration shows the medical and tantric concept of the assembly of the four subtle elements plus the space element, which form the channels and chakras. They compose the body from the nuclei of elemental particles (*jungwé dültren*), starting in the umbilical chakra. *Lung dzinpa* thus acts as the sustainer of the subtle mind, the center from which the five mental poisons and the resulting subtle and gross elements arise.

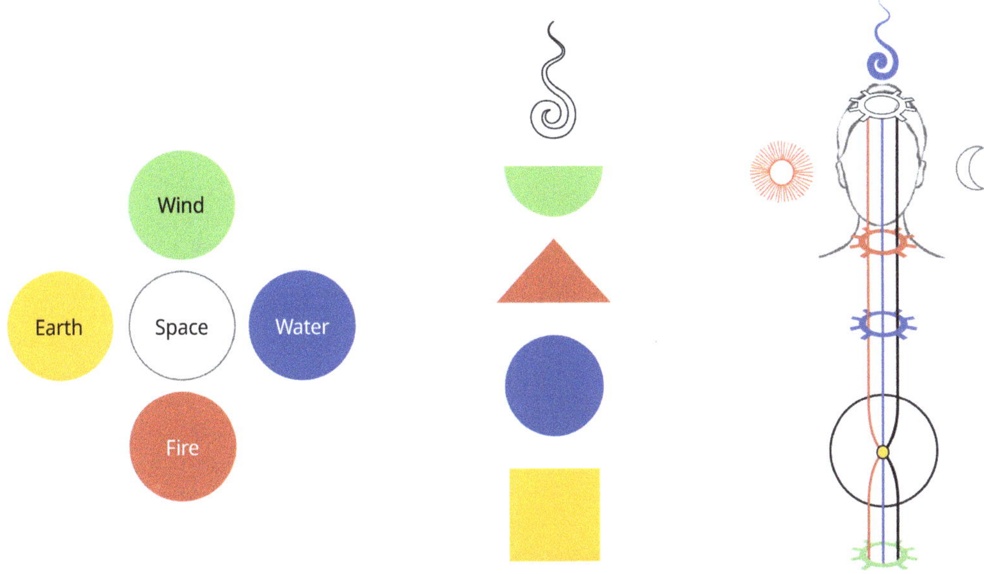

FIGURE 13.2 The five subtle elemental energies, astrological symbols, and the five chakras formed by the corresponding psycho-emotional powers

The first element in the formation process is space, which has existed from the beginning of time. Space consists of invisible particles that are the basis of all the other elements, as described in Buddhist cosmology. Space is filled with material yet subtle space element particles (*namkhé dül*). The movement of these particles produces wind element particles (*lung dül*), which are less subtle, and the wind element particles in turn produce fire element particles (*mé dül*). The fire element particles then produce water element particles (*chu dül*), which, lastly, produce earth element particles (*sa dül*). Throughout this sequence, from space to earth, the elemental particles (*jungwé dül*) transform into less subtle particles until they form earth, which is the most solid element. The earth element holds the center of the world and the foundation for the existence of manifold things and organisms, just as ice cream rests upon a cone. Similarly, the spleen and stomach, which are earth element organs, hold the center of the body as they give nutrition to the body-mind. According to Tibetan Buddhism, space particles will remain until the collective karma of all beings has been consumed in universal apocalypse. This ensures the Earth's continuing existence for eons upon eons.

Ancient scholarly explanations of the origin of life have some parallels with modern explanations of DNA as the carrier of human characteristics. Whereas the former see with a meditative eye, biomedicine approaches it through scientific experimentation. The fundamental difference between modern science and Tibetan medicine on this matter is that of the elements being activated by the mind and *lung trawa*. They together revitalize the energy that comes from the parents' sperm and ovum in order to give life to a new being. In the absence of the mind, the elements may grow like a flower, but it cannot give rise to human consciousness.

The five gross elements

The subtle elements transform into five basic or gross elements (*jungwa chenpo nga*): earth, water, fire, air, and space. The physical body is produced from both the subtle and basic elements, through the parents' energies. Tantra teaches us that the body, the elements, and consciousness are of the same nature:[3]

> The water element manifests from consciousness; therefore, the mind is of water nature. If not, why can a dead body not produce liquid?
> The consciousness is of the fire element, therefore the body has heat; otherwise, why does a body whose consciousness has left has no heat?
> Wind, the body of consciousness, breathes

---

3 Sa skya pa rgyal mtshan dpal bzang, 1991, 48. A similar passage can be found in the *Vajrāsana Sādhana* (*Rdo rje gdan gyi sgrub thabs*) of the Tengyur.

TABLE 13.2 The five elements in the body

Element	Color	Chakra	Solid and hollow organ	Sense organ, faculty, and object	Components	Extremity
Space (*namkha*)	White	Crown	Heart and small intestine	Ear, auditory, sound	Orifices, channels, hollow spaces (pervasive)	Head
Fire (*mé*)	Red	Throat	Liver and gallbladder	Eyes, visual, form	Body temperature, digestive heat	Right arm
Water (*chu*)	Blue	Heart	Kidney and urinary bladder (plus brain, glands, and reproductive organs)	Tongue, gustatory, taste	Blood, lymph, hormones	Left leg
Earth (*sa*)	Yellow	Navel	Spleen and stomach (plus pancreas)	Nose, olfactory, smell	Flesh, bone, hair	Right leg
Wind (*lung*)	Green	Secret	Lungs and colon	Skin, tactile, touch	Breath, skin (pores), nerves	Left arm

like spreading smoke; but when the
consciousness has left, the body has no
more breath.
The mind is of the earth element because
it is heavy; when the consciousness leaves,
a corpse floats in water.
There are five body elements, which are
one in nature,
Yogis should know this and contemplate.

Gyüzhi medicine and tantra consider body and mind to be two sides of the same coin, as two aspects of the same thing. Body and the mind each express different levels of gross and subtle energy, yet are interdependent. Therefore, changes in behavior and lifestyle effectively act on both. Balance in the body's elements is essential for conception and a child's physical and mental development. If the subtle elements are in disharmony during conception, or if the gross elemental energies are disturbed, congenital disorders may arise. The five basic or gross elements are concentrated in the parents' two energies of the ovum and the sperm. In this regard, the embryology chapter in the *Explanatory Tantra* states:[4]

From earth, flesh, bone, the nose, and the
faculty of smell are produced.
From water, blood, the tongue, moisture,
and taste.
From fire, heat, color, the eyes, and sight.
From air, breath, the skin, and touch.
From space, the passages, ears, and sound.

2. Karmic connection (*lé drel*)

Karmic connection is a key concept in Tibetan Buddhism. Karma binds the relationship between the body-mind and samsara. It is the power that instigates the reunification of mind and matter, that binds a child and its parents, and that connects all aspects of life. The accumulated favorable karma of one's past life establishes the connection with one's future life, and one's fortune. Karma directs the consciousness towards the future parents. Without a karmic connection, conception will not take place, despite a couple's high-quality relationship and the presence of other favorable conditions.

3. The bardo consciousness (*bardö namshé*)

The bardo is a mental state of transition, which also takes place between past and future lives. During this time, consciousness is clothed in an illusory, dream-like body, and is able to experience joy and suffering. After death, the mind begins to travel in an unknown world. The bardo consciousness can pass through material objects and move to any place instantly, propelled by its desires for a maximum duration of 49 days. Some bardo beings attain their new life several days after death, while others do so within a much shorter time span. This depends on its mental state, which is in turn governed by past karmic actions. It is said that positive karma brings tranquil illusions, while the opposite produces nightmare-like experiences.

The mental body is as light as a feather and possesses a strong power of clairvoyance. It sees its future parents and is attracted to them like bees to a flower. Searching for its next parents and eventually roaming around its future mother without knowing why, the bardo being senses the menstrual cycle and the circulation of hormones, further increasing its desire. Other consciousnesses that have similar karmic attractions surround the woman, especially before and during menstruation. The strongest connection will succeed in manifesting as newly conceived human life. Because of this attraction and attention, women experience agitation, nervousness, and increased emotions. Depending on the condition of the woman's body-mind, the bardo consciousness may suffer, like when a bee is not able to suck the nectar of a flower moved by wind. Such sufferings could leave traces in the latent memory (*bakchak*) of the child.

4. The two parental energies

The quality of the parents' reproductive fluids is a primary factor influencing the conception of a child. In particular, the mother's menstruation is vital for her fertility, just as fertile soil is essential for the growth of a flower. There are positive and negative qualities inherent in the parent's energies, which determine the likelihood of conception.

Positive qualities:

- The woman's menstruation should resemble red enamel or rabbit's blood, and its stains should be removable with water

- The man's semen should be whitish, heavy, sweet, and plentiful

---

4   G.yu thog yon tan mgon po, 1993, 17.

Negative qualities related to menstruation:

- Wind disorder menstruation has a rough quality, a dark color, and an astringent taste

- Bile disorder menstruation is yellowish, has a sour taste and an offensive odor

- Phlegm disorder menstruation is sticky like mucus, has a sweet taste, and is cold

- Blood disorder menstruation is as if it were decayed

- Phlegm-wind disorder produces menstruation made up of small parts (clotting)

- Blood-bile disorder menstruation resembles pus

- Phlegm-bile disorder menstruation is knotty

- Wind-bile disorder menstruation dries up in the womb, resulting in early menopause or irregular menstruation

- Contamination caused by disruption of all the humors combined produces menstruation that resembles a mixture of feces and urine

Any of these types of menstruation do not support the conception of a child. Dysmenorrhea and amenorrhea, reproductive organ disorders, and so on can also impact fertility.

Negative qualities related to semen:

- Semen containing a small amount of spermatozoa, which occurs more often with men embodying the wind-phlegm constitution

- Deformed spermatozoa

- Lazy or weak spermatozoa

Any of the problems affecting reproductive fluids described above may prevent conception, or result in a handicapped child or congenital disease. Poor semen is like an inferior seed that cannot germinate. Poor menstruation is a barren field, unable to nourish a growing seedling.

5. The menstrual cycle

Datsen is a monthly sign of quality, which must be synchronized. This term comprises the follicle as well as ovum, which can be referred to as the "white essence egg" (*kham kar gonga*).[5] The latter, however, has received less scholarly attention in Tibetan medical literature compared to menstrual blood. Metaphorically, menstruation and the follicle are like a flower and its seed. The follicle matures, and in case there was no conception, it breaks down and exits the body during menstruation. Classical Tibetan medical sources do not distinguish between ovum and follicle. The follicle is produced in the *samséu* organ, which refers to the ovaries as well as to the male testicles. So far, Sowa Rigpa commentators did not elucidate the meaning of this term. According to the author, *sam* refers to "thinking," which together with *séu* means the "tiny fruit which grants thinking power." Many emotions, especially desire, indeed arise from hormonal circulation, in which the reproductive organs play a chief role.

The menstrual cycle is a fundamental conception factor. According to the *Gyüzhi*, the first menstrual cycle (menarche) occurs around the age of 12.[6] The cycle continues until a woman is around 50 years old, with some exceptions. Individual cycles and ovulation times differ, yet they can be viewed as a personal body clock that is likely to correspond to the lunar phases.[7] Before the age of twelve, girls use all nutritional energy for growth, which is why menses do not occur. The onset of menstruation is a sign that puberty has begun. When women enter menopause, nutrients are once again needed to sustain the body. As a general rule, ovulation occurs during the waxing moon and menses occur at the beginning of the waning moon. According to biomedicine, menstrual cycles are usually 28 days in length and commence with menstruation, which lasts for about four days. Menstruation is followed by the follicular phase, during which estrogen stimulates maturation of the ovum and thickening of the uterine lining. On the 14 day of the cycle, ovulation takes place, whereby an egg is released from one of the ovaries. Ovulation is followed by the luteal or secretory phase, which lasts for 14 days and is mainly influenced by the hormones progesterone and estrogen. If conception has not occurred, hormone levels decrease at the completion of the cycle, prompting menstruation and the commencement of a new cycle.

---

5 *Kham kar* means "white nature." It is a white-colored body essence, which is applied in this context to denote the woman's ovum and follicle.

6 Some girls experience their menarche at age 9 or 10 or even earlier, which is also attested in Tibetan medical texts. This may be explained by differences in geography, hormones, upbringing, or lifestyle.

7 The menstrual cycle is described in further detail in *Mes po'i zhal lung*, Zur mkhar blo gros rgyal po, 1991, vol. 1, 110–14.

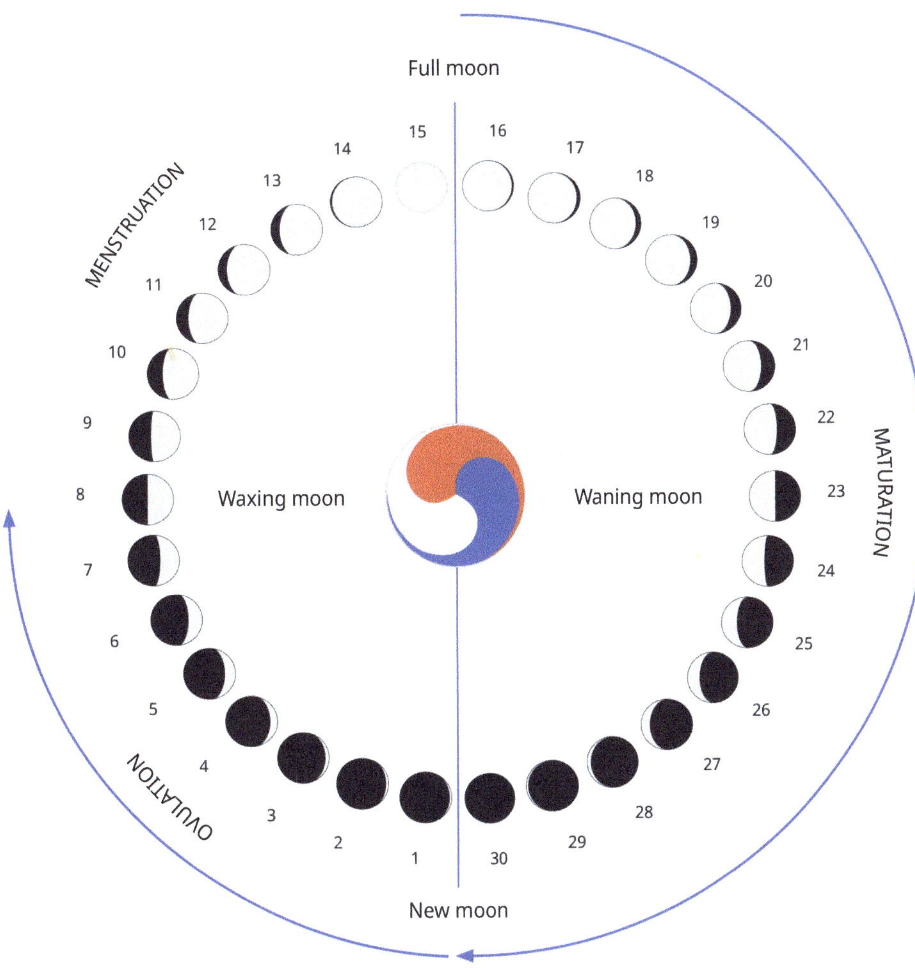

FIGURE 13.3 Lunar phases and the menstrual cycle

The Tibetan medical term *datsen* seems to match closely with biomedical understandings of menstruation, though there are some differences, as outlined below. A woman's menstrual cycle is associated with the lunar cycle because her solar energy is attracted to and moved by masculine lunar energy. This is why a woman's menstrual cycle is counted according to the lunar calendar. It has three overall phases:

- Maturation of the follicles starts after full moon (the 16th day of the lunar calendar month, when solar energy starts to increase) and continues for 14 days until the dark moon (the 30th day of the lunar month)

- Ovulation occurs from the first to the eighth day

- Menstruation occurs from the eighth to 15th day, when the moon's energy is increasing.

13.3 MODE OF CONCEPTION

When a couple's desire is at its peak and the bardo consciousness is located nearby like a bee attracted by a flower's nectar, the world experienced by the bardo being is at a point of revolution. The being's emotional state changes by attraction to either the father or the mother, resulting in a shift in perspective. Depending on its karma, it will experience entering a palace, a house, a garden, and so on. At conception, the bardo consciousness enters the mother's womb, having passed with the father's breath through his nostrils.[8] At this instant, wind energy of the father's sperm unites with the mother's egg. This unification consists of two steps: the bardo consciousness faints, whereas wind continues to work with the parents'

---

8 Sa skya pa rgyal mtshan dpal bzang, 1991, 7, offers a different explanation and states that the bardo consciousness enters through father's anus. There are various additional interpretations that are not discussed here.

two energies towards the development of the child.

From Yutok Yönten Gönpo the Younger's era in the 12th century up until nowadays, conception has been the subject of intense debate. With the progress of time and the scientific understandings of human biology, our knowledge has increased. This progress has clarified many previously hidden meanings in some areas of *Four Tantras*, while also creating new doubts. Even though Sowa Rigpa physicians previously accepted that conception occurred on the third day of menstruation, some questions remained. On this point, ancient medical literature and modern conceptions differ. Numerous books on Tibetan medicine have been published recently with an updated description of when conception occurs, while others have stuck to the original. Below, we will first cover the traditional concept, followed by the updated interpretation.

The literal explanation, as mentioned in the embryology chapter commentary of the *Blue Beryl*, is as follows. Conception will not take place on the first three days nor on the 11 day after the start of menstruation. Conception takes place from the fourth day. Conception on odd days (1, 3, 5, 7, 9) will result in a male child; conception that takes place on even days (2, 4, 6, 8) will result in a female child. The womb will close its door after the 12 day like a lotus blossom closing after sunset. Note that the system for counting days begins after the third day of menstruation, which entails that the fourth day is considered the first day of possible conception. This traditional interpretation maintains that during the first three days of a woman's menstrual cycle (when menstruation occurs), sexual intercourse should be avoided.

These conception days are also given in the Buddhist saint Vāgbhaṭa's *Ashtāngahridayasaṃhitā*, which provides less detail on the subject. Tantric literature confirms the same information. It can be inferred then that this concept is shared by several ancient Asian spiritual and medical sciences. According to these, conception cannot take place during ovulation.

As mentioned above, a new understanding of when conception occurs was more recently introduced. The new interpretation goes as follows. Conception will not take place in the first three days of menstruation and the 11 following days. After the 14th day (from the start of menstruation), conception can occur. If it takes place on odd days (1, 3, 5, 7, 9) a male child will be born, while conception on even days (2, 4, 6, 8) will produce a female child. In short, the updated theory accepts that conception can occur during ovulation, which is closer to modern medicine.

TABLE 13.3 The traditional interpretation of male or female conception

Sex	Conception day				
Male	First day (the fourth day after menstruation)	3rd	5th	7th	9th
Female	Second day	4th	6th	8th	

TABLE 13.4 General factors that influence the sex of the child

Mental factor	Element	Essence	Humor	Sex
Attachment + strong anger	Fire and wind	Female	Bile	Female
Attachment + less anger	Water and earth	Male	Phlegm	Male
Attachment + confusion	Space	Mixed		Intersex

Signs of conception (*ngel dzinpé tak*)

During conception, women experience feelings of satisfaction, heaviness, tiredness, shivering, increase in heartbeat, as well as involuntary movements of the limbs. One or two months later, pregnancy symptoms begin with the cessation of menstruation and food cravings. These symptoms are considered normal, are called *tri né* (which translates as "attachment disease"), and may include nausea, vomiting, vertigo, sleepiness, bad digestion, and headache. Pregnancy signs such as morning sickness are more severe for women with a bile constitution and women who suffer from gallbladder complaints. These symptoms can therefore equally be labeled bile symptom pregnancy signs. Pregnant women should be offered psychological support. Light medical treatment should be given only if absolutely necessary (such as Zhiser or Serdok 11 in case of severe headache and vomiting). Generally, it is safer to avoid any treatment or surgery.

Twins

After conception has taken place, multiple childbirths may result if the mother's wind humor was agitated, dividing the united ovum and sperm. According to the number of dispersed pieces, the mother will carry twins, triplets, or more babies. It is not specified if several consciousnesses are involved before this division, but according to the law of cause and effect, this is probable.

Congenital disorders

Even if the conditions for conception are favorable and successful fertilization has taken place, an imbalance in the parent's united reproductive elements, contamination by disease, wind disturbance by improper diet, psychological imbalance, or other negative factors may cause handicaps or congenital abnormalities in the child. These traditionally include blindness, deafness, limping, dwarfism, and intersex individuals (*tsen nyi maning*). Poor sperm quality may result in skeletal disorders, neurological conditions, or brain damage. Poor ovum quality may result in blood disorders or organ malformation.

Precautions during pregnancy

A pregnant woman should avoid eating types of meat which are not customarily eaten in her culture or for which she does not have an interest, such as beef in India, or horse, donkey or dog meat in Tibet. Eating such meat is said to produce a negative psychological effect that could influence the child. Tibetan medicine specifically advises that a pregnant woman should avoid eating horse, donkey, numerous types of seafood, and the meat of various birds. Generally, a pregnant woman is said to be sensitive. Harmful emotions should be avoided, and a harmonious environment is preferable.

13.4 FETAL DEVELOPMENT (*NGEL PELTSÜL*)

Fetal development begins immediately following conception. Pregnancy lasts 38 weeks and goes through three significant stages in which the fetus resembles a fish, a turtle, and a pig. The primary source of development is of course the mother, as she gives nutrition to the fetus through the umbilical cord, via the placenta (*shama*). The umbilical cord is called *tétak*, which literally refers to the "navel thread" that joins with the placenta. Another term used is *butak*, *which* means "fetal thread."

In his *Six Dharmas of Nāropa* commentary, Peljor Döndrup clarifies several points of early fetal development. He states: [9]

> After conception, apart from the *künzhi*
> the seven other consciousnesses become
> unclear like a drunk man.
> At the center of the five elements, inside
> the *künzhi*, the mental affliction mind
> (*nyönmongpé yi*) arises.
> Instantly, life force wind is generated from
> the white and red *dangma*, and karmic
> wind (*lé kyi lung*) arises.
> It turns milk into yoghurt, which becomes
> elongated in shape; mixing, binding,
> stabilizing, preserving, and then growing.
> This is the formation of the mental
> afflication mind from the *künzhi*.

First month

The first day of the first week after conception is the time of fertilization. The mixing of sperm and ovum is like a drop of yeast added to milk. The mixture is activated by a subtle wind called *sogklung a*.[10] This wind is promoted by *nyönmongpé yi*, the deluded mind that derives from the *bardo* consciousness. S*oklung a* is the source of all physical causes of the body-mind. It is like

---

9 Dpal 'byor don grub, 1995, 73.

10 The letter "a" refers to "the source," a metaphor for the life-sustaining wind arising from the *künzhi*. "A" is also the mother of all letters and sounds, and stands for *ama*, the mother figure as the generator of life.

the transcendental sound "A" that brings forth all other sounds; like a bean that produces a sprout; like the root that supports all parts of a flower; like a mother giving birth. Different aspects of this wind manifest under different names in the following weeks and months of fetal development. All manifest from the *soklung* of the *künzhi. Soklung a* also represents *lung uma*, the central or neutral wind energy and its continuation from the past life. It produces *tsa uma*, the central channel, and the two lateral channels. These three channels become the core of the physical body, humors and gross mind development, supporting the body like the pillars of a house. To obtain in-depth knowledge on this subject, detailed information from Buddhist tantra is required. In medicine, a simple correspondence with the respiratory (the wind system, including the nervous system), blood (bile) and lymph and endocrine systems (phlegm) of the body is a good starting point.

Second week: a subtle wind (this and all following subtle winds are branches of *soklung a*) called *küntu düpa* manifests and begins to mix the two energies (sperm and ovum) together. The fertilized ovum becomes a little thicker and longer.

Third week: a subtle wind called *dzöka* manifests and helps the two energies to fully merge. The fertilized ovum's consistency resembles curd.

Fourth week: a subtle wind called *lé kyi lung ngönpar düpa* manifests. The fertilized ovum begins to develop into a round, oval or elongated shape, according to the child's gender (male, female, or intersex respectively). During this week, pregnancy symptoms such as nausea and food cravings may occur. According to Tibetan medicine, these symptoms manifest from the child's needs for his/her development; therefore, the mother should not suppress food cravings or any particular emotions, even if these are challenging. Preventing the consumption of desired food and drinks may harm the child's development.

Second month: the beginning of the fish stage

Fifth week: a subtle wind called *yangdakpar düpa* manifests, growing the child's umbilical cord and navel chakra in the center of its body. This week is the beginning of the fish stage as the fetus develops into a fish-like shape.

Sixth week: a subtle wind called *gya chenpo* manifests and helps develop the central channel from the navel, much like a sprout develops from a germinating bean.

Seventh week: a subtle wind called *khyilwa* manifests, developing all three channels. The left channel

(*tsa kyangma*) first forms the eyes and organs in the head, as well as the crown chakra together with the other two channels. The right channel (*tsa roma*) forms the heart, and the central channel (*tsa uma*) forms the secret chakra along with the right and left channels.

Eighth week: a subtle wind called *dokching gyurwa* manifests and helps form the throat chakra, and shape the head.

Ninth week: a subtle wind called *nampar jépa* manifests and helps develop the upper and lower abdomen. This week ends the first stage of development and is therefore called "completion of the fish stage."

Third month: the beginning of the turtle stage

10th week: a subtle wind called *sawar jépa* manifests and helps form the protuberances of the shoulders and hips. This week is called the "beginning of the turtle stage" because the fetal body's shape resembles a turtle.

11th week: a subtle wind called *buga nangwa* manifests and helps form the nine internal orifices of the body. They are the eyes, ears, nostrils, mouth, and anal and urinary passages.

12th week: a subtle wind called *yönpö go* manifests and helps form the five solid organs.

13th week: a subtle wind called *bur gyüpa* manifests and helps form the six hollow organs.

Fourth month

14th week: a subtle wind called *küpé kha* or *küpé go* manifests and forms the upper arms and thighs.

15th week: a subtle wind called *péma* manifests, helps form the arms, and makes the calves protrude.

16th week: a subtle wind called *dütsi drowa* manifests, helping the twenty fingers and toes to form.

17th week: a subtle wind called *dridong* manifests and supports the development of the three principal channels and the connective branches of nerves, blood, and lymph vessels. This week is called the "completion of the turtle stage."

Fifth month: the beginning of the pig stage

18th week: a subtle wind called *drima mépa* manifests and helps mature the fleshy and fatty tissues. As this stage marks the beginning of the period when the fetus develops fatty tissues, this week is called the "beginning of the pig stage." From this week, the fetus desires food and experiences hunger, but lacks knowledge on what is edible.

19th week: a subtle wind called *shintu trawa* manifests and helps develop all ligaments, tendons and nerves.

20th week: a subtle wind called *shintu tenpa* manifests and helps construct the bones, bone marrow, and white matter.

21st week: a subtle wind called *yangdakpar kyöpa* manifests and helps develop the skin as well as the tactile constituents.

Sixth month

22nd week: a subtle wind called *küntu gyelwa* manifests and helps open and shape the nine external orifices.

23rd week: a subtle wind called *yongsu dakpar dzinpa* manifests and helps to develop the head and body hair and nails.

24th week: a subtle wind called *küntu chöwa* manifests and contributes to the maturation of the five solid and six hollow organs. The fetus begins to feel joy and sorrow and comfort or discomfort during its slumber.

25th week: a subtle wind called *drongkhyer dzinpa* manifests, and respiration starts.

26th week: a subtle wind called the *kyéwa ngönpar drupa* manifests; the child begins to awaken from their unconscious state and remembers past lives.

Seventh month

27th–30th weeks: each week manifests a different subtle wind. These winds are called *menyön chenpo, métok dzinpa, métok trengwa,* and *chak kyi go*. They develop and strengthen the organs, tissues, and channels. In short, all body parts, gross and subtle, complete their development. The body becomes like a well-built palace and the mind begins to function.

Eighth month: the competition stage

31st–35th weeks: during these five weeks, one subtle wind called *métok düpa* manifests, supporting the infant's growth. This period is called the "competition stage of the mother and child," because they compete over the energy of *dang*. The child's and mother's radiance and complexion dominate alternatively. This is not considered an ideal time to give birth, but under certain conditions delivery may occur. If this is the case, the health of the mother or the child may be compromised. During these weeks, the child completes its development, and its hair and nails grow.

Ninth month

36th week: the child experiences five unpleasant feelings related to its situation in the womb:

1. A sense that the womb is unclean
2. That there is an unpleasant smell
3. Like being locked up in prison
4. It is dark
5. Claustrophobia

These feelings condition the child's mind to develop further and become independent.

37th week: because the child experiences the unpleasant emotions described above, it wishes to leave the womb and therefore begins to turn downwards.

38th week: a subtle wind called *tokpé kyen* manifests and with the help of descending wind (*tursel lung*), the child moves downward. Delivery indicates that the body of a new human being has been completed. The growth of the child's body-mind now needs to be fostered with food, care, clothing, education, and experience to become a complete person who is able to live a conscious and healthy life.

Giving birth

The appropriate time to give birth is after a normal period of pregnancy, lasting around nine months and 10 days (counted from the last menstruation). According to *Gyüzhi*'s embryology chapter, there are three obstacles that can delay childbirth or create other difficulties:

- Delivery may be delayed if the mother has lost blood during pregnancy

- Delivery may be delayed, and the mother or child's life may be at risk, if the child has grown too large

- Delivery may be hindered if descending wind is disturbed.

Presence of any of these obstacles requires the aid of a physician or midwife to lessen the potential risk to mother and child.

Determining the child's sex through pulse reading

Although experienced physicians can read a mother's pulse to determine the sex of a child two months into a pregnancy, a more accurate reading can be made later. A pregnant woman's pulse is thicker, stronger, and more taut. A more prominent right kidney pulse in the mother indicates that she will give birth to a boy, and a strong left kidney pulse indicates a girl.

If the child resides more in the right side of the abdomen and if the right side of the belly appears higher, it is the sign of a male child. A pregnant woman may be carrying a boy if she feels physically lighter, if she dreams about men more frequently than women, and if some milk exudes from her right breast. A pregnant woman may be carrying a girl if she has an increased desire for men; if she wishes to sing songs, dance, and wear ornaments, and if she shows signs opposite to those described above for a male child. Twins may show a higher belly on both sides.

How to help the pregnant woman

Some women experience changes in emotions and moodiness when they get pregnant. This should not concern the family, as these are natural processes. From the second month of pregnancy, the mother is advised to avoid surgery, bloodletting therapy, or strong medications. In particular, she should not use toxic or purgative substances. As described above, pregnancy syndromes such as cravings for sour or other specific foods or drinks should not be inhibited as they derive from the child's developmental requirements. From the seventh month until the very end of pregnancy, sesame or mustard oil massages of the lower back, thighs, legs and feet are useful to smooth the descending wind and to harmonize the elements in the lower abdomen. The woman should move during the eighth month as it helps to make delivery easier. She should see a doctor or midwife regularly for check-ups.

Once labor is established, when the woman begins to experience rhythmic contractions (for example, every two hours), Tibetan physicians prescribe Agar 35 and Zhijé 11, to be taken alternatively with strong black tea especially in case of prolonged delivery. These medicines stimulate contractions, reduce labor pain, and relax uterine tension. They regulate the descending wind, which can be disturbed by the woman's fear and pain or by other minor obstacles related to labor. After the baby is born, Zhijé 6 helps clean the uterus and aids in delivering the placenta. If the medicines mentioned above are not available and/or if the child has not descended into position, this indicates that the descending wind is blocked. In this case, moxibustion should be applied to the mother's two little finger points to stimulate the downward positioning of the infant.

Post-delivery advice

The mother should relax and recover from the exhaustion of giving birth with the support, care, praise, and solidarity of her family. Medical treatment is only indicated in case of infection or excessive pain, for instance. After birth, the child should be given a name chosen by the family, and should be brought up with love and care.

A new mother is advised not to: take cold baths, touch cold surfaces with her bare hands and feet, eat hard foods, or to be exposed to cold wind for the first week after giving birth. This will prevent the advent of early osteoporosis, arthritis, chronic kidney illness, lower back pain, and other illnesses associated with cold.

Three chapters in the *Oral Instruction Tantra* are dedicated to women's disorders and pediatrics, including general and specific gynecology as well as common complaints. Numerous gynecological disorders could manifest as a result of imbalance in the humors, hormonal imbalance, poor hygiene, or psychological influences. The *Gyüzhi* further includes one chapter on childcare (*jipa nyerchö*) in which eighteen practices are described, including name giving, the birth ceremony, and so on.

13.5 BODY SIMILES (*LÜ KYI DRAPÉ*)

The body can be viewed as a house for the mind. This simile is often referred to in Buddhist literature and particularly in Tibetan medicine, where the body is described as similar in shape and function to a house. One chapter of the *Explanatory Tantra* is dedicated specifically to such metaphors (*drapé*).

The hip bones are like the foundations of the body house. The spinal vertebrae are like a pile of golden coins. The life channel is an agate pillar. The sternum is the main supporting beam of the house. The 24 ribs are wooden crossbeams. Rib cartilage acts as walls.

The channels, ligaments, and tendons are like a network of roof laths. The flesh and skin which cover the body are like cement. The two collarbones are like the outside parapet of a mansion. The scapula is like the corners of the house. The head is like the top-story shrine of a temple, with the skull acting as the roof, and the skull's central crown point operating like a chimney. The five sense organs are like windows. The ears on the head's two sides are like flying *garuḍa* birds. The nose is like an exquisite crown ornament. The hair is like tiles. The two hanging arms are like pendent banners. The upper and lower abdomen are like courtyards, with the diaphragm acting as the curtain screen that divides them.

The similes for the organs of the body are as follows: The heart is like a king seated on a throne. The five mother lungs (the posterior lobes) are like a minister, whereas the five son lungs (anterior lobes) are like a prince. The liver is like a crown queen and the spleen is like a junior queen. The kidneys are like powerful foreign ministers; they carry the weight of the body. The *samséu* (testicles and ovaries, including seminal vesicles and fallopian tubes) are like a treasury. The stomach is like a cooking pot. The small and large intestines are like the queen's attendants. The gallbladder is like a bag containing condiments. The urinary bladder is like a tank filled with water. The urinary tract and rectum are like the sewage pipes of the house. The two legs are like an arched doorway at the entrance, where horses are dismounted. The various vital parts of the body such as the brain, nerves, ligaments, and bones are like a governor or general who has received his authority from the king.

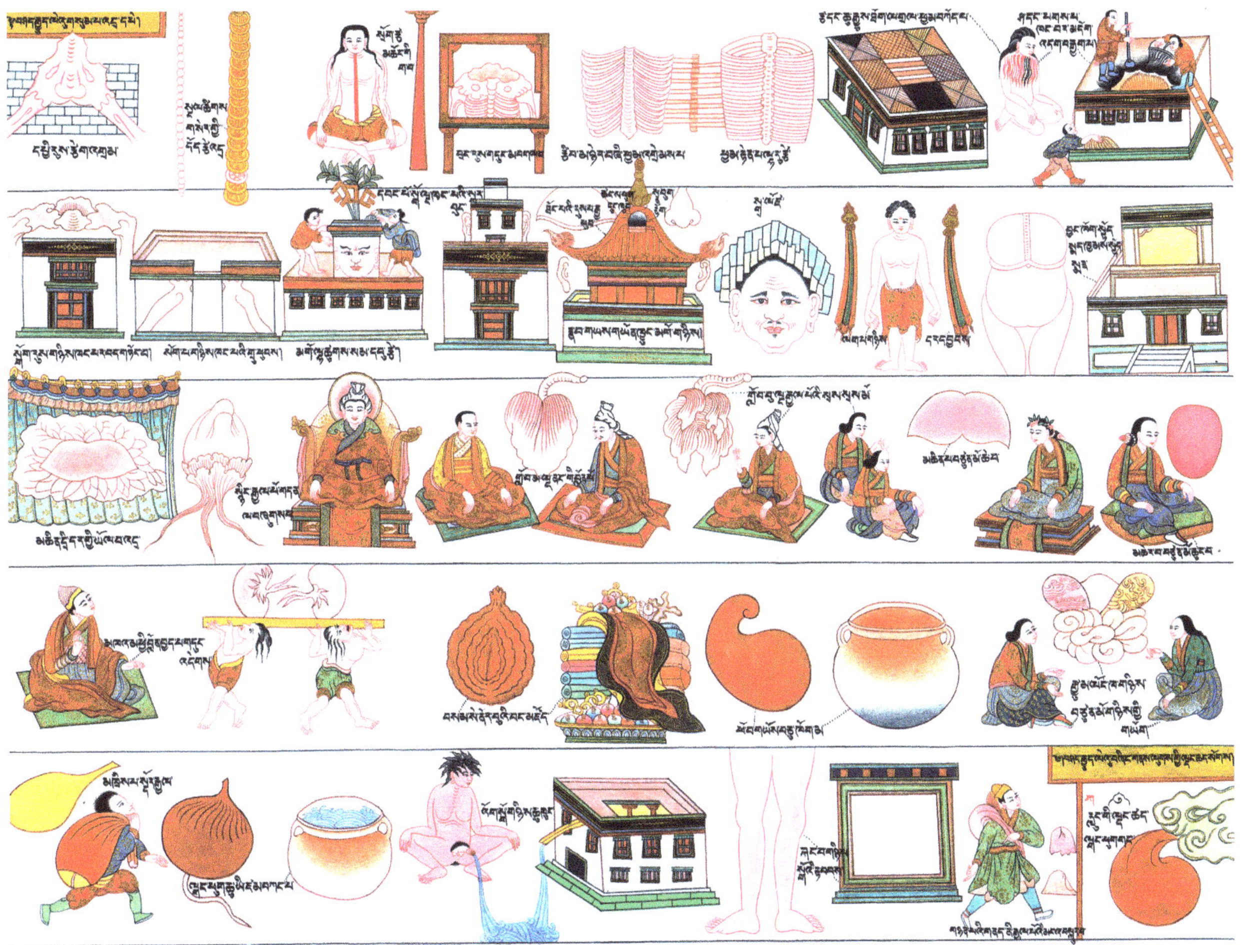

FIGURE 13.4 The bodily metaphors

PART 5

THE ORGANS

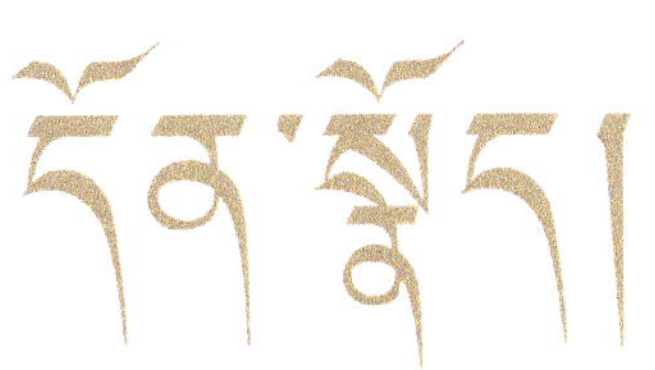

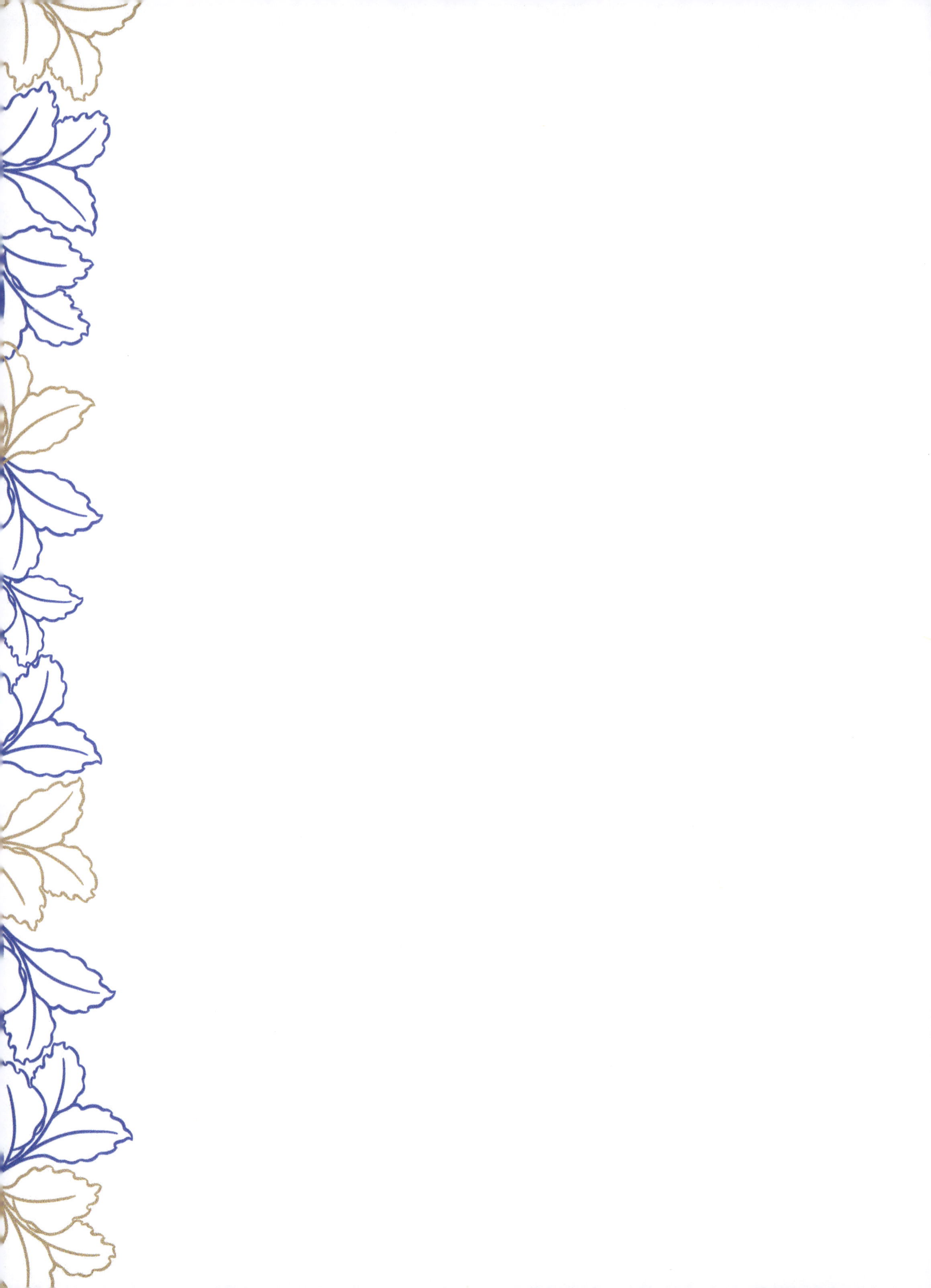

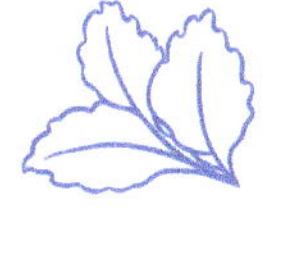

CHAPTER 14

THE FIVE SOLID ORGANS (*DÖN NGA*)

14.1 GENERAL INTRODUCTION TO THE ORGANS

The body is a house for the mind, and it of course houses the organs as well. If the body is construed as a tree, the hollow organs are its roots and leaves, the sense organs its flowers, and the vital organs fruits. The five solid or vital organs are called the five functionaries (*dön nga*). They are bases of the five elements. Each vital organ is furthermore linked to one or more of the "six containers" or hollow organs (*nö druk*) through inner pathways.

The author is somewhat hesitant to write on anatomy (*rotra*), since it has been in decline in Sowa Rigpa for centuries. Some basic anatomical knowledge comes from ancient texts such as Bici's *Yellow Book*,[1] which describes the names of organs, body parts, and *turma* surgery along with other aspects of health and pathology. The style of composition tells us that it is a synthesis of a larger volume on these topics. It is possible then that Tibetan medical anatomy started to develop around 1,000 years ago. Unfortunately, there is scant further evidence. The *Gyüzhi*, first composed in the 12th century, lists the organs in the *Root Tantra* and provides analogies for them in the *Explanatory Tantra*. There are no chapters dedicated exclusively to organ physiology, yet the chapter on wounds in the *Oral Instruction Tantra* focuses on pathology and treatment. Vāgbhaṭa's *Ashtāngahridayasaṃhitā* also remains silent on the topic.

There is scant evidence available on teachings of dissection and anatomy in ancient times. It appears that after Dési Sangyé Gyatso (1653–1705) there are hardly any accounts of anatomical study based on the dissection of human or animal bodies. This is probably not because of taboo, because sky burial was and is still fairly widely practiced in Tibetan and Himalayan regions. There must be other reasons for its neglect. Nonetheless, the Dési's medical *tangka* paintings demonstrate great advancements. The *tangka* are unique for their clear and lively representations of the human body and organs, which are comparable to a certain extent to modern anatomy. It is said that human corpses were used for this purpose. The descriptions of the organs' nature, names, size, and the measurement of their location in the body are also informative. These *tangka* represented a leap forward after medicine suffering for a long time from political instability in Tibet.

In 1974, during the author's second year of Tibetan medical studies at Men-Tsee-Khang, an elderly inpatient without any family died. The author recounts that:

> I was able to observe a dissection of his body, undertaken by the preeminent female physician Lopsang Dolma Khangkar. I still vividly remember watching her remove the abdominal organs.

It is an exceptionally rare chance for students of Sowa Rigpa to witness a dissection in traditional society. Given the lack of materials on anatomy in the 1970s, the study of organ physiology proved to be challenging. In recent times, modern technological innovations have provided a new space for practitioners to better understand Tibetan medicine, especially when it comes to the physical body and organs.

The organs, mind, and emotions

Gross mind cannot exist without the support of a physical body. Emotions are interdependent body-mind expressions. In both tantra and medicine, *lung* is posited as the subtle material link that provides the condition for consciousness to manifest emotions. For the deep-seated mental poisons to transform into day-to-day feelings, it is thus necessary for wind to create a structural interface that mirrors and cooperates with mental impulses.

---

1   Bi ci, 2005.

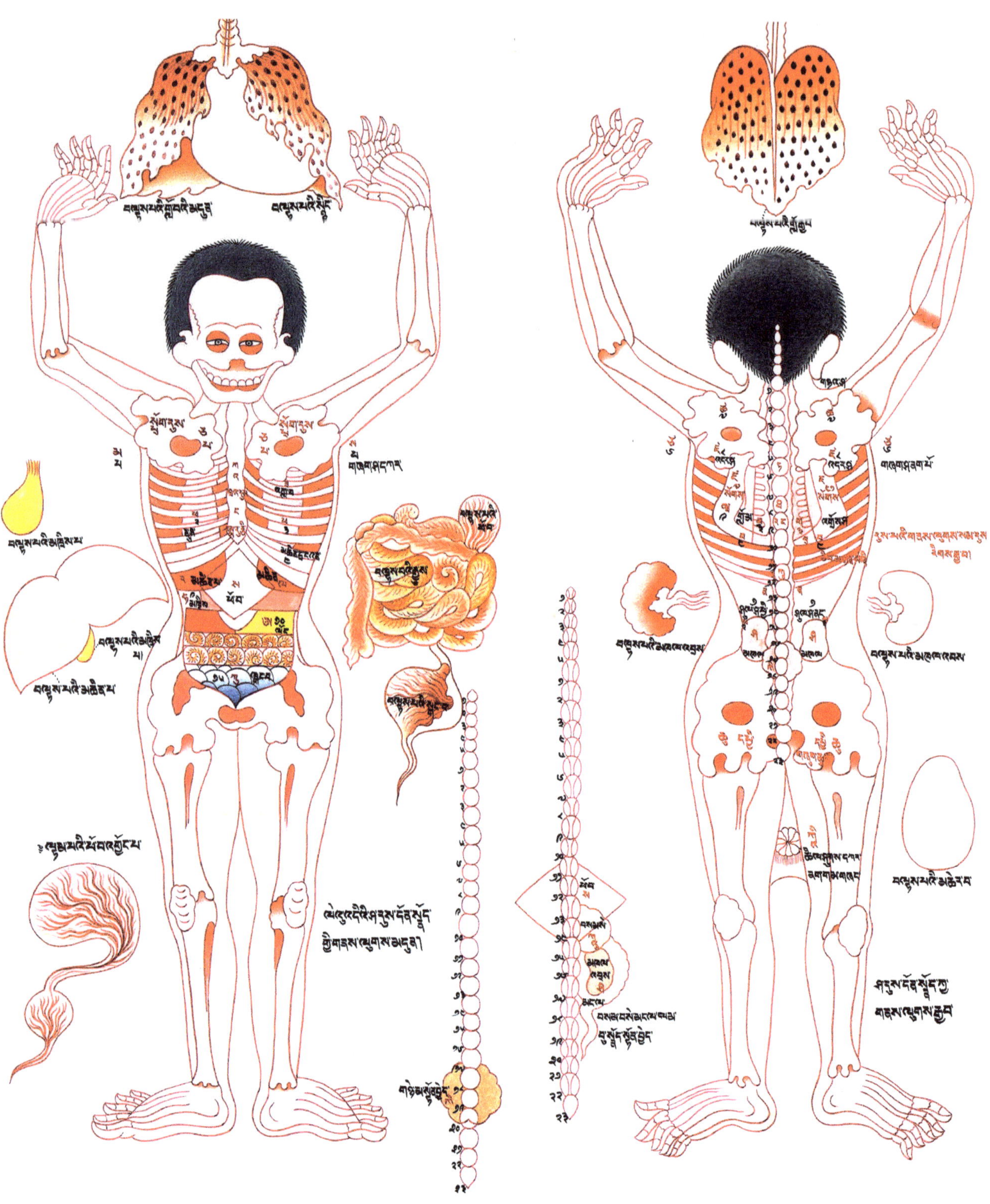

FIGURE 14.1 Traditional anatomical depictions of the organs

Organs are not just mechanical parts of the body; they are equally physical bases of emotions that are generated through wind-mind connections. Moreover, the body not only contains solid, hollow, and sense organs but also constituents, waste products, and countless microbes (*sinbu*). Each has its role, and all have an impact on the gross mind (*sem rakpa*) and its emotions (*sem tsor*). Even though it may come across as if there is an independent mind ruling the body, here we maintain that all body components collectively produce the gross mind, its thoughts, and feelings, like an umbrella that can protect from rain because of its many parts functioning as a whole. Or like an elected president who represents the people of his country. Even though a president may act based on his own nature and personal interests, the influence of his party and supporters is undeniable. A person's constitution, organs, and humors influence their psychology. Although there is a subtle causal link between this gross mind and the subtle mind from which it developed, most emotions are in fact bodily products.

We easily forget how much the organs influence our minds. The *Gyüzhi* also does not clearly lay out the links between organs and emotions. However, when we get ill, the relationship becomes clearer. Paying attention to these hidden connections is a promising avenue for deeper knowledge on emotional wellbeing and the body-mind interface.

All organs are nourished by blood through connecting blood vessels (see Section 17.5). Using a pine tree as a metaphor, one can view the solid organs as hanging fruits, the hollow organs as leaves and roots, and the channels such as the blood vessels (*traktsa*), nerves and lymphatic channels, as the trunk branching into the boughs and branches of the tree.

Through analogies it is also possible to get a succinct understanding of Tibetan medical physiology (see Section 13.5). More detail on this subject can be found in the chapters on organ pathology and trauma in the *Oral Instruction Tantra*. The primary explanation for the vital organs as a group relates to a political system, where the heart is said to be like a king, the

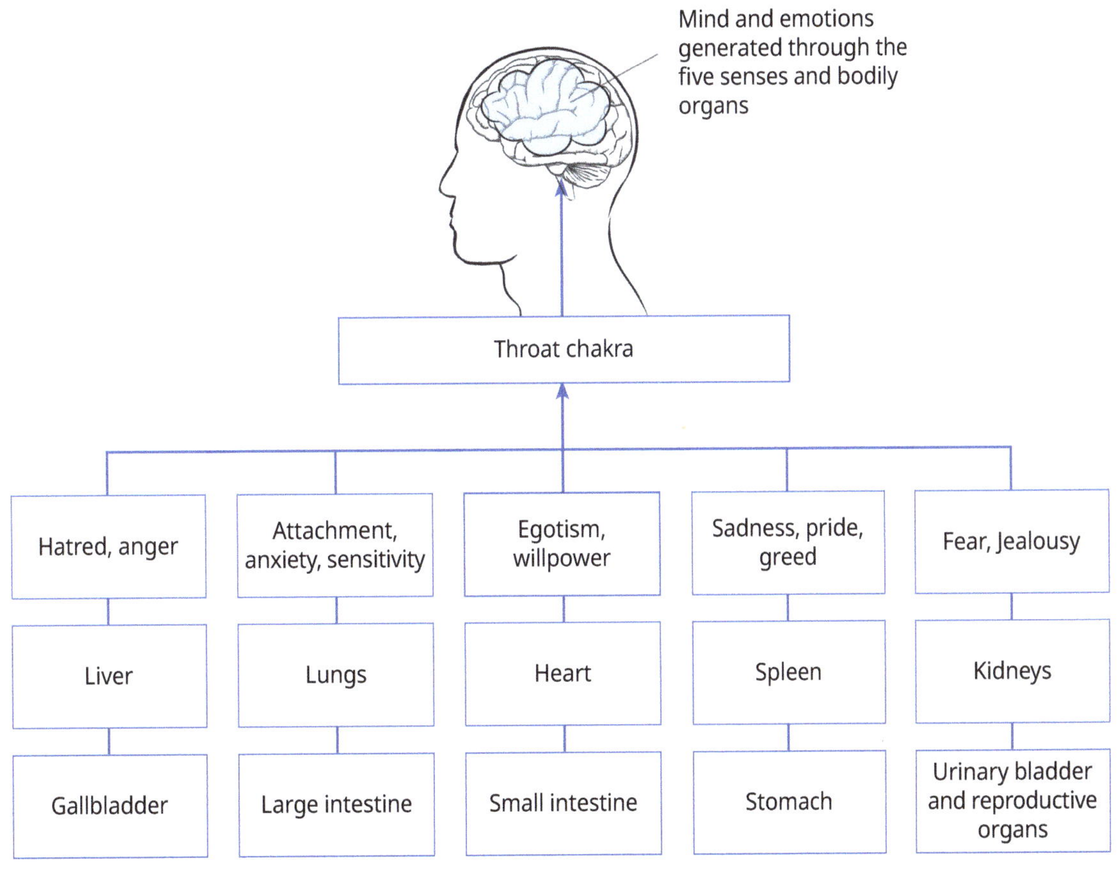

FIGURE 14.2 Gross mind, emotions, and the organs

lungs like interior ministers, the liver like a queen, the spleen like a junior queen, and the kidneys like powerful foreign ministers. Another analogy states that the body's parts are like citizens, the body like the country itself, and the humors are the country's rulers. Sowa Rigpa has no meridian concept for the vital and hollow organs, unlike Chinese acupuncture. However, friend/foe and mother/son relationships are noted in the chapter on pulse diagnosis in the *Subsequent Tantra*. This framework cannot be taken as fundamental since it is only found in this one section.

Generally, the organs are healthy at the beginning of one's life. They develop their activities in harmony and naturally support each other to maintain health. They digest food, absorb and distribute nutrition, and sustain the body-mind both physically and emotionally. The organs should interact harmoniously with each other, yet they equally have destructive capacities through the humors when unbalanced.

An unhealthy organ refers to one that is malfunctioning or functioning weakly. This manifests in cases where there is disharmony between the humors and/or from poor digestion, which produces deficient *dangma*. In some cases, the organs are defective from birth. This is called *lhenkyé né*. Many congenital diseases are connected to the parents or to *soklung* imbalance (see Section 13.2).

The solid organs

The five vital or solid organs (*dön nga*) are the heart, lungs, liver, spleen, and kidneys. They are the seats of the five gross emotions and the five elemental and nutritional energies. The heart receives and stores the space element essence from the *dangma* that is transformed into blood by the liver, whilst the lungs do the same for the air element essence. The liver receives the fire element, the spleen receives the earth element, and the kidneys receive the water element. These organs sustain the bodily elements, consume the gross and subtle nutrients, and transform them into vital energy for the function of body and mind. Metaphorically, they are the fruits of the channel trees, whilst the sense organs are their flowers. They support the mind to sense and produce emotions through impressions of the five external objects of form, sound, smell, taste, and touch. In Table 14.1 below, the negative emotions associated with the organs are mainly based on the author's experience with patient symptoms.

TABLE 14.1 The correspondences of the five vital organs

	Organ	Analogy	Element	Emotional base[2]	Function	Flower	Object
1.	Heart (*nying*)	King	Space	Egotism, willpower	Consciousness	Tongue (*ché*)	Taste
2.	Lungs (*lowa*)	Interior ministers	Wind	Attachment, anxiety, sensitivity	Respiration	Nose (*na*)	Smell
3.	Liver (*chinpa*)	Queen	Fire	Hatred, anger	Metabolism	Eyes (*mik*)	Form and color
4.	Spleen (*cherpa*)	Junior queen	Earth	Sadness, pride, greed	Body structure	Lips (*chu*)	Tactile sensation
5.	Kidneys (*khelma*)	Foreign ministers	Water	Fear, jealousy	Flow of liquids	Ears (*nawa*)	Sound

---

2 Healthy organs produce corresponding positive emotions. The heart, for instance, radiates happiness when wishes are fulfilled, whereas the spleen generates satisfaction.

14.2 HEART (*NYING*)

- Location: chest
- Color: brown
- Element: space
- Physiology: seat of the all-ground consciousness (*künzhi*)
- Psychic function: egotism, willpower, hatred and anger (via the blood)
- Root: small intestine
- Waste product: space element waste products derived from the channels and hollow organs, including intestinal mucus
- Flower: the tongue, which gives satisfaction to the heart

The heart is called *nying* or "essence." It is described as "precious," "fruit," and "center of the body." The heart is space element and empty by nature. Analogically it is like the king of a country, being the seat of the mind and mental consciousness. It is brown-red, and its principal function is to govern the kingdom of the body-mind from the center. The heart is located in the upper left side of the chest, at the level of back vertebrae BV6–7 (thoracic vertebrae 5 and 6). It is principally derived from the mother's blood energy and the space element. The *Oral Instruction Tantra* describes it thus:[3]

> The heart is the king, the seat of the body's lifeforce and mind.

Master Taktsang Lotsawa defines the heart as follows:[4]

> The heart is the seat of the self-grasping mind and of memory.
> It resides at the vena cava of the upper chest, and is like a coconut fruit.
> It is called *nying*.

---

3   G.yu thog yon tan mgon po, 1993, 432.
4   Dbang 'dus, 1982, 196.

The Indian physician Chandranandana said this of the heart (quoted in the same source):

> It is like a closed lotus flower facing down, with an empty space inside.
> It sustains mind and emotions.

The heart is the root of the blood channel (*traktsa*) system and its main arterial and vein trunks run alongside the vertebrae, standing straight like a pine tree (see also Section 17.5 on the arteries). The heart itself has four root blood channels that branch out to the lungs, hands, neck, and the heart itself, which correspond with the four coronary arteries and veins. These four channels sustain the heart and nourish the body through the circulation of blood. These channels (and the four smaller channels, the coronary artery branches) are like the four gates of the heart mandala that enable the heart chambers to empty, facilitating psychic balance and symbolizing emptiness as well as the seat of the mind. Tibetan medical anatomy paintings depict the heart as turned downward. This is not intended to be literal. Instead, it indicates the Tibetan Buddhist concept where, when human beings achieve bodhisattva states, the heart turns upwards. This is achieved by the practitioner's highly developed wisdom and loving-kindness. Not many further details are given on the anatomy and physiology of the heart.

In tantra, the heart is also known as the heart chakra, which can be visualized as a flat wheel or disc. It is formed by channels that are referred to as "the essence of the channels." In its center, there is a subtle channel called *yi zangma* (see Figure 17.4), surrounded by the other four channels. These heart channels are said to be as fine as horse hairs. Five-colored lights shine from its core. All five channels are empty and transparent, like glass tubes, and connect with the *yi zangma*. They transport light of different colors in each direction. The lights manifest from the *tiklé* and the corresponding dominant energy of the channel, blood, air, and heat. According to

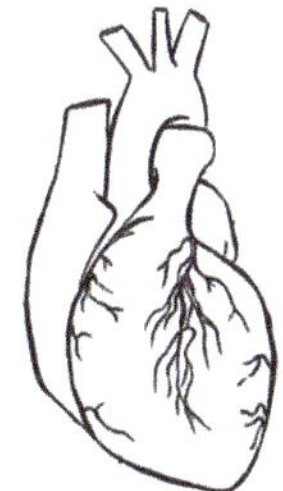
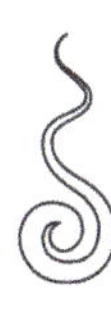
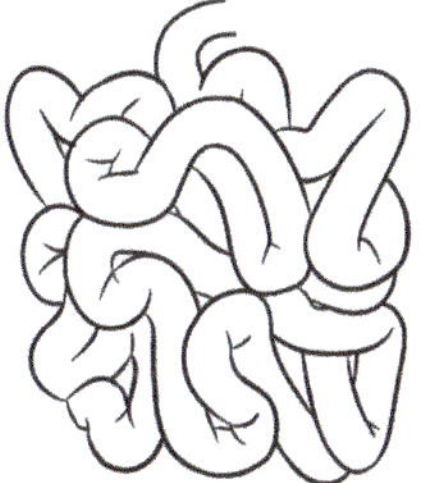
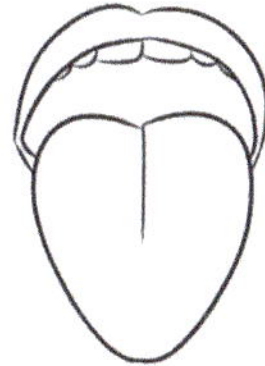

FIGURE 14.3 The heart and its functional links

Sumtön Yéshézung, these form the central spokes of the middle channel.[5]

Nying, in all its complexity and with its various functions, is considered a primary center of mental operations. The subtle physiology of the heart is challenging for many to grasp. The heart is said to house the *künzhi*, where mind and emotions manifest in the morning and return during sleep and the dying process. The *künzhi* mind, by means of *lung* as its vehicle, involuntarily regulates the ecosystem of the heart and communicates emotions to the brain and the rest of the body. The term "psychic center" can therefore be utilized to refer to this subtle mind (*sem trawa*). The *künzhi* is regulated by the force of mental affliction wind (*nyönmongpé lung*), which produces the gross mind and emotions throughout the brain and body. Tibetan Buddhist philosophy explains that the mind's nature is selfless and empty. It is subtle and without solid form, an energy that continues to function through a system of echoes in the empty heart. It is a luminous, aware, knowing and thinking energy. This mind functions through the heart, which produces the "I" of the self-grasping mind like a rainbow.

The *künzhi* receives all the information perceived and transmitted by the six gross mental and sense consciousnesses. In the heart chakra, the subtle mind records all experiences in the memory bank and transmits them to the very subtle mind (*shintu trawé sem*), which is located below the navel in a dormant state. The traces of the positive and negative deeds that are eventually stored in the very subtle mind are what is called karma. This karma is carried on to future lives where it will produce karmic results.

The heart is the center of wisdom, but it is also the seat of anger, love, compassion, fear, happiness, joy, desire, profound ignorance, and depression. It enables the memory to function, induces sleep, facilitates laughter, nervousness, and the taking of responsibility, among other characteristics. In men, the door of the mental consciousness in the heart faces the left side, while in women it faces the right side. In consideration of this psychic connection, Tibetan physicians start reading the pulse of men on their left wrist, and of women on the right.

The heart sends its waste products to the small intestine, where they become mucus which lines and protects the intestine. The flower of the heart is the tongue and its contact with the world is through taste, speech, and the tongue consciousness.

14.3 LUNGS (*LOWA*)

- Location: chest
- Color: grey
- Element: wind and water
- Physiology: respiration, distribution of air and moisture
- Psychic function: attachment, anxiety, and emotional sensitivity
- Root: large intestine
- Waste product: mucus of the throat and large intestine
- Flower: nose

The lungs are called *lowa*, which has several meanings: intimate friend, supporter, attendant, or assistant. These signify that, physiologically speaking, the lungs are the heart's main support. The lungs are sometimes described as the wind bags of the body. They are whitish grey, consisting of tubes and soft tissue. The root of each lung connects to the larynx, and their blood channels connect to the heart and vertebrae. The lungs hang in two lobes, on either side of the trachea. They are derived principally from the father's energy and are one of the principal wind humor organs. The 85th chapter of the *Oral Instruction Tantra* states:[6]

---

5   Sum ston ye shes gzungs, 1999a, 136.

6   G.yu thog yon tan mgon po, 1993, 432.

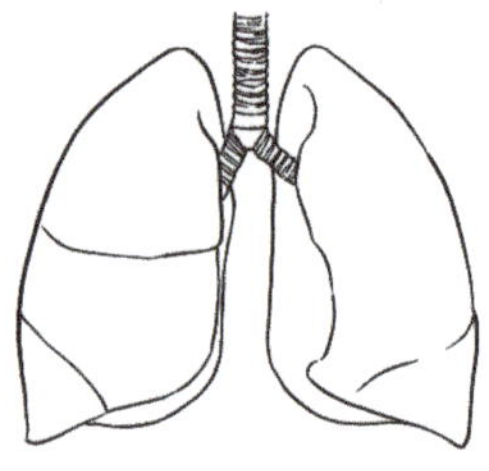 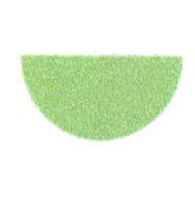 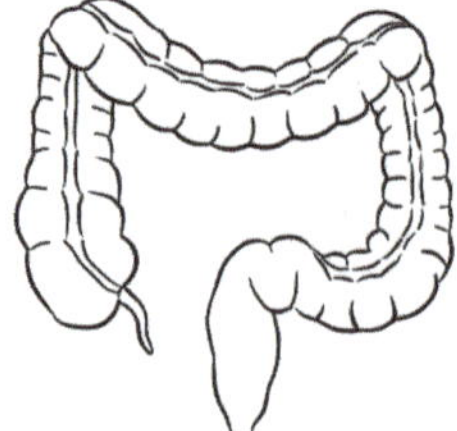 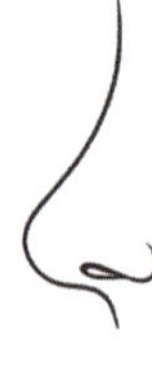

FIGURE 14.4 The lungs and their functional links

The five sons are like princes and the five
mothers are ministers.
The mother lungs hold the heart in their lap
like a child.

Lowa are located in the chest at the level of BV4–5
(thoracic vertebrae 3–4). According to Tibetan anatomical descriptions, they have two main components:
mother lungs and son lungs. The mother lungs are the
external lobes. They are said to function like an interior minister to the heart, protecting it from behind.
The son lungs are the inner parts of the lungs that surround the heart. They support the heart and are delicate by, like a prince. The mother and son lungs have
five subdivisions each, making a total of 10 lung parts.
The five outer mother lungs (*lowa ma nga*) are:

1. *Tak go*, literally "tiger head," referring to the
   tips of the right and left lungs
2. *Gangtö gangmé*, "upper and lower" (cf. the
   right and left lung), lateral to the spine

3. *Tsip* ("spokes"), referring to the right and left
   upper middle lobes
4. *Sham*, the "lower" middle lobes
5. *Zak na*, the "dropping edge" lobes

The five inner son lungs (*lowa bu nga*) are:[7]

1. *Dzo na* ("yak-cow hybrid's nose"), located
   above the heart
2. *Ja gap*, name of the shoulder blade's front
   muscle, at the upper right and left side of the
   heart
3. *Tuk khap* ("heart castle"), an empty protective
   area around the two sides of the heart
4. *Té mik* (meaning unclear), supporting the
   lungs from the bottom
5. *Dra ché* (meaning unclear), supporting the
   lungs from the bottom

---

7   Future research should aim to retrieve and elaborate the
    traditional anatomical meanings and functions of the son lungs.

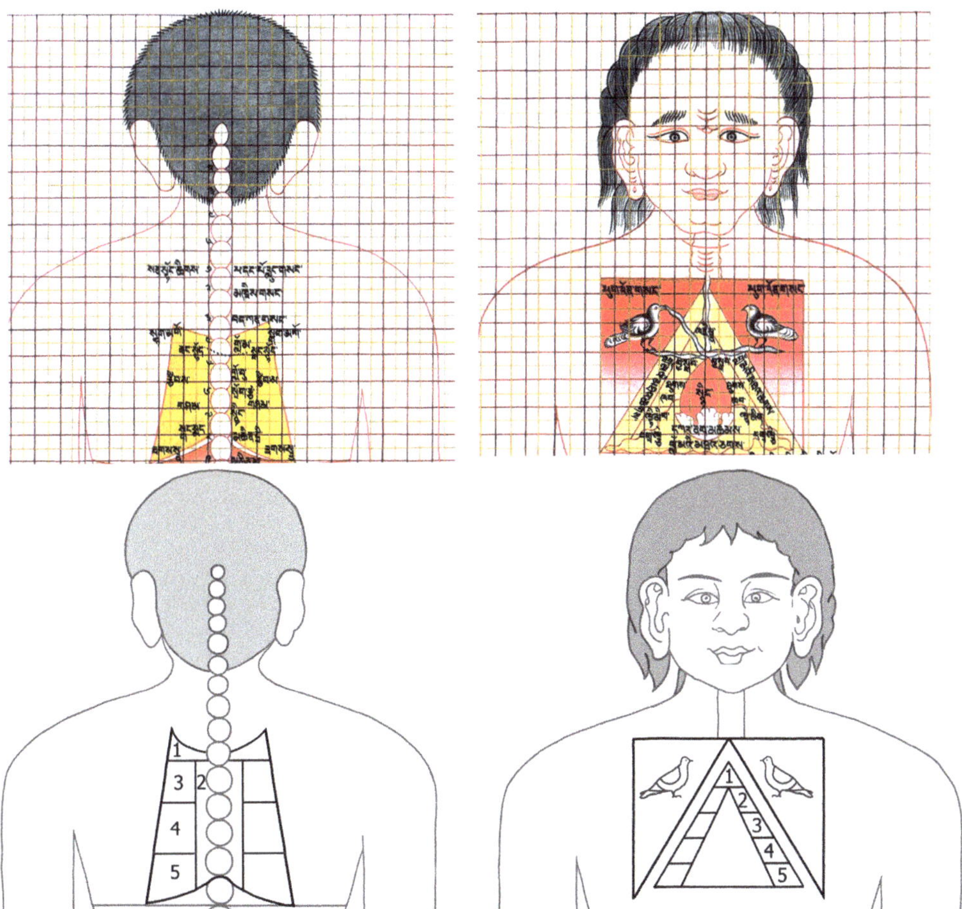

FIGURE 14.5 The mother longs viewed from the back and the son lungs viewed from the front

The lungs receive oxygenated air (water-earth wind) and transport it through the bronchial tubes to the bronchioles, and eventually to the body's blood cells. They also remove carbon dioxide (impure fire-air wind) by expelling it through the nose. The *lowa* regulate the body wind system, protect the heart, and cool down bile heat. They govern respiration (by means of ascending wind), circulate blood and wind, and thus maintain the life of the organs, tissues, as well as the body's microbes (*trasin*). The lungs aid in speech, give strength and radiance, keep the body straight, and remove toxins from the throat through the breath. They are the main organs that purify air and supply the body with oxygenated blood. The lungs keep the mind clear, inducing movement of the physical and subtle energies.

The lungs' nature is of the phlegm and wind humor. They cool down bile heat by sustaining the movement of cooling energy and the circulation of humidity, which they receive from the brain (the phlegm seat). The lungs are particularly vital organs, sustaining life through respiration. Psychologically, the lungs produce fear, restlessness, and anxiety. They keep the physical body upright and help to balance its weight. The wind energy's waste product is sent from here to the large intestines, regulating descending wind. The flower of the lungs is the nose, and the method through which the lungs contact the outer world is through smell and the nose consciousness.

14.4 LIVER (*CHINPA*)

- Location: upper right abdomen
- Color: brown
- Element: fire
- Physiology: regulates the blood, maintains the bile humor and fire element
- Psychic function: hatred and anger

- Root: gallbladder
- Waste product: bile secretion
- Flower: eyes

The liver is ruled by the fire element. In Tibetan it is called *chinpa*, which also means "precious," "delicate," and "dear." The liver is red-brown and located on the right side of the ribcage, at the level of BV8–9 (thoracic vertebrae 7 and 8). It is like a fruit hanging from the vena cava trunk, in front of the vertebrae. *Chinpa* is the principal organ derived from the mother's blood energy and fire nature. The 85th chapter of the *Oral Instruction Tantra* describes it thus: [8]

The liver is like a rock arching over a cliff.

The liver receives food essence (*dangma*) via the portal veins from the digestive organs and transforms it into blood. It plays the role of the queen to the heart-king. It produces blood and supplies it to the heart. It is an extremely important organ as it governs metabolism and is the gate for the transformation of the body constituents, as well as processing the waste products. It governs digestion through the digestive fire and regulates temperature. *Chinpa* also gives strength to the upper and lower back, the spinal vertebrae, and the legs. It induces yawning and sleep, increases appetite, generates digestive heat, and clears bile, blood, and skin. In addition, it regulates the functions of the intestines, balances weight, rules eyesight, and maintains the blood vessels. The liver digests the fire element in foods in particular, absorbing it via the duodenum, thus sustaining the bile system. It also derives blood constituents from each of the five elements of the *dangma*, distributing these throughout the whole body.

Psychologically, the liver gives intelligence, a sharp mind, anger, aggression, jealousy, and fear. The waste product of the blood becomes bile juice (bile salts).

---

8 Ibid., 433.

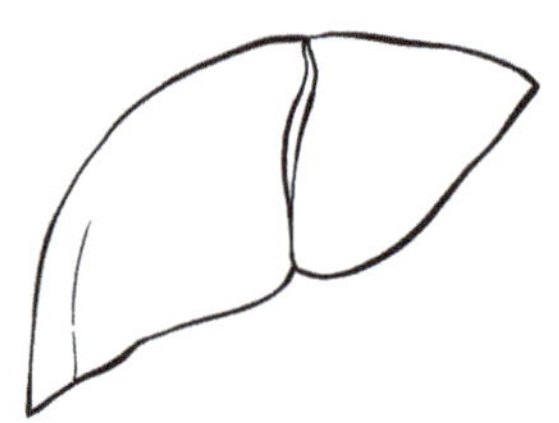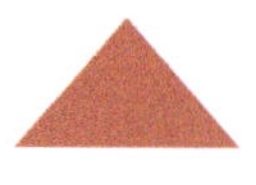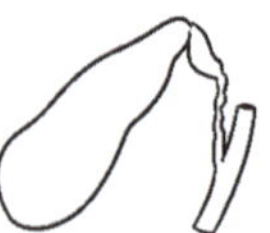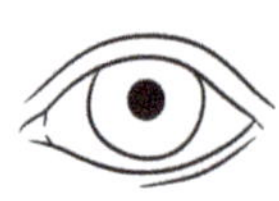

FIGURE 14.6 The liver and its functional links

Bile juice's *dangma* becomes *chuser* and goes back into the blood, becoming an important substance that sustains the blood function. Bile juice flows to the intestines to aid digestion and regulates bowel movement. The eyes are the flowers of the liver. They receive visual impressions through the eye consciousness.

14.5 SPLEEN (*CHERPA*)

- Location: upper left abdomen (under the ribs)
- Color: dark purple-brown
- Element: earth
- Physiology: digestion and intestinal gas formation, maintenance of phlegm
- Psychic function: sadness, pride, and greed
- Root: stomach
- Waste product: stomach mucus
- Flower: lips

The spleen is called *cherpa*, which implies it is a shy, timid, sad, and delicate organ. It is of the earth element, and functions like a junior queen to the king. It is greenish dark brown. It is a flat organ of a round, bread-like shape, located on the left side of the rib cage at the level of BV11 (the 10th thoracic vertebra). The spleen, like the liver, is derived principally from the mother's blood energy. The 85th chapter of the *Oral Instruction Tantra* describes the spleen as follows:[9]

> The spleen is thick at the edges and thin in the center, like bread.

Cherpa helps digest food into nutrients (*dangma*) and transports these to the liver and the heart. It sustains the function of the lymphatic system and produces weight, lymph, fat, and dampness in general.

It maintains the functions of the lips and stomach, and intestinal wind flow (gas). The spleen absorbs the earth element present in food and utilizes it to sustain phlegm as well as the stability of the body-mind. The spleen also supports the energetic base of the other elements. It is of a cool and heavy nature.

The digestive function of the spleen is not mentioned in biomedicine. The spleen is said to be a blood reservoir and blood filter (removing old red blood cells, transforming hemoglobin into bilirubin that is then sent to the liver), and has an immunological function (creation of antibodies). Although spleen physiology is barely mentioned in Sowa Rigpa, spleen pathologies are associated with gastric and intestinal symptoms. In pharmacology, a lot of digestion-improving medicines are indicated for the spleen.

Psychologically, the spleen produces a phlegm personality and emotions, fear, sadness, depression, melancholy, a slow mind, patience, tolerance, stability, concentration, love, compassion, pride, and greed. The spleen's waste products are accumulated in the stomach in the form of mucus (decomposing phlegm), which aids digestion. Its flowers are the lips of the mouth, and it contacts the world through speech and the tactile consciousness.

---

9   Ibid.

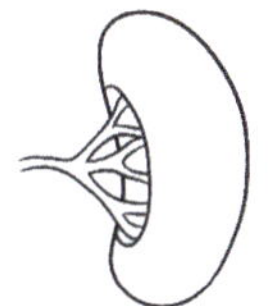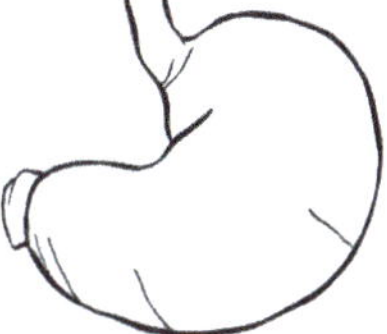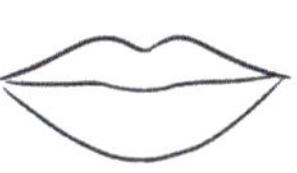

FIGURE 14.7 The spleen and its functional links

14.6 KIDNEYS (*KHELMA*)

- Location: lower back
- Color: brown
- Element: water
- Physiology: regulates the water system and element
- Psychic function: fear and jealousy
- Root: urinary bladder
- Waste product: urine
- Flower: ears

The kidneys are called *khelma*, which signifies "transporter," "carrier," "strength," or "animal pack." The kidneys are seen as the carriers of the body's weight load. *Khelma* are water element organs that control the water system of the body. The kidneys are said to function like a powerful foreign minister. They are located in the BV14–15 area (lumbar vertebrae 1 and 2). They are brown and resemble ears in their size and shape. The kidneys are also sustainers of blood energy. The 85th chapter in the *Oral Instruction Tantra* describes them in the following way:[10]

> The right and left kidneys are like strong men carrying the beam of a house.

Khelma protect the body kingdom from the external and internal enemies of fever, infection, inflammation, and heat. This defense may be compromised by taking on too many responsibilities, leading to backache and stress. The kidneys and heart function together to circulate blood and water from the head, along the spinal column, and down to the legs. Blood and water reach all parts of the body, then returning to the kidneys and urinary bladder to be filtered. The kidneys nourish the body with the water element, help digest food, and transport food essence. They are the main water organ of the body. The kidneys rule sexual activity, urination, menstruation, ejaculation, and the power of the back and legs.

Psychologically, the kidneys govern sexual desire, fear, jealousy, pride, attachment, and love. The waste product of the kidneys is urine, which is collected in the bladder and eliminated by descending wind. The flowers of the kidneys are the ears, which contact the world through hearing and the ear consciousness.

---

10 Ibid.

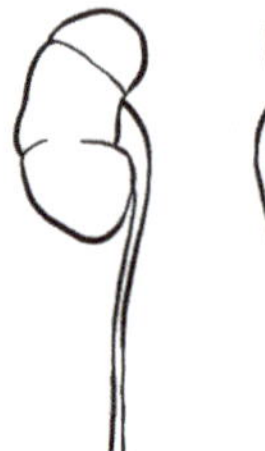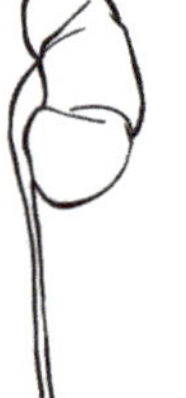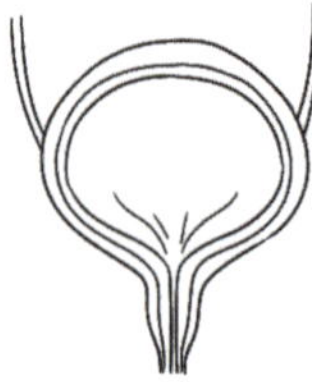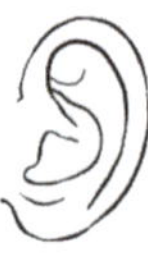

FIGURE 14.8 The kidneys and their functional links

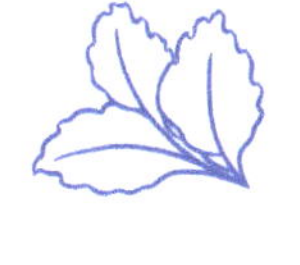

CHAPTER 15

THE SIX HOLLOW ORGANS
(*NÖ DRUK*)

The six hollow organs or "containers" (*nö druk*) are energy producers, like factories or workers. The stomach mixes food. The small intestine digests and absorbs the *dangma* while the rest is transformed into stool in the colon. Each digestive organ contains an intestinal flora of countless bacteria (*zé drülwé sinbu*), which help with digestion (*zé juwa*). Digestion takes place through the contribution of phlegm in the stomach, bile in the small intestine, and wind in the colon. The gallbladder produces the digestive fire. The urinal bladder collects the liquid waste products. The reproductive organs collect the final body essence consisting of reproductive fluids, the treasure of the body. *Dangma* is transported via the portal veins to the liver and transformed into blood, which nourishes the organs and the whole body. Eventually, the refined part of the reproductive fluids becomes radiance (*dang*). *Dang* is a product of the hollow organs that is further refined by the vital organs. The *nö druk* also collect waste products and clean the body. This not only comprises physical waste products but also the elimination of more subtle aspects such as undesired experiences, stress, and tension. A tense stomach could impact the chest area, heart, and shoulders, for

TABLE 15.1 The correspondences of the six vessel organs

	Hollow organ	Analogy	Element	Emotional base[1]	Functions
1.	Stomach (*powa*)	Cooking pot	Earth	Sadness, stress, anxiety	Digests food, especially earth element
2.	Small intestine (*gyuma*)	Attendant to liver	Space	Anger, fear, desire	Further digests food, absorbs nutrients, especially bile and fire element food
3.	Large intestine (*long ga*)	Attendant to spleen	Wind	Sensitivity, internal conflict	Further digests food, especially wind element food
4.	Gallbladder (*nötri*)	Nutrient or spice sachet	Fire	short temper, aggression	Collects bile juice, regulates metabolism and the intestines, produces chuser
5.	Urinary bladder (*gangpa*)	Sewage tank	Water	Impatience, fear	Collects wastewater, urine
6.	Reproductive organs (*kyépel wangpo*)	Treasure house	All five (male water dominant, female fire)	Lust, jealousy, aggression	Produces reproductive fluids, transmits heredity

---

1   Healthy organs produce corresponding positive emotions. Sexual stimulation of the reproductive organs is a source of bliss.

instance, whereas anger and impatience accumulated in the small intestine may cause headache and diarrhea. Long-term worries and fear can manifest as colitis, leading to further mental instability. Strong dissatisfaction and aggression may provoke a gallbladder disorder. Excessive fear could disturb the urinary bladder. In this way, the condition of the hollow organs impacts our state of mind, while emotional instability may also cause physical disorders.

The six vessel organs are called *nŏ*, "sacs" or "containers," because of their storage properties. They remain empty when they are not filled with food or other substances, expanding when filled with food, beverages, or waste products. The hollow organs are the servants, helpers, attendants, and workers of the vital organs:

1. The heart is linked to the small intestine
2. The lungs are associated with the colon
3. The liver is linked to the gallbladder
4. The spleen is related to the stomach
5. The kidneys are connected to the bladder
6. The reproductive organs are 'common hollow organs': phlegm nature but associated with all organs, which cooperate to produce the reproductions fluids

15.1 STOMACH (*POWA*)

- Location: below the diaphragm
- Element: earth
- Color: greyish pink
- Physiology: stores and digests food
- Psychic function: accumulates sadness, stress, and anxiety when out of balance
- Fruit: spleen
- Waste product: food residue
- Flower: lips

Powa means "spilling," "passing" or "transferring" a substance from one place to another. The stomach receives food through the mouth and passes it to the intestine. The 85th chapter of the *Oral Instruction Tantra* explains the appearance of the stomach in this way:[2]

> The stomach, the food container, is like a withering radish with four folds.

The stomach lies at the level of BV12 (11th thoracic vertebra) and is linked to the vena cava as well as the back of the aorta. The stomach is connected to

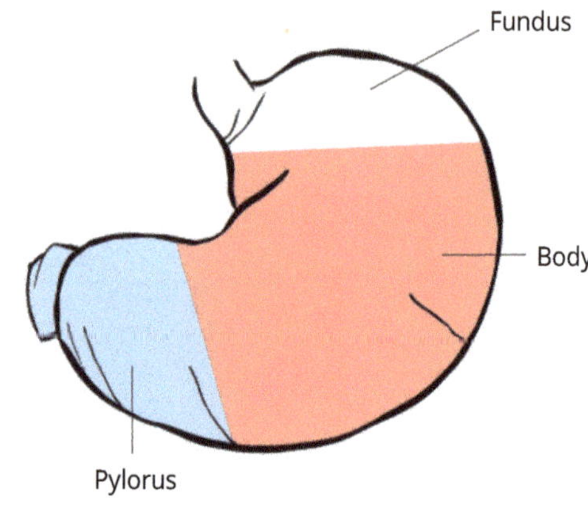

FIGURE 15.1 The three sections of the stomach

the esophagus and ends at the duodenum. It is also described as a hanging bag or a stale radish, since it is small and folded when empty, and expands when filled with food and liquid. The stomach has three regions: upper, middle, and lower, where the phlegm, bile and wind humors prevail respectively. The size of the stomach is said to be eight fingers in height and 12 fingers in width. The stomach receives food and passes it to the right side into the duodenum, and then to the small intestine. *Powa* is related to the spleen. As an earth element organ, it holds and centers the energy of the body.

The stomach is like a cooking pot because it keeps and digests food. All three humors are active in the stomach (see Chapter 10 on general digestion). The first is decomposing phlegm, mainly in the stomach's upper part. It functions like water in a cooking pot, in the form of a liquid secretion similar to saliva. It makes the bolus smooth, helps break down food, and supports absorption of the sweet-tasting nutrients of the earth element through the stomach's pores. This increases the phlegm humor and its constituents. The second humor is digestive bile, *médrö*, which is the digestive fire. It is mainly located in the duodenum, but also actively functions from the center of the stomach. It digests the fire element, absorbs sour-tasting nutrients, and sends them to the liver via the portal vein channels. This increases the bile humor and its constituents. The third is fire-like wind. It is mainly located in the lower stomach and colon. It functions like gas, fueling the flames of *médrö*. It further digests food and absorbs bitter-tasting nutrients, sending them to the liver via the portal veins. This increases the wind humor and its constituents. The stomach also contains phlegm-associated bacteria and parasites (*bésin*) that usually support digestion. Disharmony of these

---

2 Ibid.

organisms may lead to many disorders, including peptic ulcers induced by *Heliobacter pylori*. In short, when the humors are in harmony in the stomach and the body as a whole, they produce healthy energy for the body-mind, which results in good overall health and wellbeing.

Psychologically, the stomach is the seat of sadness, melancholy, and suffering due to stress, tension, depression, and trauma. There are two stomach waste products. The solid waste products pass down through the intestines and become stool, while the liquid waste matter is absorbed by the intestines and becomes urine.

15.2 SMALL INTESTINE (*GYUMA*)

- Location: below the stomach
- Element: space
- Color: grey
- Physiology: digests food and absorbs nutrients
- Psychic function: anger, fear, and desire
- Fruit: heart
- Waste product: food residue
- Flower: tongue

Gyuma refers to a long tube or tunnel, to something that is lazy, slow, and curved like a long meandering river. It is a hollow organ located at the level of BV17 (4th lumbar vertebra), linked energetically to the heart, and ruled by the space element. The upper small intestine is attached to the end of the stomach, and its end joins the ascendant colon on the right side of the abdomen. The 85th chapter of the *Oral Instruction Tantra* states:[3]

> The upper and lower small intestine are like a filled irrigation canal.

The small intestine has three parts in which nutrition is absorbed by means of villi (*powé pu*, or *gyumé pu*). Gastro-intestinal villi are described in Tibetan medicine as "stomach hairs." These can be destroyed by hidden fever (*gaptsé*), becoming the cause of chronic digestive disorders such as celiac disease. The upper part of the small intestine is where the duodenum (*zangtsak lugu go*, or *gyusor chunyi*) joins the stomach; this part is dominated by digestive bile. The pancreas, which is described metaphorically as the burner on a gas stove, is attached here. The middle part or jejunum is under the control of the wind humor. It transports foodstuffs but is otherwise empty. The bottom part or ileum is joined to the large intestine,

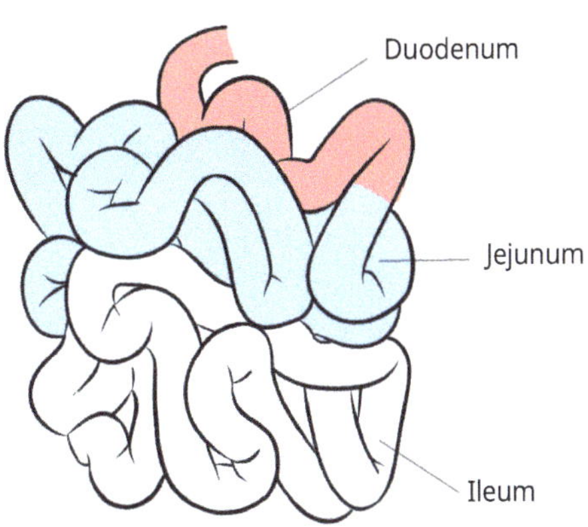

FIGURE 15.2 The three sections of the small intestine

and is governed by the phlegm humor. This is where stool is kept. The small intestine contains bile bacteria and parasites (*trisin*) that aid digestion.[4] The small intestine is described analogically as an attendant to the crown queen (the liver). It is where digestive bile actively functions. The majority of the food essence is digested and absorbed here before being transported to the liver via the portal veins. The small intestine is responsible for digesting food of the space element in particular, such as foods that are empty inside like peppers. It also processes foods associated with the fire element such as spicy ingredients, alcohol, oils and fats, and foods possessing sour, salty, or pungent tastes.

Psychologically, the small intestine is the seat of anger, stress and tensions that originate from hatred. The small intestine collects the waste products of the heart, the space element, and the bile humor.

15.3 COLON (*LONG GA*)

- Location: four fingers to right and left side of the navel
- Element: air
- Color: grey
- Physiology: digests food and separates nutrients from stool
- Psychic function: sensitivity, internal conflict
- Fruit: lungs
- Waste product: food residue in the form of stool
- Flower: nose

---

3   Ibid.

4   These include parasites such as pinworms (Oxyuridae), which may attack the digestive system, anus, genitals, etc.

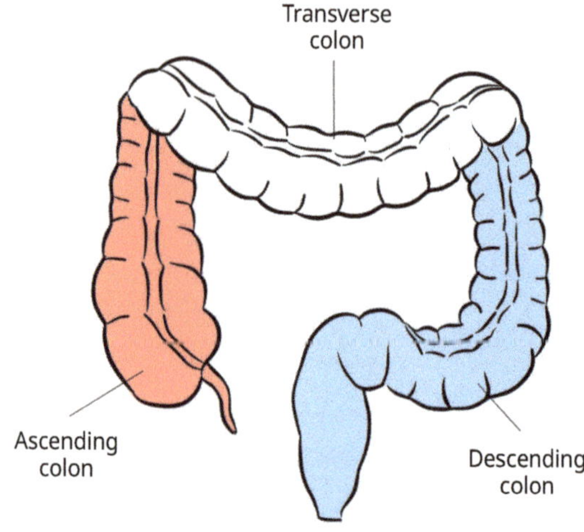

FIGURE 15.3 The three sections of the colon, and the rectum

The large intestine (*long*, or *long ga*) is a horse-shoe-shaped organ that is also said to resemble a leisurely moving gas-filled balloon. More comparisons are found in the 85th chapter of the *Oral Instruction Tantra*:[5]

The colon is connected to the small intestine and ends at the rectum (*nyéma*). Energetically, it is linked to the lungs. It is located above the navel, at the level BV16 (the 3rd lumbar vertebra), and consists of three parts: ascendant, transverse, and descendant. Bile dominates the ascendant or first part of the colon, while the transverse or middle colon is dominated by phlegm. The descendant colon joins with the rectum, which is referred to as a pouch or storeroom for stool. All three sections are generally governed by wind, and the rectum especially is controlled by descending wind (*tursel lung*), which controls the elimination of stool. *Long* is ruled by the lungs' wind energy. Analogically, it functions as attendant to the queen because it absorbs wind element nutrients (with bitter, astringent, and certain spicy flavors) and transports them to the liver and spleen. The large intestine digests food, thus sustaining the wind humor and its constituents. Related to this, it is sometimes described as the fan of the wind humor. The colon and rectum are islands on which various communities of bacteria and intestinal parasites reside. These parasites (*long sin*) help digest foodstuff and transform it into stools. Psychologically, the colon is a seat of emotional sensitivity. It is easily blocked, and cramps may follow

strong feelings. The colon is the organ that collects gross waste products from food and subtle waste products from the lungs. The rectum is the final part of the colon, which stores fecal matter. The 85th chapter describes it as follows:[6]

The three hollow organs described above represent the three stages of digestion and are the principal seats of the three humors. The stomach is a phlegm organ, where phlegm energy principally functions. The small intestine is the seat of the bile humor. The colon is a wind humor organ. Each of the three digestive organs contains different types of microorganisms, which multiply naturally and aid in the transformation of foodstuff into stool and urine. Such beings may also constitute an important factor that influences the mind, whereas the mind can equally impact and disturb their functions. Together, these three hollow organs are the basic energy factories that sustain and regulate the humoral system. They are also the first organs to become ill if the relationship between the humors becomes unbalanced or is disturbed by poor quality food, stress, or tension.

15.4 GALLBLADDER (*NÖTRI*)

- Location: under the right-side ribs, below the liver
- Element: fire
- Color: dark greenish
- Physiology: digests food and produces *chuser*
- Psychic function: anger and resentment
- Fruit: liver
- Waste product: collects blood residue, of which the essence becomes *chuser*; its waste product colors the urine
- Flower: eyes and skin

Nötri refers to the gallbladder, the bile container. It is a fire organ that is located at BV10 (the 9th thoracic vertebra), below the liver, at the level of the elbow. It is a dark greenish, hanging organ approximately six fingers in height and three in width. *Nötri* is a hollow organ attached to the liver, from which it collects bile.

---

5 Ibid.

6 Ibid.

7 Darmo sman rams pa blo bzang chos grags, 1991, vol. 2, 397, states that *yangzhak* (*g.yang gzhag*) is like a ritual cake, with melted butter poured on it.

The 85th chapter of the *Oral Instruction Tantra* offers the following description:[8]

> The gallbladder lies aside the liver, like a hanging, golden pouch.

The gallbladder collects blood residue, produces heat, and secretes bile juice (*trikhu*), which becomes an important fluid that digests nutrients in the stomach, intestines, and other body parts. Practically, it is the material source of digestive bile. Tibetan medical texts do not explicitly mention bile salts or acid, but explain that bile heat produces body temperature and the digestive fire (*médrö*). Yet, the term "bile salt" also makes sense from a Sowa Rigpa perspective, as salt is considered warming, heavy (aiding downward flow), and a digestive aid. *Nötri* also refines bile juice into blood plasma (*chuser*, "yellow fluid") and sends this back to the blood through the liver. This process produces and sustains the bile humor. Plasma nourishes the blood, organs, and skin. The gallbladder is likened to a hanging bag of nutrients or spices because it gives vital energy to the blood and body constituents. Bile enters the digestive organs, supporting metabolism, gas flow, blood circulation, and the skin. The gallbladder digests food by neutralizing fat and food toxins, regulates intestinal functions, and changes urine's color. Malfunction of the gallbladder is a major source of chronic indigestion, (cold) bile disorders, bile-phlegm disorders, chronic brown phlegm, metabolic disorders, allergies and food intolerance, colitis, Crohn's disease, and other ailments. Malfunction of the gallbladder disturbs the bile parasites of the small intestine.

Psychologically, the gallbladder manifests hatred, anger, aggression, impulsiveness, impatience, fear, doubt, indecisiveness, and laziness.

15.5 URINARY BLADDER (*GANGPA*)

- Location: four fingers below the navel
- Element: water
- Color: grey
- Physiology: collects and expels urine
- Psychic function: impatience, fear
- Fruit: kidneys
- Waste product: liquid residues (urine)
- Flower: ears

The urinary bladder, located at the level of BV18 (the 5th lumbar vertebra), is compared to a sewage tank. The 85th chapter of the *Oral Instruction Tantra* further states:[9]

> The bladder mouth faces down like a water sack.

The bladder is linked to the kidneys. It is a sack for urine and its nature is of the water element. It is called *gang pa*, which means "expanding," as it enlarges when filled with urine. The bladder collects and expels the body's wastewater, acting as a sewage system. Pure water energy is absorbed and becomes the foundation of the water element in the body. It is a very sensitive organ and is connected psychologically to fear and stress.

---

8   Ibid.

9   Ibid.

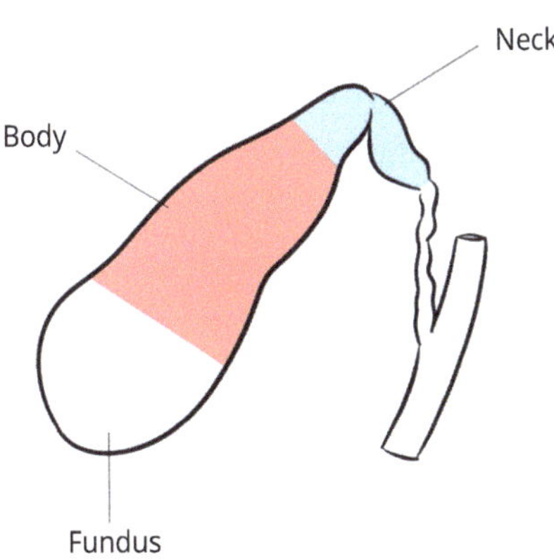

FIGURE 15.4 The three sections of the gallbladder

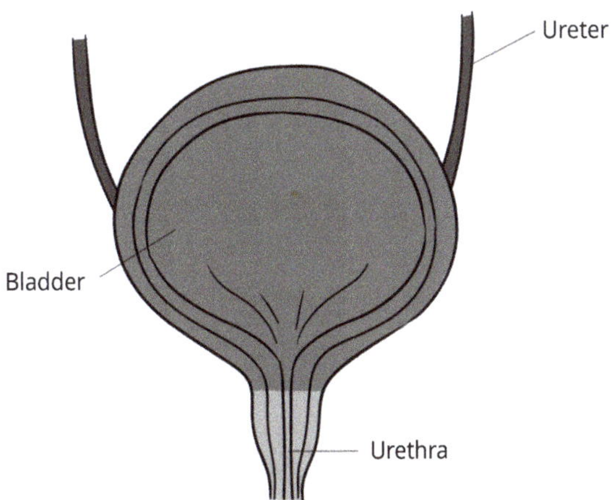

FIGURE 15.5 The urinary bladder

15.6 REPRODUCTIVE ORGANS (*KYÉPEL WANGPO*)

- Location: genital area
- Element: all elements, ; water (male) or fire (female) predominates
- Color: mixed
- Physiology: generates sexual desire and transmits heredity
- Psychic function: lust, jealousy, and aggression
- Fruit: all organs, but mainly the kidneys
- Waste product: sperm and menstruation
- Flower: the entire face

The reproductive organs are called *kyépel wangpo,* "the faculty that generates birth," or alternatively *samséu.* They are located at BV19 (the 1st sacral vertebra), and include the seminal vesicle and testicles for men, and the ovaries and uterus for women. The 85th chapter of the *Oral Instruction Tantra* notes:[10]

Samséu is a knot of channels, like a fleshy gland.

Samséu consists of *sam,* referring to thinking, and *séu,* a small berry. This implies that the reproductive organs are "small thinking organs" that give rise to emotions. These hollow organs expand in size when semen or menses are restored, reducing in size again after their expulsion from the body. Their functions include sexual intercourse, conception, and the maintenance of bodily strength. *Kyépel wangpo* produce semen and menses as well as giving the body radiance, power, impatience, nervousness, anger, and courage. The male *samséu* organ produces semen in the testicles seminal vesicles. The female *samséu* organ produces eggs in the ovaries and menstrual blood as the lining of the uterus, which leaves the body as monthly menstruation. The *samséu* organs are the roots of the body's subtle power. They are described as treasures are the final product of food energy, and because they contribute to the radiance or body light called *dang.*

---

10 Ibid.

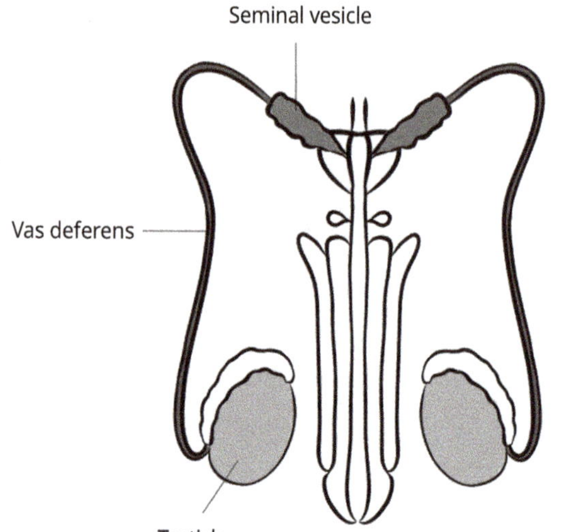

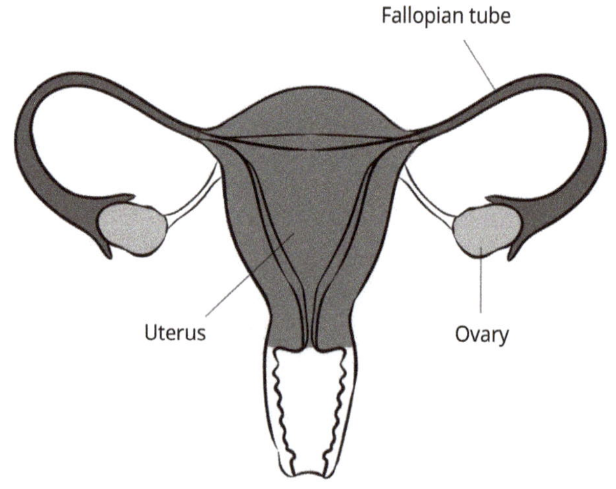

FIGURE 15.6 The male and female reproductive organs

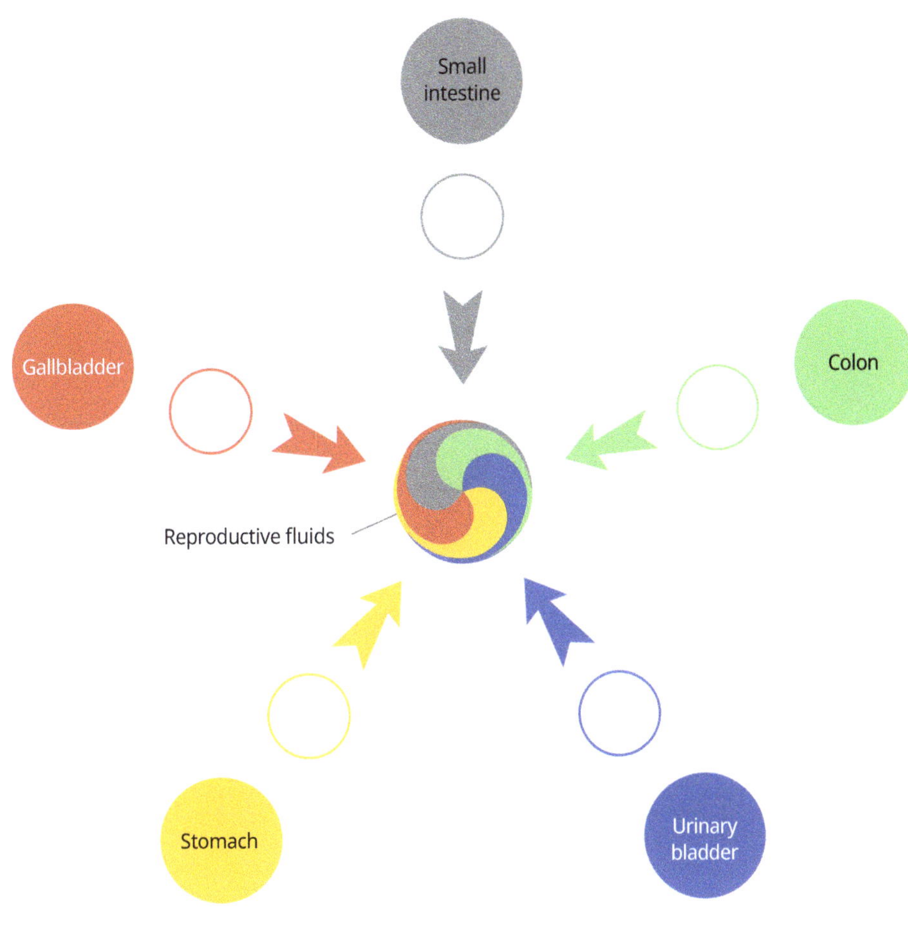

FIGURE 15.7 The reproductive fluids incorporate vital essence energy (*dang*) from each of the five hollow organs, which correspond to the five elements

Summary of the solid and hollow organs

The hollow organs are the main centers for the production and distribution of *dangma* throughout the body and channels. They also produce the physical body's subtlest energy. The solid organs receive nutrients from the hollow organs, refining and utilizing them to sustain body-mind activity. Therefore, the hollow organs are described in analogical form as resembling, factories, storerooms, containers, or transportation channels. The hollow organs are where substances are gathered in the body, and where the alchemical transmutation of food energy occurs. This transmutation enables the highest levels of the mind, such as intelligence, improved awareness, and heightened frequency of thoughts and emotions. All these processes are determined by the *dangma* that is processed via the functions of the hollow and vital organs.

CHAPTER 16

THE HEAD AND THE FIVE SENSE ORGANS

Having described the vital and hollow organs, we now come to the five sense organs (*wangpo nga*). They act like rooms and windows to the sense consciousnesses. The sense organs are the flowers of the five vital organs. They ornament the body and are its instruments of contact and communication. The head is like the roof of the house, and is shaped like a bamboo ball. It is composed of the scalp bones, brain, glands, sense organs, and three channels. The scalp is covered with 21,600 hairs, a number that corresponds to the average number of breaths a person takes each day. There are five sense consciousnesses connected to five sense organs: the eyes, nose, ears, tongue, and skin. The chapter on similes in the *Explanatory Tantra* states:[1]

> The five sense organs are like open windows.

There are six exterior objects: forms, sounds, odors, tastes, tactile objects, and mentally perceived phenomena. Each is associated with a sensory organ (mind being the sixth sense), which operates through the sense faculties or consciousnesses with the help of the five minor winds. The functioning of the sense consciousnesses brings balance, distributes inner *lung*, perceives external phenomena, and nourishes the body-mind. All information, feelings, and experiences are processed through the sense faculties before being transferred to the mental consciousness in the heart. There, the *künzhi* processes the positive, negative, and neutral actions, tallying or omitting them from the karmic memory bank depending on the importance of the action's result.

16.1 HEAD (*GO*)

The head is the seat of the gross mind. It contains all sensory consciousnesses and organs. Therefore, the head is referred to as the house of the sense organs. The similes chapter in the *Explanatory Tantra* describes the head thus:[2]

> The head and crown are like the roof of a multi-storied mansion.

There are seven head shapes or types that bear seven different brain qualities as described in chapter 83 of the *Explanatory Tantra* and the *Blue Beryl*.[3] These brain types have varying qualities and resistance to head injury. The brain's memory has to develop in each new life, requiring education and training. In the author's understanding, this typology also relates to the memory and strength of the mind as they can be linked to the seven body constitutions (see also Section 9.3):

1. A wind constitution head is generally elongated, ; wind types are mentally more creative, but have instable memory

2. Bile people's heads have a protruded occiput; they have sharp memory, are rational and intelligent, yet impatient

3. A phlegm head is shaped like a shoulder blade; phlegm people are slow in thinking and remembering, their thoughts are initially unclear but can also be profound

4. Wind-bile heads are rectangular; this type comes with fast and sharp memory, but forgetting easily what is not repeated

---

1   Ibid., 20.

2   G.yu thog yon tan mgon po, 1993, 20.

3   Sde srid sangs rgyas rgya mtsho, 1994, vol. 2, 916–17.

5. A bile-phlegm person's head is round; this type of people is pragmatic and has good memory, but also many conflicting thoughts

6. Phlegm-wind people's heads are flat; they have poor memory, and much confusion

7. The most balanced person's head is flattened and oblong; it has the memory and mind of the three humors in balance

The *Four Tantras* do not clearly lay out the relationships between the sense organs, nerves, and the brain. Except for descriptions of the major blood vessels, scalp bones and nerves of the head, there is little information to be found, especially on brain anatomy. As classical texts lack detail on these important connections, there is a need to accommodate details from modern biomedical anatomy and physiology. Despite these shortcomings, head injuries, headaches, and their remedies are well-described in the *Oral Instruction Tantra*.

Bones and muscles

The head is said to consist of 59 different bones. The skull bones are divided into those of male, female, and neutral bone quality. The nature of male skull bones is thick, small, and spongy yet hard. Female skull bones are thin, smooth, and gentle. Neutral skull bones are large, spongy, but not very resistant to injury. The head has many muscles; four of them are of foremost importance. They are listed here with their respective analogies:

1. The crown head muscle is like coiled fat (*zhakgor khyil dra*)

2. The occiput (including neck) muscles are like hanging fishes (*nya dang ship dra*)

3. The fontanel muscle is shaped like a slackened bow (*zhushül tang dra*)

4. The temporal muscles are like piled sheep's kidneys (*luk khel tsek dra*)

There are numerous other muscles in the neck, throat, temporal region, cheeks, mouth, and sense organs.

Connecting channels

The connecting blood, nerve, and lymphatic channels (*tsa*) of the head are complex. They are described in detail in the sections on wounds in the 83rd chapter of the *Oral Instruction Tantra*. A selection of *tsa* groups will be discussed below.

1. Blood channels

The head blood channels are collectively called *tsojé dartsa*, the "life-supporting silk threads." This term traditionally refers to the external veins (and arteries) covering the scalp. There are also blood vessels inside the skull, covering the brain. *Lépé gyadar*, which literally means "Chinese silk of the brain," is a protective layer covering the brain that corresponds to the meninges. Branches from the major blood vessels connected to the heart become the four external and internal vessel trees of the ears (*nawé chinang jönshing zhi*). They ramify further and converge at the top of the scalp. There, the four most conspicuous veins are called *nyen gyi rétak zhi*, the "four head-binding cords."

These channels branch from the neck's left and right blood channels and go up to the head and around the front and back of the ears. They branch further and connect in and out of the brain, resembling the leaves of a tree that covers the brain. The channels run from the occipital bone to the cheekbones, then join the brain, and again join at the anterior fontanel (*düso sum*). Essentially, these blood channels stitch the skull bones together. They are associated with the channels from the muscles, bones, and brain, which all converge in the crown point of the head. The main arterial and venous channels branch countless times inside the head, and are also connected with the inner organs.

2. Nerve channels

There are two types of nerve channels: the 13 hidden nerves connecting to the inner organs, and the six peripheral nerve channels connecting to the extremities. These are illustrated in the chapters on channels (see Section 17.5).

3. Bone channels (*rü tsa*)

The three main skull bone channels are:

- *dungtsuk* ("piercing spear") channels in three locations: the crown, the fontanel area, and the occiput. They are also called *zertsa* ("pain-causing channels"); they correspond to the skull blood channels.

- The *trényel* ("lying on one's side") channel, also called *bönpö tö* ("Bönpo's top knot," referring to a dreaded knot of hair on top of the head); It is located two times four fingers above each of the two ears.

- The *khyampo* ("wandering") bone channel has three subtypes that pervade the entire head.

Hairs cover the scalp, and the scalp covers the skull. The skull covers the brain, and the brain is covered by a silk-like membrane and blood vessels. The brain encompasses the glands, so metaphorically it is like a jewel box kept inside a pagoda.

16.2 BRAIN (*LÉPA*)

The brain is located safely inside the skull. It is similar in shape to a walnut. It is covered with a grey membrane, the meninges (*gya dar*). It has two lobes and is the size of two cupped hands. The healthy brain generates gross mind, thoughts, memory, and physical actions. The two brain hemispheres correspond to the body's two lateral channels and the brain's center corresponds to the middle channel. Symbolically, the brain can be understood through the functioning of these two channels. It is like day and night or sky and earth. In tantra, it may correspond to *tapshé*, skillful means and wisdom. In a Tibetan medical context, we can say "male" and "female," or phlegm and bile. Without question, the brain produces gross mind and emotions. It has a memory bank of this life just as the heart has a karmic one. The head stores life memories, some of which are transferred to the heart chakra. The sensory organs are considered the doors or windows of consciousness. The head is of the

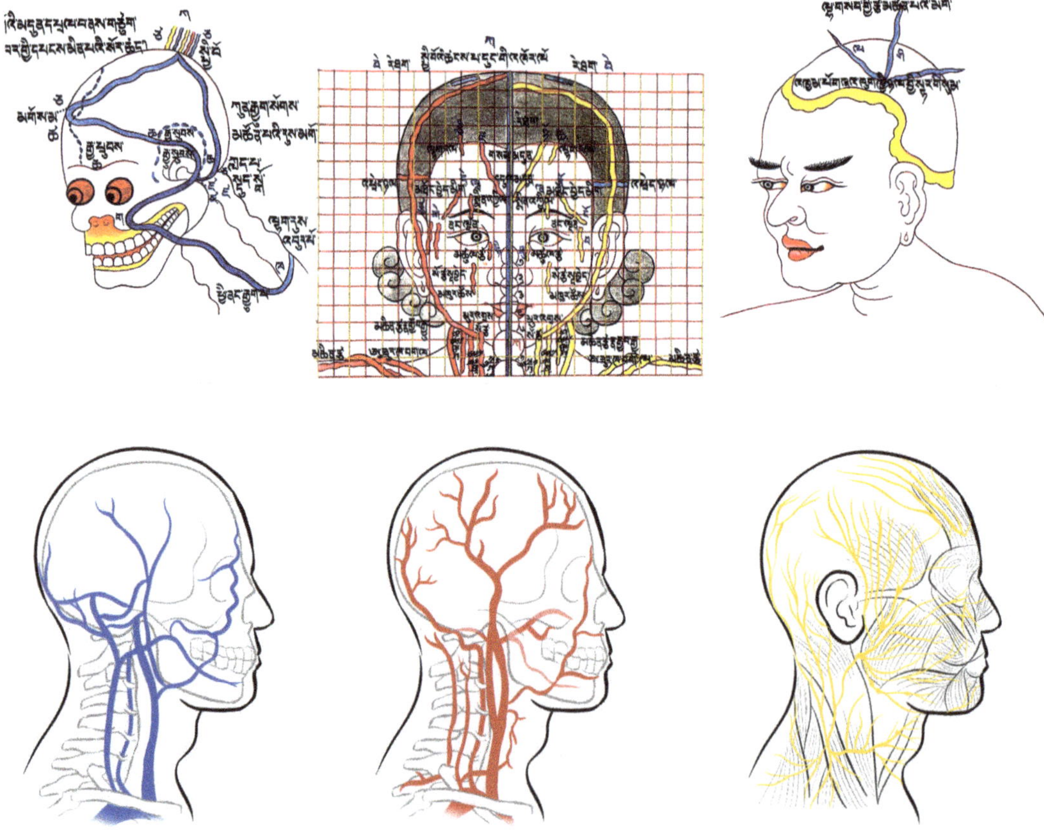

FIGURE 16.1 Comparison of traditional illustrations and biomedical anatomy of the head's veins, arteries, and lymph vessels

phlegm humor and is one of the heaviest parts of the body. It resembles a pagoda; it is the roof of the body house. The tip of the pagoda is *chitsuk*, the central crown point (ZH1).

The brain is made up of phlegm-energy grey matter and is seen as the mother of all glands. The cerebral fluid around the brain is an ocean of phlegm. This energy flows down through the spinal column, to the coccyx, and then to the feet. Bile and wind heat warm up and circulate the water up through the body and again to the brain. This process is like water from a snowy mountain that runs down and reaches the ocean. Bile heat causes water to evaporate, which becomes clouds, then rain, and then snow again. The brain is the root of the nervous, lymphatic, and endocrine systems. The lymphatic system is the body's cooling irrigation system. Like rain, its water streams down and cools the bile heat from the head to the lungs and abdomen, nourishing the constituents and organs. The brain receives blood and nutrition via the throat's right and left channels, including the basilar and anterior cerebral arteries (*nyen gyi rétak zhi*). Toxins are evacuated via the temporal and external jugular veins.

The sense organs have both automatic and voluntary components. All processes take place in the head, which is the seat of life-sustaining wind. This wind branches into five minor winds (*yenlak gi lung nga*) that function in each sense organ, acting as memory collectors. To summarize, the brain has the following functions:

- General control of bodily functions
- Sensory perception and processing
- Maintaining the mind and mental functions
- Regulating the *lung* humor
- Regulating the lymphatic and endocrine systems

Life-sustaining wind receives energy from transcendental wind (*yéshé kyi lung*) as a result of the breathing process. Its consumption is like burning fuel, which produces energy while reducing the remaining lifespan. Damage to or a malfunctioning of life-sustaining wind may cause psychological and even psychiatric disorders. Another important subject related to the head is that the brain is the base of satisfying phlegm, an important product of the glands. Satisfying phlegm gives the mind a sense of satisfaction, which is brought about by contact of the sense organs with their associated objects. A malfunction in this phlegm branch may lead to a dissatisfied mind, manifesting disorders such as bulimia, memory loss, and depression.

As described above, the brain is the house of the glands and channels. However, it is also the house of the five sense faculties and their channels, and the dwelling place of the five sense consciousnesses. The development and functions of the *yenlak gi lung nga* is illustrated in Section 6.3 The sense faculties, minor winds and consciousnesses perform the functions of seeing, hearing, feeling, smelling, and tasting, whilst the sixth sense is the mental consciousness that assists in analysis and decision-making. The development of the power of the sense consciousnesses is strongly supported by the six external object sources (*kyéché druk*). Buddhist logic tenets explain the relationship that exists between sense consciousnesses (subject) and external sources (object). They define functional characteristics, but do not explain the nature of the mind and consciousnesses. This interpretation is like a camera reflecting an image.

Tibetan medical texts describe the brain as the seat of ignorance and the base of phlegm in the body. Yutok made it clear that the ignorant mind functions from the brain, and that the body develops and is controlled through the brain. What is lacking, however, is precise knowledge on these topics relating to brain structure and function. Perhaps this lack of precision is due to the fact that Tibetan Buddhism does not consider the brain as equivalent to the mind. The brain is a complex system, a tool that coproduces the gross mind (*sem rakpa*) and sense consciousnesses, which in turn generate emotions. During sleep, consciousness dissolves in the heart, but the brain machinery continues to operate the nerves and filter memories. In this process, the neck and throat also play a vital mediating role.

16.3 FACE (*DONG*)

The face is the mirror or flower of the body, where all signs of positive and negative health and emotions appear. The forehead, especially between the eyebrows, is where *dang* blossoms and radiates its light. The sensory organs are positioned on the face for optimal functioning. The face is divided into three parts: the forehead is phlegm in nature, the middle of the face is bile, and below the nose to the jaw belongs to wind.

16.4 EYES (*MIK*)

The eye organs are flowers of the liver and have a fire nature. Their shape is said to resemble the liver. The eye's three main parts are the sclera, pupil, and iris. The eye is a ball-like organ with an intricate structure. It is referred to as the inner light of the body-mind that is emitted from the liver and gallbladder. The light channel is called *gyangjé ser gyi drönmé*, "the golden lamp seen from a distance". This inner light connects with outer light, enabling the eye consciousness to perceive and recognize objects. The eyes' heat consumes the eye secretions that are released by the brain's satisfying phlegm, especially when the liver is hyperfunctioning.

Different types of eyes are distinguished:

- Wind constitution: black or dark irises, sharp eyes
- Bile constitution: yellow or brown irises (generally)
- Phlegm constitution: big and dark eyes; white people have grey or whitish eyes
- Bile-phlegm constitution: dark or brown irises
- Wind-bile constitution: light bluish-yellow irises
- Phlegm-wind constitution: green eyes (if white-skinned)

The three components of the eyes correspond to the three humors: phlegm (the white sclera), bile (the iris), and wind (the pupil). The eyes perceive images and qualities such as size and color with the help of seeing bile. A deficiency in this humoral branch may cause color blindness or manifest as other eyesight diseases. The eye organs are like a camera, the consciousness is like the photographer, and seeing bile functions like a battery. The *lu* minor wind acts as a vehicle for the eye consciousness and transfers visual information to the mental consciousness.

16.5 NOSE (*NA*)

The nose is the flower of the lungs, functioning in respiration as a wind door. It is also associated with phlegm mucus and is therefore of the earth element. *Na* has two nostrils, corresponding in shape and number to the lungs. The nose is referred to as an empty house that is connected to the nasal cavities. The *Subsequent Tantra* explains that the nose is the door to the brain.[4]

The nasal cavities are connected to the brain, eyes, ears, and the entire face. It is the body's breathing valve that eliminates toxins from the upper body. Its other important function is to perceive smell, which is analyzed by the nose consciousness. Like the eyes, the nose has three components. The tip of the nose is associated with wind, the middle with bile, and the base belongs to phlegm. Experiencing and satisfying phlegm both function in the nose, enabling feelings

associated with good and bad smells. People of the wind constitution have long noses with down- or up-facing tips. Bile type noses are medium in size. Phlegm constitution people have flat, big noses. The *tsangpa* minor wind resides in the nose and helps to perceive smell. Imbalance of this minor wind produces a nervous and violent mind.

16.6 EARS (*NAWA*)

The ears are the flower of the kidneys. Externally, they bear a shape similar to a kidney. They are of the space element, allowing for the perception of sound via the ear consciousness. The ears consist of outer, middle, and inner chambers, which receive sound and speech via the eardrums. The ear consciousness analyzes and records sounds in the ear memory of the mind. The outer circle of the ear is wind-dominated, the middle is ruled by bile, and the inner or root part belongs to phlegm. Experiencing and satisfying phlegm both function in the ear, perceiving pleasant and unpleasant sounds. Those of wind constitution generally have a smaller ear size, bile types have medium-sized ears, and phlegm people have big, flat ears. The *Rübel* minor wind resides in the ears. It regulates the functions of hearing as well as movement of the extremities of the body.

16.7 MOUTH (*KHA*) AND TONGUE (*CHÉ*)

The mouth comprises several structures, such the tongue, teeth, gums, uvula, and upper and lower palates. It is the entrance gate for solid and liquid foods and a breathing passage. It is formed by a number of intricate anatomical components, including muscles, ligaments, nerves, bones, cartilage, and cavities. The mouth is connected to many other organs, including the nasal cavities, ears, and eyes; essentially the entire head. The gums (*so nyil*) or gingiva are a soft tissue that supports and holds the teeth. Gums are said to be connected to the liver and to be strongly related to blood circulation. The *Gyüzhi* describes 32 teeth (*so*):

- Eight precious front teeth (*chépé dün so gyé*) or incisors
- Four beautiful fanged teeth (*dzéjé kyi chéwa zhi*) or canines
- Eight cutting and grinding teeth (*chöjé kyi dram so gyé*) or molars
- Four junior peripheral teeth (*ta zhi so chung*) or wisdom teeth

---

4   Ibid., 620.

Teeth are waste products of bone and thus reflect the body's bone strength; weakened bones result in loss of teeth. The teeth are of wind and phlegm nature. The first teeth are called milk teeth (*o so*); they are lost at around eight years of age. The following teeth that grow remain for one's whole life, until they begin to fall out in old age. From about 45–50 years old, gum and teeth strength start to weaken.

The tongue is the flower of the heart. It is one of the wet sense organs that produce much saliva through their associated glands (*shermen*). The tongue is also divided into three parts. The tip of the tongue is wind, the middle bile, and the root phlegm. Information relating to the condition of specific organs is reflected in the tongue, which allows for diagnosis. Experiencing and satisfying phlegm both function in the tongue and sense the taste of good and bad food. The tongue consciousness observes these experiences and transmits them to the mental consciousness of the heart. People with wind constitutions have a bigger tongue whereas those with bile constitutions have medium-sized tongues. Phlegm people have smaller tongues. The *lhajin* minor wind functions in the tongue, supporting sensation and the experience of taste. This minor wind also makes one yawn and eliminates subtle toxins from the upper part of the body.

16.8 NECK AND THROAT (*KÉ DANG DRÉWA*)

The neck and throat, *ké* and *dréwa*, are included here as they are an important link between the head and chest regions. All three channels, the trachea, and the esophagus pass through them. In this manner, the throat resembles a narrow highway. The neck's main organs are the thyroid glands, and the neck is where ascending wind (*lung gyengyü*) functions. It flows through the chest, throat, mouth, and nose. This wind helps to expectorate mucus and saliva, removes toxins, and produces voice by means of the breath. It gives physical strength, improves the body's complexion and vigor, and clears the memory. The 84th chapter of the *Oral Instruction Tantra* describes the delicate gross anatomy of the neck in detail, covering the cervical bones, veins and arteries, nerves, muscles, tendons, and cartilage.

16.9 SKIN (*PAKPA*)

The skin is the flower of the spleen. It is the common body of the five elements. The body's main organ is the skin and tactility its main feeling. The skin is very sensitive, especially in the genital area. Experiencing

and satisfying phlegm both allow for the ability to experience good and bad sensations. The body consciousness observes and experiences these feelings, and sends them to the mental consciousness in the heart. People with a wind constitution have a thin and dry skin. Those of the bile constitution have an oily skin and face. Phlegm types have a smooth skin. The *norlhagyel* minor wind resides in the skin and experiences tactile sensations. It remains in the body even after death, until the body decomposes completely.

Conclusion on the organs

Tibetan medical researchers ought to undertake deeper study on the traditional explanations of the organs and their functions alongside biomedical anatomy, with the aim of expanding Sowa Rigpa.

Nevertheless, working on this subject has surprised the author and given great satisfaction. The *Gyüzhi* has described the organs, their shape and locations, their blood channels, and general anatomy and physiology through enlightened insight. The psychophysical dimension of the body-mind has been especially well-researched. In this regard, we can quite confidently declare that the Jangpa and Zurkhar schools are like the sun and moon in the Sowa Rigpa universe, and that Gongmen Könchok Delek was a great master and surgeon whose knowledge shines even brighter than the stars.

What is described in the *Gyüzhi* is generally sufficient for the practitioner of medicine. However, to specialize in certain organs or pathologies, we require more detail on anatomy. Sowa Rigpa's development has sadly been hampered by the recurrence of unfortunate political calamities, leading to a decline in the study of anatomy across the Tibetan plateau. Nevertheless, expertise in this field is as important as the chapters on humors, the mind, and emotions.

CHANNELS AND CHAKRAS

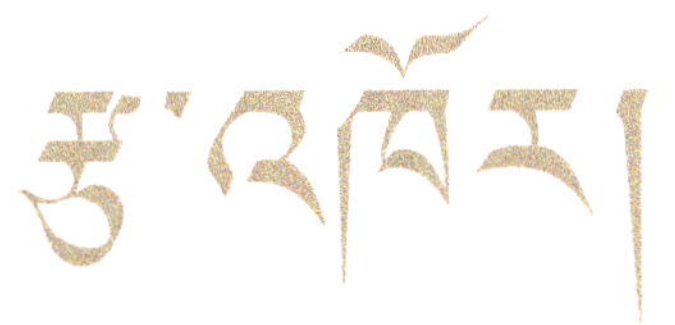

CHAPTER 17

CHANNELS

This chapter discusses the channels by dividing them into two main categories: nutritional passages (*gyulam buga*), and the networks of channels—nerves, blood, and lymphatic vessels—that are usually referred to when the term *tsa* is used. In general, *tsa* comprise all channels whilst *buga* are tube-like structures that distribute nutrition. They are pathways for *dangma*, blood, water, wind energy, and consciousness, thus carrying out essential sustaining functions. The structure of the *buga* and *tsa* is compared to that of a leaf's lines, where the midrib branches into lateral veins. The channels in the body have various shapes and sizes. Some channels such as the aorta are thick, and others like the capillaries are tiny. Some are micro-channels like the fine nerves and ductless lymphatic channels. Some *tsa* are longer than the body in length, and others are short and invisible to the eye.

In *Gyüzhi* medicine, *tsa* connotes the meaning "root" due to their function as sustainers of life. Life depends on the channels like a tree depends on its roots. Channels function on physical, subtle, and mental levels, with each system consisting of countless branches. All channels develop from the sixth week of fetal development onwards, as indicated in the embryology chapter of the *Explanatory Tantra* (see Section 13.4):[1]

> In the sixth week, the life channel forms from the navel.

17.1 NUTRITIONAL PASSAGES (*GYULAM BUGA*)

The nutritional passages (*buga*) have two subsections: internal passages and external orifices. The internal passageway begins with the mouth, continuing with the esophagus, stomach and intestines, and ends in the anus and urinary tract. *Dangma* travels to the liver and then to the blood and lymph channels, being subdivided into countless branches in the organs and tissues. The fourth chapter in the *Explanatory Tantra* on *buga* states:[2]

> Increase of *dangma* depends on the *buga*.
> Engaging in unwholesome diet and
> behavior harms the passages and produces disorders,
> resulting in excess and blockage of the
> waste products, and entrance or disruption of other channels.
> Unimpaired, clean channels give rise to good health.

Unwholesome conduct may lead to excess of the three humors, *dangma*, and waste products. This may cause a blockage, or may force fluids into other channels, which in turn attacks the other humors, causing disturbance. The direct cause of disease can be said here to be unclean food passages. The internal *buga* are divided into three groups: (1) the life-holding channel (*sok*), (2) the seven *dangma* passages (*zung*), and (3) the three waste product passages (*drima*).

13 internal passages (*nang gi buga chusum*)

There are 13 internal tubular channels where general and specific digestive processes as well as the transportation of d*angma* throughout the body take place. Elimination of waste products occurs through the nine external orifices.

1. The first *buga* is the *soktsa*, the principal life-holding channel of the body. It comprises the channels (including blood and lymph)

---

1 G.yu thog yon tan mgon po, 1993, 18.

2 Ibid. 25.

that transport the vital energy that fuels life: *soklung*. This energy flows out partially through the windpipe and nostrils.

Buga of *dangma*

2. The second *buga* consists of the digestive organs and the liver. It begins at the stomach, continues through the small and large intestines where nutrition is absorbed, and ends at the liver. It is called the *zung* or *dangma* passage.

3. The third is the blood passage between the liver and muscles.

4. The fourth exists between blood and fat, and is called the muscle passage.

5. The fifth is between muscles and bones. It is called the fat passage.

6. The sixth is between fat and bone marrow, the bone passage.

7. The seventh is the bone marrow passage between bone and the reproductive fluids.

8. The eighth channel is the reproductive organ channel that produces reproductive fluids and takes care of the transformation into *dang*.

Waste product *buga*

9. The ninth is the gross food product passage that transports waste from the stomach to the rectum. It carries waste products in the form of feces.

10. The 10th is the water waste product passage, which runs from the stomach and intestines to the urinary bladder, eliminating liquid waste in the form of urine.

11. The 11th waste product *buga* are the body's pores or perspiration channels, which eliminate waste products in the form of sweat.

Food pipe and liquid *buga*

12. The 12th channel transports the liquids absorbed from the digestive organs, which

travel to the bladder after being filtered by the kidneys.

13. The 13th channel is the food pipe. It starts from the mouth and finally reaches the colon.

Nine external orifices (*chi yi buga gu*)

There are nine external orifices: the mouth, the two eyes, the two nostrils, the two ears, the anus, and the genitals. These orifices are the body's doors to external contact with the environment, through which sensation occurs, including perceiving taste, visual stimuli, smells, sounds, and touch. They also serve to clear the body of waste products. The mouth, anus, and urinary tract are the basic passages for the elimination of gross waste products such as vomit, feces, and urine. Women have three additional *buga*: the entrance to the uterus (the vagina) and two breast channels.

17.2 INTRODUCTION TO THE THREE PRINCIPAL CHANNEL SYSTEMS (*TSA CHEN SUM*)

There are three principal groups of life-holding channels (*soktsa*): wind channels, blood channels, and water channels. These correspond approximately to the nervous, circulatory, and lymphatic systems. To know about the channels and chakras (*khorlo*) on a more profound level, however, one should study tantra and fulfill the spiritual requirements. Only then, one is prepared to perceive the human body-mind's subtle physiology. In the *Four Tantras*, Lama Yutokpa has indeed incorporated tantric conceptions of anatomy, physiology, and *lung*. It is said that whoever knows the channels also knows the body.

The *tsa* are the pathways, tubes, and vessels that enable the body to digest food, to transport nutritional essence to the body parts, and to eliminate waste products from pores and orifices. In short, all physical and mental functions of growth, maintenance, and decay are made possible by the channels. A Tibetan Buddhist description of channel development and degeneration goes as follows: [3]

> From two months of gestation until the age of 12 months, a child produces 200 new channels daily, totaling 72,000 channels. From one year onwards, each day two channels wither until one reaches 100 years.

---

3   Sa skya pa rgyal mtshan dpal bzang, 1991, 11.

72,000 channels are mentioned, in which circulate the same number of winds and emotions throughout life. Conversely, degeneration of channels reduces sensation and memory, becoming a cause for change. The tantric concept of channel degeneration is closely aligned with the process of aging. Aging causes veins and arteries (and also the lymph and nerve channels) to weaken and even close, which is referred to as the channels "drying" or withering in tantric texts. When the tiny blood vessels (*traktsa trawa*) malfunction, the channel walls become hard and thicken, causing various circulatory diseases. As the lymphatic channels deteriorate, liquid retention may occur. Weakening nerves may result in loss of feeling, failing memory, shrinking organs, and increased lethargy. To summarize, the process of aging allows the main channels to continue functioning, but the channel walls may thicken, which causes narrowing of the channels along with increased pressure. The resulting reduction in supply then causes the body to deteriorate. Another analogy is that channels flow like the river Ganges: many tributaries flow into the river, which swells and breaks its banks in countries downstream before flowing into the ocean.

Gyüzhi describes the basic channels clearly, while Tibetan medical scholars such as Zurkhar Lodrö Gyelpo and Dési Sangyé Gyatso elaborated on this subject in their commentaries. The Dési's *tangka* paintings and *Gyüzhi* commentaries, with illustrations of the channels and chakras, are mostly drawn based on a tantric perspective. In Tibetan medicine, the *tsa* are divided into three groups: wind, bile, and phlegm. From an energetic viewpoint, the right side of the body is dominated by bile channels, the left side by phlegm channels, and the central and lower parts of the body by wind channels. In actuality, the channels, whether gross or subtle, horizontal or vertical, are completely intertwined like a net branching throughout the whole body. As a result, there is no difference between the right and left sides, or any "cold" or "hot" channels per se. It is the humors that saturate these with movement, heat, and moisture in the form of wind, bile, and phlegm respectively. They are one in three aspects. The three groups of channels exist on a physical level as *traktsa*, known as blood vessels; *chutsa*, known as lymphatic ducts; and *lungtsa*, which correspond with the respiratory tract and nervous system. They may be understood as passages in the body for humoral forces and consciousness, like a valley through which rivers flow.

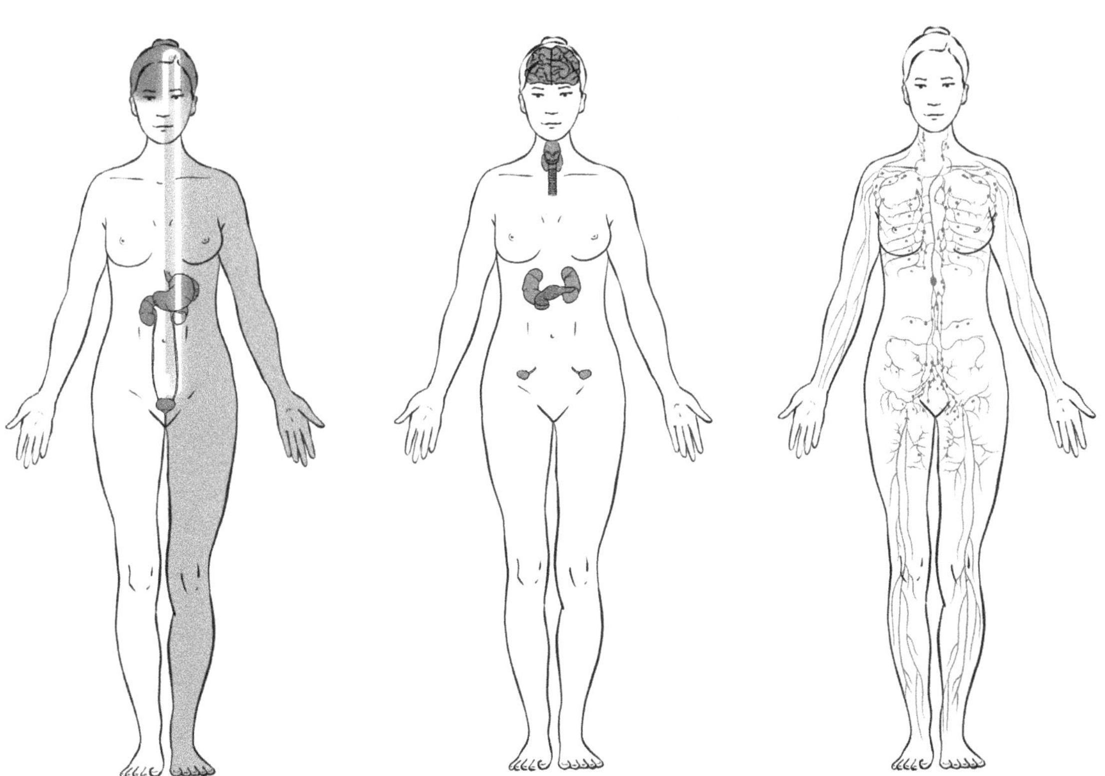

FIGURE 17.1 Different aspects of *chutsa*, which include the endocrine and lymphatic systems

All channels can be traced back to these *sokt-sa*, which are also called the three principal or root channels (*tsa chen sum*). The three mental poisons of the bardo consciousness, together with subtle wind energies, produce the three channels. These in turn produce the three humors. This is the cause and effect relationship that produces the body. The channels develop the body, which then becomes a house for the three humors, where they function to sustain the body. *Tsa* are located in all parts of the body, but generally speaking the upper body and the head (and especially the brain) are dominated by phlegm or water channels (*bétsa, chutsa*), the middle (liver and gall-bladder) and heart are dominated by bile channels (*tritsa*), and the lower body (including the kidneys and reproductive organs) are dominated by *lungtsa*.

Water channels (*chutsa*)

The body's water system consists of the lymphatic and endocrine systems, which support phlegm. It is white in color and originates from the brain and spinal column, its root and trunk. The trunk branches out in all directions, reaching the four limbs. This water network is said to resemble a radish in that the main channel penetrates deep inside the body through the vertebrae like a taproot. Lymphatic vessels collect water and bring it from the lower body to the chest and neck, where it rises to the brain like earth vapors rising into the sky. There, the brain refines it. The essence of this water becomes vital fluid or *tiklé*, also known as *kham karpo* (a group of hormones), which is secreted from glands and distributed to the organs to nourish and revitalize them. The brain not only filters but also cools, balancing the bile heat. The purified water and wastewater both circulate back to the body, where the kidneys filter the latter, which is then excreted as urine or through perspiration. The underlying cause of the lymphatic vessels is *timuk* (closed-mindedness), which has a heavy nature. The *chutsa* dominate the left side of the body and the head, where *timuk* is said to predominate. It is associated with masculine energy, patience, tolerance, stability, tranquility, and carefulness, but it also provokes a slow, unclear mind, selfishness, confusion, as well as sluggishness. Summarized, *Chutsa* have the following characteristics:

- Mental causal factor: closed-mindedness
- Physical base: the brain
- Humor: *béken*
- Dominate the left side of the body

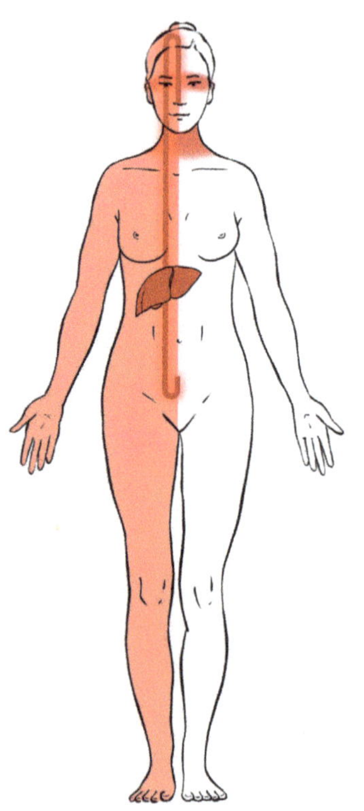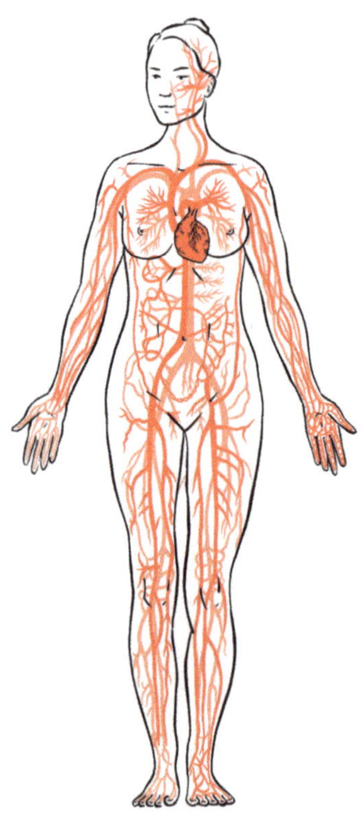

FIGURE 17.2 The *traktsa*, which include the blood circulation system

- Correspond to masculinity, the moon, the water element, and night
- Consist of the lymphatic and endocrine systems
- Produce secretions from the glands (*tiklé*)

Blood channels (*traktsa*)

Traktsa are also known as *tripa* channels because these vessels circulate both blood and bile (in the form of *chuser*, plasma). Its main trunk consists of the aorta and vena cava, which start at BV13 and go up until CV1.[4] The circulatory system is shaped like a pine tree, developing from the liver and gallbladder, and the heart. All organs grow from this root channel like fruits on a tree. It has a dark reddish color and circulates bile heat, blood, wind, and food essence. There are countless *traktsa*, which can be divided into two: the venous and arterial systems that sustain the body-mind with blood. Venous blood is the main carrier of *dangma* to the heart, from where it is distributed to the body. The *traktsa* (also

---

4 BV13 refers to the back vertebra connected to the vital energy of the reproductive fluids (12th thoracic vertebra), and CV1 stands for the first cervical vertebra.

referred to as *soktsa* in some contexts) dominate the right side of the body, and are associated with intelligence, pride, a self-centered mind. They provoke anger, hatred, and impatience. *Traktsa* have the following characteristics:

- Mental causal factor: hatred
- Physical base: liver, gallbladder, and heart
- Humor: *tripa*
- Dominate the right side of the body
- Produce blood and bile
- Correspond to femininity, sun, the fire element, and day
- Consist of the blood circulatory system

Wind channels (*lungtsa*)

Lungtsa are the primary life-holding channels. Their origin is located below the navel, from which the trunk rises like a pillar between the lateral channels. Its tip reaches the crown chakra. It is therefore called *tsa uma*, the middle or central channel. This channel is rooted in the reproductive organs, and the trunk reaches from the lower abdomen towards the crown

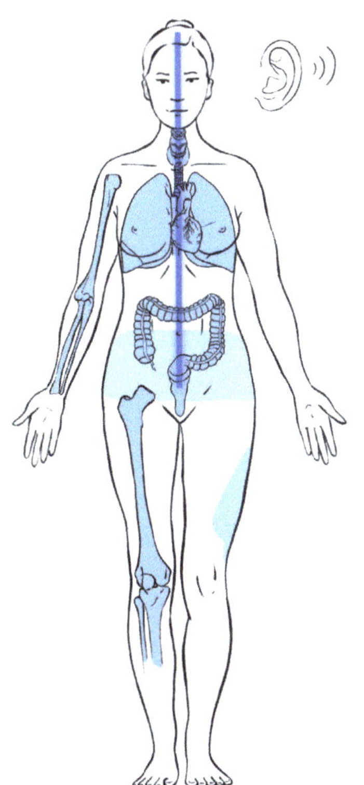
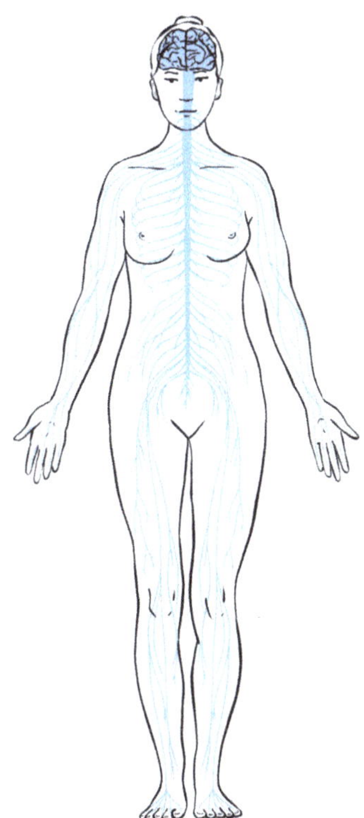

FIGURE 17.3 The *lungtsa* and the nervous system

chakra via the heart. It is also called the life rod (*sok gi yukpa*). This system is responsible for distributing life-sustaining wind to the limbs and the smallest body parts. Countless *lungtsa* carry wind energy and consciousness, regulating the functions of the nervous system. The wind channel is a fundamental subject in medicine, but even more so in tantra. It manifests forms of attachment, desire, jealousy, and fear. *Lungtsa* have the following characteristics:

- Mental causal factor: attachment
- Physical base: reproductive organs
- Humor: wind
- Dominate the central part of the body, the lower abdomen, and the lumbar-sacral area
- Comprise the nervous system
- Correspond to neutrality, equinox, and the wind element

17.3 FORMATION CHANNELS (*CHAKPÉ TSA*)

The channels discussed in the rest of this chapter are the same as described in the previous section: the *tsachen sum* and its branches. They are like the fibers of a woven bamboo basket, countless in number. All channels can be approached from four perspectives:

1. Formation channels (*chakpé tsa*)
2. The four great channels of existence (*sipé tsachen zhi*)
3. Connecting channels (*drelwé tsa*)
4. Life force channels (*tsé yi tsa*)

The *chakpé tsa* are the first of the four channel groups. They explain the process of channel formation during fetal development. In theory, the body's blueprint is already established in the bardo, which dictates the subtle winds to shape the body according to its karma.

The formation channels start to develop from the center of the umbilical cord in the sixth week after conception. The three main channels are the trunk from which smaller channels branch that then produce connections to the vital and hollow organs according to their causal mental poisons. The brain and phlegm humor channel is shaped by closed-mindedness, heart, liver, and bile by hatred, while the reproductive organs are generated through desire.

Brain channels

During the sixth week of fetal development, the central channel develops. Next, the brain channel originates from the embryo's umbilical center like a shoot germinating from a bean. The brain channel has several synonyms: single channel (*tsa kyangma*), white life-holding channel (*soktsa karpo*), and water channel (*chutsa*). This channel and its branches are formed from the qualities of heaviness of the child's mind. Closed-mindedness is the distant cause, the brain is the condition, and the phlegm humor is the result. The channel is white, and its water energy is derived from the father. During fetal development, the channel passes up to the chest and then to the head, where it first forms the eyes. From the eyes, the channel begins to form the head and brain as the first major organ. All the white substances and tissues of the body such as the brain, bone marrow, spinal cord, tendons, ligaments, and lymphatic vessels are connected to the head, where phlegm is most active. After forming these, the brain channel generates the mental functions of the six sense organs and creates their consciousnesses (gross mind).

The brain manifests ignorance, closed-mindedness, selfishness, and stupidity. It also contains many glands,

TABLE 17.1 The causal factors of the three channels

Distant cause, mental causal factor		Condition	Body location	Resulting humor	Channel name
Ignorance	Closed-mindedness	Brain (crown chakra)	Upper	Phlegm	*Chutsa*
	Anger	Liver (heart chakra)	Middle	Bile	*Traktsa*
	Desire	Reproductive organs (secret chakra)	Lower	Wind	*Lungtsa*

the cerebrum, and is the source of the body's liquids. The brain channels' main function is to circulate fluids through the lymphatic system, to filter, and to transform these into water essence (*chü kham nyingpo*) in the brain, producing glandular secretions. The brain is the source of the lymphatic and endocrine systems.

Heart channels

The second formation channel is the bile and blood system, principally governing the heart organ. It is called *soktsa marpo*, the life-holding red channel, and it develops from the right side of the point where the umbilical cord originates during the sixth week of fetal development. Blood channels (*traktsa*) consist of dark and red channels, corresponding to the veins and arteries. These two channel systems develop within the body like twin pine trees that grow from their roots at the umbilical cord. The trunk of these trees grows up alongside the vertebrae and connects with the liver and the heart before branching out to the arms, throat, and head. Roots go down to the kidneys, connecting with the reproductive organs and genitals before reaching the legs. The blood channel forms the red-colored body components, organs, and tissues. The vital center of this channel is the center-right side of the body, in the chest, where the heart and liver are located.

The blood channel forms the heart and liver, both of which are said to be its fruits. This channel grants intelligence, ego, pride, while also provoking anger, hatred, aggression, and other violent emotions. Its main physiological function is to supply nutrient- and oxygen-rich blood to the body.

Reproductive organ channels

The third formation channel is called *lungtsa*, the channel of the wind energy system, which also develops during the sixth week after conception. This channel forms the root or basis of all other channels. It is the seed of the body and seat of the bardo consciousness. Other names for it include *tsa uma*, the central channel, or *sok chenpö tsa*, the great life-holding channel. It functions as a body-mind hologram that corresponds to the nervous system. Its root lies four fingers below the navel. Its principal branch travels down and forms the perineum, reproductive organs, and the secret chakra, which is the base of subtle wind and mind. The *samséu* as well as the genitals are described as the channel's fruit. Another branch travels up, where it links to the brain. This particular link is called *düpé tsa*, "the combined channel," since reproductive fluid production is a shared function of all organs.

The reproductive organ channels also sustain the mind. They allow for sexual enjoyment and orgasm, manifesting joy, happiness, overcoming fear, interest, curiosity, imagination, and creativity. On the other hand, these channels equally provoke attachment, desire, jealousy, lust, and obsession.

17.4 THE FOUR GREAT CHANNELS OF EXISTENCE (*SIPÉ TSACHEN ZHI*)

This section deals with the second group of channels. These four great channels are the same as those described above in the section on formation channels, but their explanation focuses on how they "exist in" and govern the body throughout life. After birth, this system of existence channels begins to function like an engine. There are four types:

1. Sensory perception channels
2. Memory-clearing channels
3. Body manifestation channels
4. Heredity continuation channels

1. Sensory perception channels (*wangpo yül la charwé tsa*)

The fourth chapter of the *Explanatory Tantra* describes the sensory perception channels thus:[5]

> The channels of the senses, which perceive external objects, exist in the brain, surrounded by 500 minor channels.

These sense consciousness channels are formed in the brain, but they also connect to the heart chakra. They comprise the eye channels (optic nerves), ear channels (auditory nerves), nose (olfactory nerves), tongue (taste bud nerves), and body consciousness channels (cutaneous nerves that govern the tactile sense and touch). The brain's sensory channels develop from the root center of the three main channels, which corresponds to the limbic system. This root center is called the *khyilwé tsa*, which means "coiled channel," referring to the shape of this brain area. From here, the five minor winds of the brain activate the five sense organ channels, giving rise to their consciousnesses. Each sense organ has 24 principal channels (four from the middle channel and 10 from each

---

5 G.yu thog yon tan mgon po, 1993, 22.

of the two lateral channels) and is surrounded by 500 subtle channels. Practically, this refers to countless channels. The entire brain is governed by life-sustaining wind, whereas the sense organs systems are governed locally by the five minor winds (*yenlak gi lung nga*):

- *Lu* functions in the eyes, enabling the visual perception of objects
- *Rübel* resides in the ear and supports hearing
- *Tsangpa* allows the nose to smell
- *Lhajin* promotes tasting through the tongue
- *Norlhagyel* grants the body the sense of touch

The 500 subtle channels that surround each sense organ in the brain are collectively called the great blissfulness crown chakra (*chiwo déchen gyi khorlo*) in tantra. Through them, the sense organs perceive forms, images and colors, sounds, odors, and tastes, which together contribute to one's experience. From each of the three main channels branch eight sub-channels, making 24 sense channels. These surround each of the five sense consciousnesses. The 500 subchannels can be described as follows: 200 branch from the eight branches of the *traktsa* channel, 200 branch from the *chutsa* channel, and 100 branch from the *lungtsa*. All 500 subtle channels surround the 24 channels and support the sense organs, thus producing the gross mind of the brain.

Gross memory (*sem rakpa*)

Gross memory derives from the brain. Memory is made up from the collective experiences of the five sense consciousnesses, which are recorded in the coiled channel (*khyilwa*). Metaphorically, this channel is like a computer that saves data files. Their collective functioning in the brain may be referred to as general memory. They are equally important and powerful in their influence over the mind. Salient gross memories are transferred to the heart, where the *künzhi* is located. In essence, this is what is termed "collecting karma." It is the continuation of the subtle mind's memory. However, before transferring the memory to the heart *künzhi*, the brain's memory-clearing channels scan and filter through all daily experiences. The gross or general memory operates in the brain, which acts as a precondition for more subtle memories.

2. Memory-clearing channels (*drenpé wangpo selwé tsa*)

The fourth chapter in the *Explanatory Tantra* describes these channels as follows:[6]

> The memory-clearing channel of the
> sensory organs exists in the heart,
> surrounded by 500 minor channels.

Memory-clearing channels act as a second, subtle memory located in the heart. There are 500 of these channels, similar to the sensory perception channels described above. *Drenpé wangpo selwé tsa* are collectively referred to as the heart chakra of phenomena (*nying a chö kyi khorlo*). This chakra grants the ability to discriminate right from wrong, wisdom that ought to be developed from the heart: the mirror of the world. Buddhist conceptions of the heart are highly complex and can only be properly understood if the learner unlocks the door to tantric practice.

The subtle anatomy of the heart

The heart (*nying*) is the central figure of Mahayana teachings, and of medicine as well in terms of the *künzhi* mind and memory. Life-sustaining wind's primary branch produces pervasive wind in the heart, which rules this organ's activity. Pervasive wind regulates both the circulation of blood and wind as well as the *künzhi*. The latter corresponds more to the heart chakra, which consists of memory-clearing channels (*drenpé wangpo selwé tsa*). These give awareness of this life's memories, which are transferred from the brain, and support deep memory of past lives. This secondary, more subtle memory is supported by 24 main and 500 minor channels that together produce a self-image or sense of "I."

The heart is an empty mandala of the body-mind and its emotions. In the center of this mandala, there exists a unique channel, derived from *tsa uma*: the *yi zangma*, the "noble lady" or "compassionate lady" channel. Its shape is like a lotus flower with 24 petals, surrounded by 500 smaller petals (minor channels). The *künzhi* mind resides within these petals, encircled by four channels from which the four other minds flow (as portrayed in Figure 17.4). The core of the *yi zangma* contains the *kartika*, a subtle crystalline white channel, which is surrounded by the rainbow-like lights of the five psycho-elemental forces (*ja tsön na nga*) in each direction: green (wind), red (fire), blue (water), yellow (earth), and white (space). The *yi zangma* is the actual seat of the *künzhi* as well as of

---

6 Ibid.

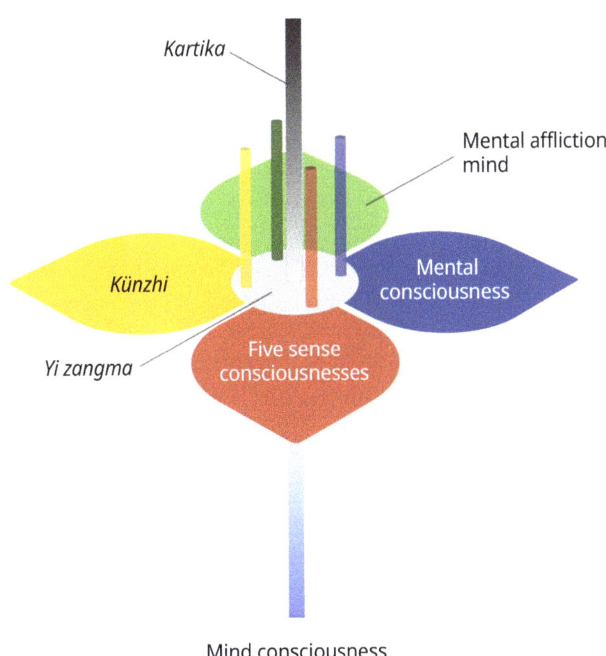

FIGURE 17.4 The subtle structure of the central channel at the level of the heart chakra

the subtle mind, which gives rise to self-grasping and subtle memory. The *Blue Beryl* states:[7]

> The sense consciousnesses flow through the front channel, which is red.
> The *künzhi* consciousness of the mind flows through the right channel, which is yellow.
> The *yi* consciousness flows through the left channel, which is blue.
> The mental affliction consciousness flows through the back channel, which is green.

The mind's subtle memory (*drenshé tramo*) is stored inside the *künzhi* (see also Section 4.4). The five sense consciousnesses experience, transfer, and record memories in the *kartika*, where the five subtle consciousness channels are bundled together. This mandala is extremely subtle, carrying memories of past as well as current lives.

The heart is also the main seat of self-grasping (*dakdzin*), a self-centered mind that produces the sense of self. According to tantra, the deep memory awareness channel is closed in ordinary people, thus creating the darkness of ignorance and delusion. If the awareness channels are opened, one becomes awakened and wisdom increases. As long as the crystal-like memory of the heart is obscured by ignorance, we cannot see the truth. On a material level, the heart chakra is filled with pervasive wind (*lung khyapjé*), the blood and wind energy which flows in the heart and through its four channel roots. Pervading wind regulates the heart and sustains the functions of the *künzhi*. Ordinary *künzhi* mind is furthermore under the control of mental affliction wind (*nyönmongpé lung*), which manifests negative emotions. One could say this is the principal channel from where ignorance flows and influences life. Mental affliction wind generates the deluded mind, yet its physical function may correspond to the electric impulses that generate the heartbeat according to biomedicine, through the sinoatrial and atrioventricular nodes. The heart has four major external blood channels (including the aorta and vena cava), and four coronary artery veins surround it. The joining of these channels can be interpreted as the *yi zangma*. They are all channels that sustain the heart and that act as pathways for consciousness.

---

7 Sde srid sangs rgyas rgya mtsho, 1994, vol. 1, 102.

In relation to this, Peljor Döndrup's work on Nāropa's *Six Dharmas* states:[8]

> The *bodhicitta* of the life-holding wind is
> the essence of blood in the center of the
> heart.
> It is the size of an egg of *jilbu lentsa*[9] in
> which a luminous sphere, the size of two
> bean halves held together,
> holds the memory consciousness in its core.

From a tantric perspective, life-sustaining wind is the inseparable essence of the blood, the center of which is located in the heart as a *tiklé*. This *tiklé* is the seat of the *künzhi* consciousness.

Besides the memories of the brain and heart channels, there also exists a minor third memory, which is the memory-activating factor that resides in the throat chakra (*drinpa longchö kyi khorlo*). It is regulated by the ascending wind branch. It gives power to the gross and subtle memories, supporting its and many other functions.

3. Body manifestation channels

The fourth chapter of the *Explanatory Tantra* describes the body manifestation channels thus:[10]

> The channel of body aggregate
> development exists in the navel,
> surrounded by 500 minor channels.

Body manifestation takes place through development channels that branch out from the umbilical cord, the fetus's connection with its mother. The navel emanation chakra (*téwa trulpé khorlo*) refers to the place of sperm-ovum union from where the new child grows. Later on, it is known as the navel, the body's center. Channels grow from this site, resembling sprouting beans. This core where the two parents' energies and the bardo consciousness gather is the basis that supports further growth. 500 subtle channels that develop the body-mind surround the 24 main channels, similar to the other chakras. The manifestation channels produce the organs, limbs, and other parts, so that the growing body resembles a tree growing from a tiny seed. After birth the navel chakra and channels become less active, like a seed casing that is shed after germination.

4. Heredity continuation channels

The fourth chapter of the *Explanatory Tantra* describes the heredity continuation channels in the following way:[11]

> The channels that ensure progeny exist
> in the genital organs, surrounded by 500
> minor channels.

The secret chakra (*sangwé khorlo*) is responsible for heredity. It generates attachment, produces male and female reproductive fluids, and manifests desire for sexual pleasure. The wind humor's root develops from here. An alternative name for this specific area is the bliss-guarding chakra of the secret place (*sangné dékyong gi khorlo*). The secret chakra functions in the lower abdomen, including the lumbar area, and is governed by descending wind.

5. Flavor enjoyment channels

Gyüzhi describes only four channel centers. In commentaries and in tantric works, however, five energy centers or chakras are often discussed. The fifth chakra, consisting of flavor-experiencing or -enjoyment channels, is the throat chakra.

The throat and mouth are made of nerves, blood vessels, cervical vertebrae, muscles, the pharynx, and larynx. These channels, delicate by nature, resemble a narrow city road. Ascending wind assists in respiration, swallowing food and beverages, and enables speech. Additionally, it activates the memory powers of the brain and the heart. The flavor enjoyment channels' main function is to experience taste and feelings of satisfaction. Therefore, they are collectively called the throat enjoyment chakra (*drinpa longchö kyi khorlo*), which increases the desire for food and life. 24 major and 500 minor channels carry out these functions, surrounding the feeling sense consciousness.

---

8   Dpal 'byor don grub, 1995, 100–101.

9   The meaning of this word (Wylie: *byil bu lan tsha*) is unclear. It
    probably refers to a bird's egg.

10 G.yu thog yon tan mgon po, 1993, 22.

---

11 Ibid.

17.5 CONNECTING CHANNELS (*DRELWÉ TSA*)

Drélwé tsa connect the body organs and tissues, supplying *dangma*, carrying blood, lymph and *chuser*. The connecting channels consist of two groups: dark life-holding channels (*soktsa nakpo*) and white life-holding channels (*soktsa karpo*).

Dark life-holding channels

These channels refer to the blood vessels, with "dark" referring to the bluish color of veins visible under the skin. There are two types of blood vessels: stable veins (*dötsa*) and pulsing arteries (*partsa*). Arteries and veins are differentiated according to their color and different functions in circulating blood and transporting *lung* through the body.

1. Veins (*dötsa*)

The veins are referred to as stable channels (*dötsa*) to distinguish them from pulsing arteries, or as *soktsa nakpo*. The dark blood network transports *dangma*, *chuser*, and bile energy. During fetal development, the main dark vein channel develops from the umbilical cord (at the level of BV13), reaching up to the chest along the front side of the spinal column. From the vena cava onwards, it extends into 24 branches like a pine tree, connecting to the various vital and hollow organs. The channels then reach to the hands and head, permeating the whole body.

After the *dangma* and oxygenated blood has been utilized, it is collected through the 24 main vein branches and countless minor veins. The heart then redistributes renewed blood with fresh oxygen (*tsolung*, life-nurturing wind or air) and food essence through the arterial channels. The heart, lungs, and liver (involved in *dangma* and blood production) all seem to operate like pumps in this system. The dark blood vein channel branches into an elaborate micro-vein system of blood vessels, carrying the bile humor and fire element that fuel the metabolism. The venous blood system contains *mélung* ("fire-wind"), which refers to deoxygenated blood containing carbon dioxide. This fire-wind mixed with blood is considered toxic, giving veins their dark color. This used, dark-colored blood is therefore called impure blood. When excessive amounts of impure blood are present in the body, diseases such as blood circulation disorders, heart, liver, spleen, skin, and many other disorders may develop over time. It also manifests negative emotions such as anger, impatience, and aggressiveness. Cleaning the impure blood and releasing *mélung* from the body calms the mind and refreshes the body.

The vena cava is the main trunk of the venous network, which consists of 24 principal blood vessel branches: eight are hidden veins (*bépé tsa*, which cannot be seen through the skin) and 16 are externally visible. The invisible veins are connected to the internal organs and the visible veins to the extremities.

Bépé tsa are internal veins that transport *dangma*, blood, heat, wind, and fluids to the solid and hollow organs. These channel branches also collect waste products from the organs and tissues. The eight hidden, internal veins (IV) are:

- IV1–3: Three vein branches exit at the level of BV3 (2nd thoracic vertebra) from the vena cava. One branch is joined to the heart and the other two to the lungs.

- IV4: One vein branch exits at the level of BV9 (8th thoracic vertebra) from the vena cava and joins the liver.

- IV5: One vein branch exits at the level of BV11 (10th thoracic vertebra) from the vena cava and is linked to the spleen.

- IV6: One vein branch exits at the level of BV13 (12th thoracic vertebra) from the vena cava and is linked to the reproductive organs.

- IV7–8: Two vein branches exit at the level of BV14 (1st lumbar vertebra) from the vena cava and are linked to the two kidneys.

16 externally visible veins (EV) are listed:

- EV1–6: Six vein channels leave the vena cava, branching to the head from the right and left sides of the neck. Each side has three main branches (totaling six for both sides) and divides into many subbranches in the head. They maintain blood and wind circulation, and collect impure blood from the head and brain.

- EV7–10: Four vein channels go to the arms, hands, and fingers from their roots in the heart and lungs. Each hand has two main vein channels from which many branches spread. These veins collect blood from the arms and hands, sending it back to the heart and lungs.

- EV11–14: Four leg vein channels, of which two branches leave from the kidneys and two from each thigh, spread down to the legs. These channels collect blood from the legs.

- EV15–16: Two reproductive vein channels exit the vena cava at the kidney level (BV14), connecting down to the reproductive organs and genitals. They maintain blood and wind circulation in the lower abdomen, sustain sexual functions and the vital energy of the reproductive fluids, and return impure blood to the heart and lungs.

In addition to the channels described above, countless smaller blood vessels in all parts of the body transport food essence, sustain life, and gather waste products. Excess impure blood leads to various health problems. For this reason, Tibetan medical practitioners perform bloodletting (*tarka*). This external therapy targets specific blood vessels to release impurities from different body parts. Releasing blood allows the fire or bile heat to escape and removes toxins. Vein points are generally used, since the veins carry impure, deoxygenated blood. Very few arterial points are considered usable. Of the countless vein blood vessels, 77 external channel points are mostly used for bloodletting as described in the venesection chapter of the *Subsequent Tantra*. Listed briefly, the 77 points consist of 21 points in the head, 34 points in the arms and hands, 18 points in the legs and feet, and four points in the abdomen.

2. Arteries (*partsa*)

The second group of dark life-holding channels comprises the pulsing blood vessels of the arterial system. These are also called the red life-holding channels (*soktsa marpo*). The arteries are filled with blood and oxygen. Their root is the aorta (*soktsa*), which is the heart's main blood vessel root, the foremost life-holding channel. These red channels are the main base of *nyönmongpé lung*, which creates the conditioned mind and generates the heartbeat, the primary sign of life. When Tibetan physicians take the pulse, they examine the deluded mind wind from the *künzhi* through the patient's heartbeat.

The function of the *partsa* is to transport water and air (oxygen), blood, as well as other essential substances to the body and organs. They sustain the life force and memory, mental clarity, a creative mind as well as intelligence. These channels help circulate water and earth-wind energy (*tsolung*, oxygenated blood), which returns through the black venous channels in the form of fire-wind that is then expelled from the body. Arterial blood and energy circulation also sustain millions of microorganisms (*sinbu*). The arterial

channel system has the same branching structure as the venous system, resembling a pine tree. The system has 24 main and many finer branches that are located deeper inside the body than the veins.

Summary

The 85th chapter on wounds in the *Oral Instruction Tantra* portrays the venous and arterial channels as follows:[12]
> Inside, there are white and dark life-holding channel trees.
> They are like pines standing alongside the vertebrae.
> From there, many branches ramify to all body parts.
> From the third vertebra, three main branches extend to the front.
> From the central branch, the heart protrudes like a fruit.
> Inside the three folds of the heart five channels exist, of which the center is wind.[13]
> In the four channels of the four directions of the heart, mixed wind and blood channels exist.
> The right and left channels of the three branches are joined to the lungs.

The passage continues:
> The life channel's two branches flow to the two hands.
> The carotid and jugular vein[14] channels extend to the head.
> From the ninth vertebra, one channel connects to the liver,
> one joins the great liver valley and the pancreas,[15]
> and one joins the spleen and each of the kidneys.
> From the 14th vertebra, the *soktsa* branches into two,
> passing through the groin and then down to the two legs.
> From the above-mentioned channels countless channels spread to the vital and hollow organs like a tangle of threads.

---

12 Ibid., 434–35.

13 The central channel here refers to the *kartika*.

14 This vein corresponds to the *nyilok tsa* or "sleeping vein."

15 The pancreas is likely the organ referred to here as *chindri nakpo*, but this remains unclear.

White life-holding channels

Both the lymph ducts and the nerves belong to this category, as they are whitish grey in color. Like the blood connection channels, these two are equally primary life sustainers. The *Explanatory Tantra* does not clearly distinguish between the lymphatic and nervous systems, whereas the endocrine system is barely covered. Commentators who have written on these channels describe all three under the same heading of "white channels" (*tsa kar*), causing further confusion perhaps due to a historical lack of anatomical knowledge. Leaving these disputes aside, the author proposes to differentiate the lymphatic from the nervous system whilst keeping them under the same general heading. *Soktsa karpo* refers specifically to the nerves, which control the body and are conduits of (sensory) consciousness. We reserve *chutsa* for the lymphatic system as well as the circulation of hormones by the endocrine system. This body water system can also be called *tsa kyangma*, the "single water channel" that balances the energies of blood and bile heat. The brain (*lépa*) is the common root of the lymphatic, endocrine, and nervous systems. Mainly consisting of grey and white matter, it is of a heavy quality, acting as a water reservoir. Brain-derived water—including cerebrospinal fluid—cools down the bile heat and nourishes the body. The fourth chapter of the *Explanatory Tantra* describes the brain in the following passage:[16]

> From the brain, which is a great ocean of channels, a channel having 19 actively functioning *chutsa* branches projects downwards like a root.

The brain's external morphology resembles a large walnut encased in a shell that is the skull. It is essentially a bunch of wires connecting via a single main cable. The brain root passes down through the neck and spinal column, up until the sacrum and coccyx. The nerves resemble the root of a long radish. The endocrine glands are mainly located in the brain but release their secretions to the blood and organs. Conversely, the lymph vessels bring up water from its countless tiny branches throughout the body.

1. Water channels (*chutsa*)

The *chutsa* circulate water and nourishment to the body's organs. They are phlegm channels which act in a similar way to the earth's hydrological cycle. Water evaporates from the earth's surface to form clouds that make rain, snow, and glaciers, which in

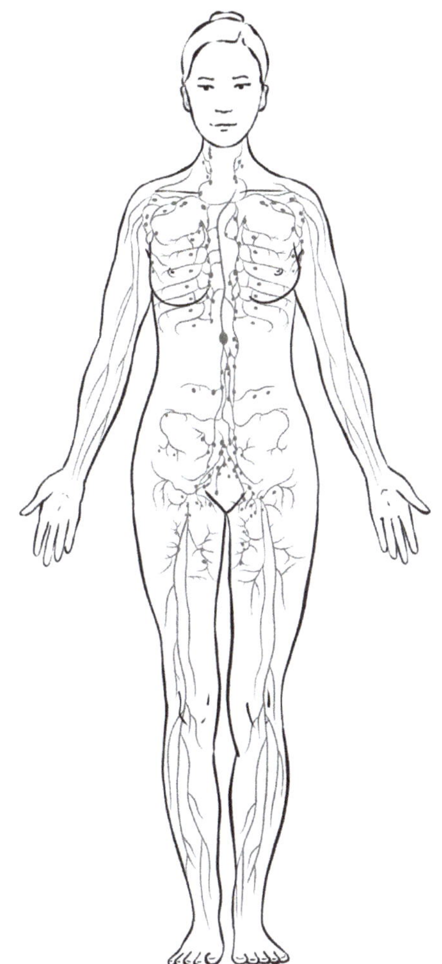

FIGURE 17.5 The water channels of the lymphatic system

turn feeds rivers and lakes. The *Gyüzhi* describes the water channels only briefly.

The lymphatic system exists in all parts of the body. Lymph vessels (*sherchü gyulam*) absorb liquid and circulates it just as the earth absorbs and circulates water, keeping the body and its organs moist, producing the liquid that is present in blood as well as allowing sweating. Lymphatic fluid is collected from various parts of the body through small vessels that unite and join larger vessels until they reach the main lymph channels. Lymph nodes filter impure water and foreign particles. The fluids flow to the root of the neck—where they enter the bloodstream via the subclavian veins—and are later pumped up to the brain.

Once in the brain, the endocrine system is in charge of transforming liquid into vital energy that is redistributed to the body through glands. According to Tibetan medicine, the lymph nodes and glands are the essence of fat; they are reservoirs of vital phlegm

---

16 Ibid., 23.

energy. The lymph nodes are found in groups: in the armpits, groin, kidneys, stomach, spleen, pelvis, and legs, and along the vertebrae, the back of the neck, the roots of the lungs, and in the area near the large abdominal veins. The connective tissues of joints as well as the vertebrae also belong to the water channels, which bind the bones and muscles together (through joints and ligaments), and store essential liquids (such as synovial fluid). There are many lymph nodes, but the following eight are the most vital to health because they collect fatty waste products, and because damage to them may be life threatening. The eight vital lymph nodes (LN) are:

- LN1–2: Two blue-headed glands (*menbu gongön nyi*) are located four fingers above the shoulders; they correspond to the cervical nodes.

- LN3–4: Two upper arm blue-headed glands (*pungpé menbu gongön nyi*) are located five fingers up from the tip of the elbow, and correspond to the auxiliary lymph nodes.

- LN5–6: Two white glands (*menbu karpo nyi*) are located twelve fingers up from the back of the knees; these correspond to the thigh lymph glands.

- LN7–8: Two glands are located three fingers above LN5–6, and are called the two cobra-headed lymph glands (*drülgo dengdré menbu nyi*).[17]

The endocrine glands (*shermen*) and their functions are not described in detail in the *Gyüzhi* and its commentaries. Nevertheless, endocrine channels (*shermen chutsa*) are vital phlegm energy vessels that secrete water essence (*sherchu*) into the body. We propose that the compounds released into the blood through various glands in different organs can be interpreted as a type of essence drops (*tiklé*). All glands exhibit phlegm nature, belonging to the water energy system that sustains the phlegm humor. The lymphatic and endocrine systems are distinct but work hand in hand. The lymphatic system receives nutritious liquid derived from digestion and circulates it around the body. Metabolism occurs in the abdomen, from where evaporated water passes through the throat and reaches the head and brain. There, the water is filtered before it becomes cerebral fluid. The brain is a seat of phlegm, a great reservoir of the body's vital

water. From this storage, water energy is sent to the glands of the brain such as the hypothalamus, pituitary and pineal glands. These in turn produce essences of water (*tiklé* and hormones) that eventually regenerate the body, radiating from the body and face. This is called *dang*, the body's aura or light.

According to tantra, there are two main *tiklé*: relative or physical *tiklé* and subtle *tiklé*. The former relate to sperm and menstruation, the latter reside in the heart and head. The gross *tiklé* are mainly produced in the reproductive organs, giving vitality to the sperm and ovum. This corresponds to the energy of the male and female hormones that are secreted by the glands, circulating in the blood and rejuvenating the organs. The overarching organ governing these processes is the brain itself, which contains several glands that regulate the release of hormones. The two physical *tiklé* can be termed masculine essence/hormone (*potsi*), and feminine essence (*motsi*). They stimulate the synthesis of reproductive fluids in the *samséu* channels.

The root of the hypothalamus extends down to the anterior pituitary gland, and joins the spinal cord via the brainstem, which finally reaches the area of the reproductive organs. According to Tibetan medicine, there is a channel called *düpé tsa*, the "combined channel" of all the organs. It extends down through the spine and enters BV13 (the 12th thoracic vertebra), from where it joins the reproductive organs, stimulating the flow of *tiklé* and feelings of pleasure during sexual intercourse. In tantra, relative *bodhicitta* is a synonym for the reproductive fluids or gross *tiklé*. Nonetheless, Sowa Rigpa would benefit from more research into endocrinology, which recognizes the following major glands: hypothalamus, pituitary and pineal glands (which are neuroendocrine organs), (para)thyroid glands, adrenal glands, the pancreas, and the reproductive glands.

2. Nerves (*soktsa karpo*)

As quoted above, the brain is said to be an ocean of channels. This is the Tibetan medical interpretation of the central nervous system, a network of countless white channels. The brain is also referred to as the mother of the bigger glands such as the hypothalamus. The root of the brain joins the spinal cord, which extends down through the spinal column and ends in the coccyx. Its extensions—the peripheral nerves—branch out into all parts of the body from the cervical, thorax, dorsal, lumbar and coccyx vertebrae. The nervous system is the vehicle that governs the body's motor and sensory functions. It coordinates vital and hollow organ activity, the muscles, digestion, defecation and urination, speech, movement, thinking,

---

17 It is difficult to compare biomedical anatomy and traditional understandings of lymph nodes. The gland identifications listed here should be regarded as tentative.

and relaxation. It is the primary network of the gross mind, which operates through cognition, sensory perception, and neuro-muscular communication.

In biomedicine, the nervous system is divided into two parts: the central and peripheral systems. There is some similarity here to the Tibetan medical perspective, which describes two general types of nerves: outer channels (*chitsa*) and inner channels (*nangtsa*). However, their attributed functions differ in several ways. Sowa Rigpa concepts of the nervous system require deeper study and elaboration, and more attention should be paid on anatomical and physiological subjects in general. In the following paragraphs, we will cover how the two main nerve divisions are traditionally taught and explained, following chapter 60 of the *Oral Instruction Tantra*. There are 19 principal nerve channels in total: 13 internal or hidden nerves, and six external or peripheral nerves.

The internal nerves coordinate systems that require involuntary activity for their regular function; in other words, they control organs that operate without conscious mental influence. The main internal nerve channels are the 13 hanging threads (*dar gyi changtak chusum*). They are also counted amongst the hidden nerves (*bépé tsa*). All these channels exit the base of the brain and extend down along the spinal cord. From different locations along the spine, they join different organs as detailed below. They are classified in three channel groups that correspond to the three humors. Each humor has four single channels that link with the 12 vital and hollow organs. In addition, there is one nerve that is called the "combined life channel" (*düpé soktsa*), which connects to the reproductive organs.[18]

There are four wind-producing nerve channels:

- Two nerves exit from beneath the occipital bone at the base of the skull and extend down to BV7. There, they join the heart organ, where they sustain its function and regulate *lung* together with the other two nerves.

---

18 Some of these wind and bile humor channels are not in agreement with the normal relationship between organ and humors. This is a topic worthy of future research.

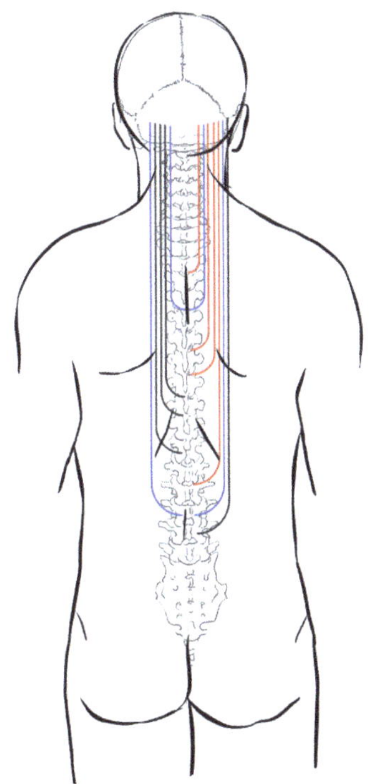
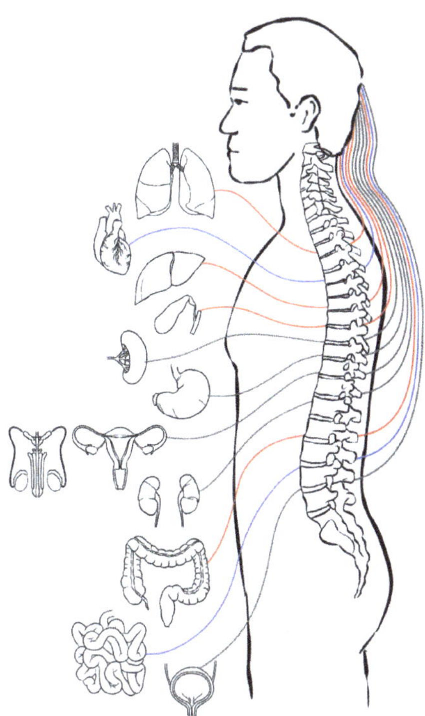

FIGURE 17.6 The Tibetan medical view on the brain-organ nerve connections

- An additional two nerves exit from the same location and extend down to link to the small intestine. They regulate the intestines.

Four bile-producing nerve channels are listed:

- One bile channel exits from beneath the occipital region and passes down to BV5, from where it joins the lungs. It produces and regulates *tripa* along with the other three nerves.

- One bile channel exits from beneath the occipital bone and extends down to BV16, linking to the colon.

- One bile channel exits from the same area and links to the liver at BV9, on the right side.

- One bile channel exits from the same area and links to the gallbladder at BV10, on the right side.

The four phlegm-producing nerve channels are:

- One phlegm channel exits from beneath the occipital bone, extends down through the cervical vertebrae, and links to the stomach at BV12. It regulates *béken* together with the other three nerves.

- One phlegm channel exits from the base of the skull and links to the spleen at BV11, on the left side.

- One phlegm channel exits from the same area, extends down through the cervical vertebrae to BV14, and branches out to the kidneys.

- One phlegm channel exits from the same area and links to the urinary bladder at BV18.

The single combined channel exits the brain from beneath the occipital bone and extends down to BV13, where it connects to the reproductive organs. It sustains sexual, reproductive, and hormonal functions.

There are six main external or peripheral nerve channels (*chi yi tsakar*) that branch out from the root of the brain. These nerves act under voluntary control and therefore largely belong to the somatic nervous system. They control and regulate the head, bones, muscles, extremities, as well as the sense organs.

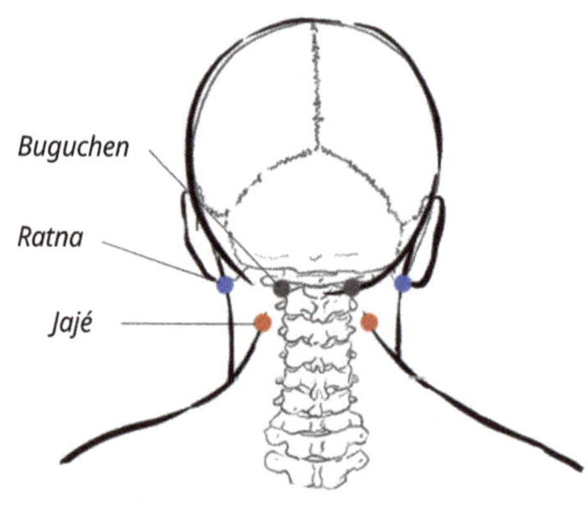

FIGURE 17.7 The exit points of the three sets of principal external nerves

Buguchen refers to "hollow" or "tubular" nerves. They are phlegmatic in nature, so people with phlegm constitutions tend to experience impaired function. Apart from one's constitution, body-mind behaviors may influence these nerves, leading to depression, sadness, or a confused mental state.

The two major *buguchen* nerves exit the right and left side of the skull base below the occipital bone (*takpé dügo*), descending straight along the two sides of the neck until they reach BV1 (the 7th cervical vertebra). From there, they extend further down through the central spinal cord until the level of BV5. They then continue down until BV12 (the 11th thoracic vertebra), at which point they ramify into three main branches and many tiny subbranches.

The first *buguchen* branch enters from BV12 into the lower abdomen and connects to the intestine, kidneys, urinary bladder, and reproductive organs. The second branch continues down from BV12 to BV14 (1st lumbar vertebra), where it exits and crosses the iliac crests towards the inguinal area. It then continues down to the interior parts of the thighs, the lower legs, and passes behind the medial malleolus, before reaching the big toes. From there, it turns downward, ending at the sole of the feet. The third branch continues down from BV14 to the sacral plexus (BV17, 4th lumbar vertebra) and then turns outward on both sides towards the hip joint. It passes down the latero-posterior side of the thigh and covers the leg and knee. It then passes behind the lateral malleolus and branches to the little and middle toes. Then it turns downward and ends at the sole of the feet, where it joins with the other nerves. This branch is the sciatic nerve channel that controls the posterior muscles of the legs.

Phlegm energy circulates down through these channels to the back, regulating the flow of fluids. These nerves control the back vertebrae and discs, the back muscles, and the posterior and interior sides of the legs. They are responsible for holding the contents of the lower abdomen in place and for maintaining the strength of the lower back, as well as for bone functions, and the hip, thigh, knee, leg, and feet muscles. Each nerve branch has thousands of subbranches that together cover the lower back, lower abdomen, legs, and feet. If these nerves become inflamed, damage and impairment may occur, leading to immediate neurological symptoms or even paralysis of the legs.

Jajé means "[nerve which] causes paralysis." The *jajé* channel is of a bile nature. Those with bile constitutions tend to experience impaired function of these nerves. Excessive hatred and anger as well as an excess of the bile humor also provoke disorders. There are two principal *jajé* nerve channels in the right and left shoulders, which lead to numerous subchannels that branch throughout the shoulders, neck, back, and legs.

The principal *jajé* nerves are called shoulder *jajé*, which exit from the occipital bone on the right and left sides at the *takzur pukhyil* point (corresponding to acupuncture point GB20 in Chinese medicine). It then passes down through the lateral sides of the neck and to the two shoulder joints. From there each channel separates into two further subbranches. On each side, the first subbranch turns to the back of the arm from the shoulder joint and crosses the elbow. It then crosses the thumb and turns inside to the palm, where it ends. The second subbranch enters the shoulder mass, passes down through the armpit and alongside the inner arm muscle, before ending inside the inner elbow joint.

The occiput *jajé* channel exits from below the occiput bone and turns upward, branching up the back

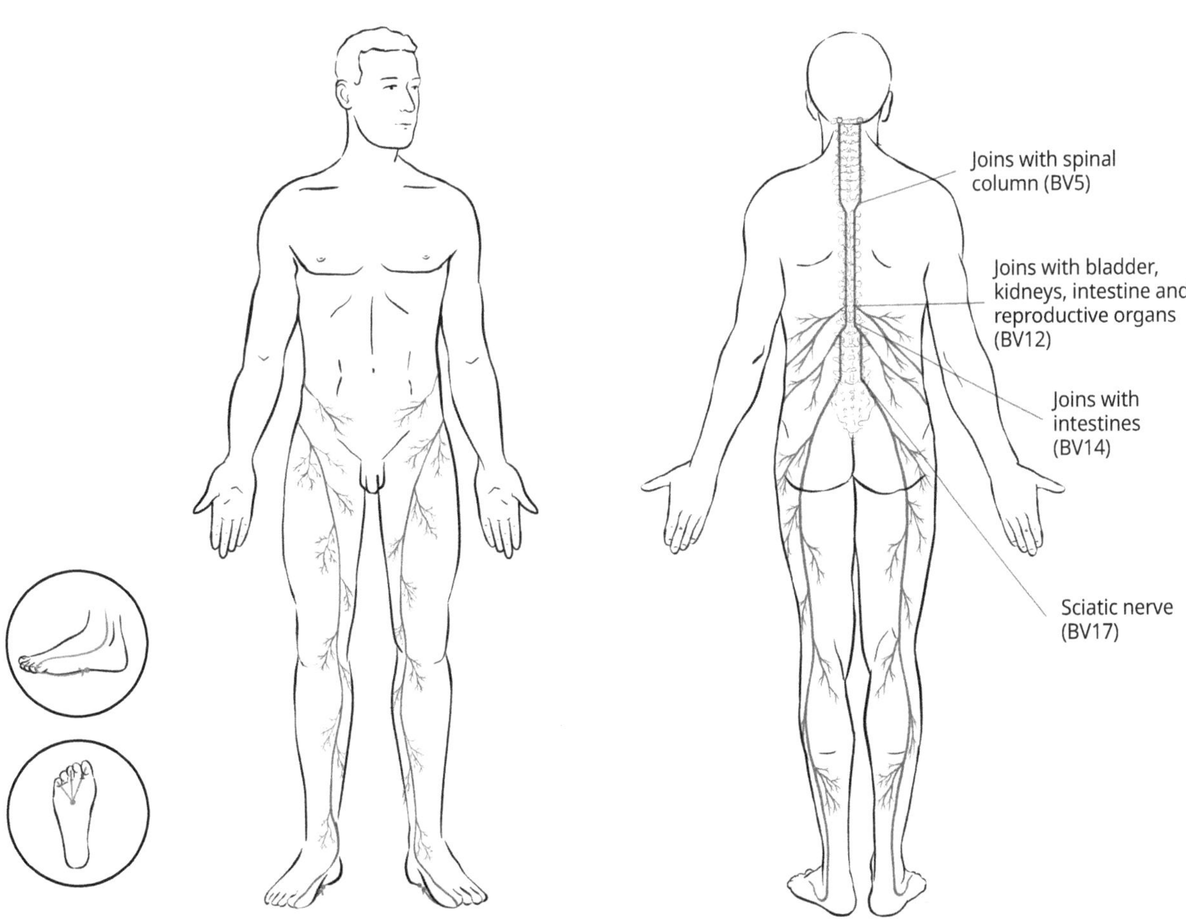

FIGURE 17.8 The *buguchen* nerves

of the head on the right and left sides. It controls the back of the head, the fontanel, and the temporal areas. The leg *jajé* passes straight down from the neck to the level of BV14 (the first lumbar vertebra), where it branches out on either side of the sacrum. Its primary and secondary branches reach the hip joints and then continue inside the thighs, down the backs of the knees, and toward the heels. From there, they turn inside towards foot soles and join with the *buguchen* nerves.

The *jajé* nerves control the head, shoulders, neck, upper back, chest, arms and fingers, as well as thighs and legs. Cuts, injuries, or inflammation affecting these nerves may cause severe pain, impaired function, and may even lead to paralysis.

The *ratna* or "jewel" channels are named thus because their functions are considered precious like a jewel. Damage to them may result in unpredictable neurological symptoms. This is a wind nature nerve channel. Those with a wind constitution have a tendency to experience impaired function. Excessive psychological and emotional disturbances may provoke wind disorder that affects this channel. This nerve has two principal channels and two subbranches.

The two main *ratna* channels exit from beneath the slope of the ear lobes. The first main branch reaches down through the right and left sides of the neck below the ear lobe, continues under the clavicle bones, and turns to the inner side of the shoulder. It continues down to the inner side of the arms, crosses the elbows, and extends to the forearms to reach the ring fingers. These channels end at the center of the palm where they join with the *jajé* nerves. The subbranches of these nerves branch across the throat, the chest, and the front of the ribs. A second branch innervates the jawbone and teeth. Its subbranches extend across the cheeks and temporal area, representing the facial nerves.

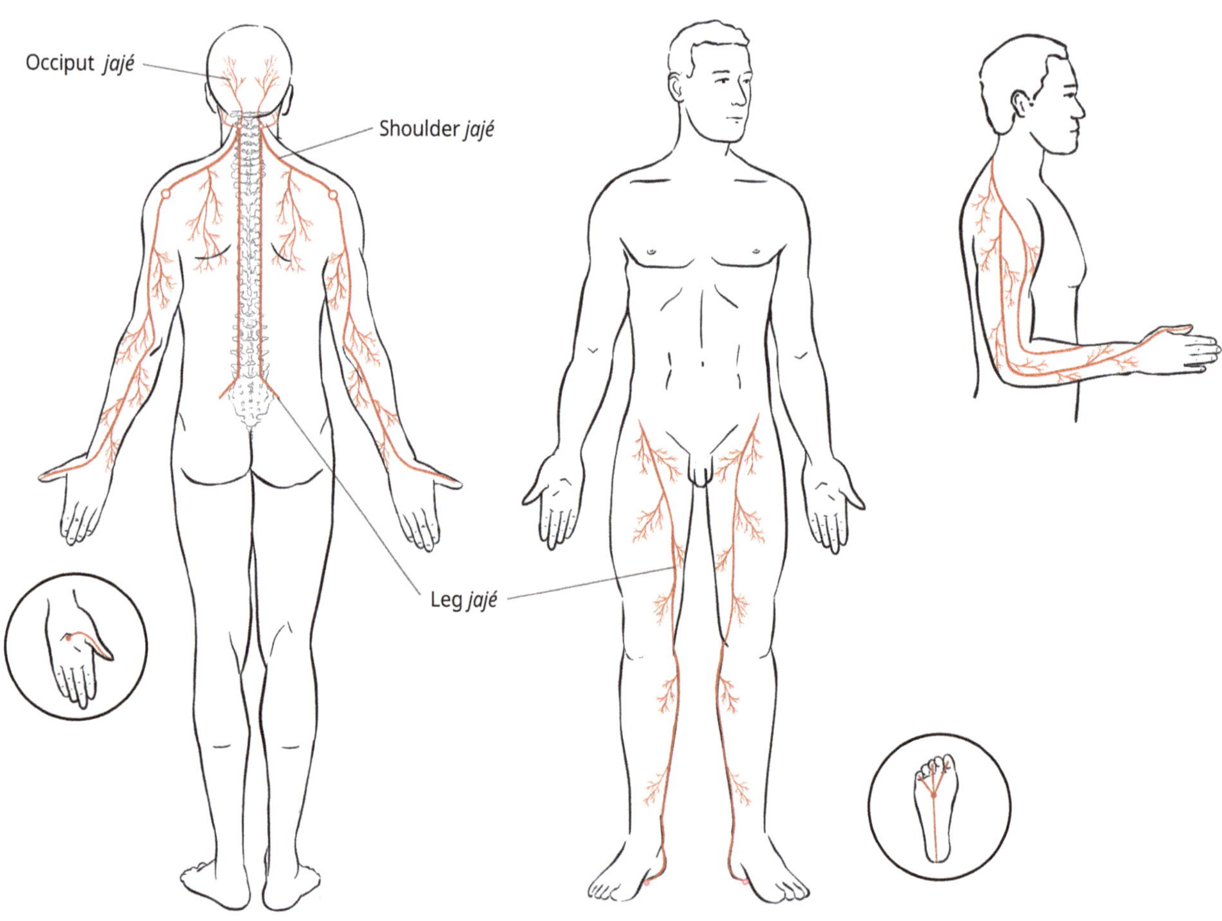

FIGURE 17.9 The *jajé* nerves

These nerves control the sensory and muscular functions of the face, including the mouth, eyes, nose, ears, jaws, and so on, as well as the chest, shoulders, inner arms, hands, and fingers. Damage to these nerves may impair the function of the face, sense organs, and neck, as well as the shoulders, arms, and hands, which may become numb or even fully paralyzed.

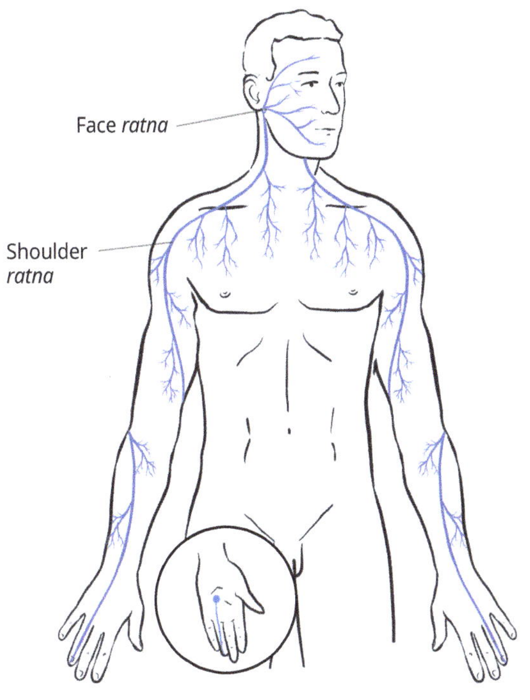

FIGURE 17.10 The *ratna* nerves

16 minor external channels (*chutsa trengbu chudruk*) branch from the three major external nerve groups described above. They locally connect with muscles, tendons, ligaments, and lymph channels:

- Two jawbone and teeth channels (*sotsa déjé*)
- Two elbow channels (*drumö chutsa*)
- Two wrist channels (*trikmé chutsa*)
- Two thigh channels (*belgö chutsa*)
- Two thigh channels (*la yi chutsa*, which are *buguchen* branches)
- Two inferior extensor retinaculum channels in the feet (*sélong chi longwar gyi zhungtsa*)
- Two Achilles tendon channels in the heels (*tingpé chutsa*)
- Two big toe hair-growing point channels in the foot (*tébong pukyé chutsa*)

17.6 LIFE FORCE CHANNELS

The life channel (*tsé yi tsa*) is where the life force flows in the form of *soklung*. It is the body's subtle breath or life-wind. The life force channel chapter of the *Explanatory Tantra* describes three types:[19]

> Humans have three life channels:
> one channel pervades the head and the whole body,
> one flows together with the breath,
> and one wanders around like the *la*.

Put simply, the first type carries *lung* and *tiklé*, which flow in the brain and throughout the whole body. Commentators disagree on its exact interpretation. The second type is called the breath (*uk*) channel that allows for air to move in and out. The third holds subtle *la* energy, which shifts from place to place.

Whether animate or inanimate, each object has a lifespan. Human beings share this characteristic with all other creatures, with each person having a unique lifespan in accordance with their individual and collective karma. A person's lifespan is equally called *tsé*, and it is supported by the *soktsa*. The difference is that *soktsa* refers more to physical channels such as vital blood vessels, whilst *tsé yi tsa* is the name given to the collective function of the channels which sustain life. Like the functioning of a car, our body-mind is dependent on its many components. A major influence on a person's lifespan is the metabolic heat produced by the three humors, their channels, and organs. Kongtrül Lodrö Thayé explains that lifespan, heat, and consciousness are intimately interdependent: if any of these three is missing, life cannot be sustained.[20]

Historical and contemporary *Gyüzhi* commentators have provided complex interpretations of the life channels. Here, we instead provide a more accessible explanation. The living body operates through the collective functions of its components, whether they are winds or channels. All are interdependent by nature. The body is like a car. The heart is like the car's engine, the breathing channel system is like the car's petrol, and mind is the driver. There are many other more and less important parts, but the prime factors enabling the body to work are the channels, winds, heat, *tiklé*, and consciousness.

Lung and *tiklé* life channels

The life channel pervades all parts of the body, especially the head. It consists of life-sustaining channels

---

19 G.yu thog yon tan mgon po, 1993, 23.

20 Karma ngag dbang yon tan rgya mtsho, 1991, 207.

in which oxygen (*tsolung*), blood (bile), water (phlegm), and nerve (wind) energies flow. These provide the basis for life to continue as well as a place for the mind to dwell. There is a disagreement between commentators on the topic of the life energy channel. Zurkhar Lodrö Gyelpo (1509–1579) describes the debate and lays down his own interpretation in his *Mépö zhélung*.[21]

Breathing life channels

A second group of life channels relates to the breath and lifespan wind (*sok gi lung*). It includes the channels for the inhalation and exhalation through nose and mouth.[22] The root of the subtle breath is lifespan wind, which is deposited in the middle channel (see also Figure 4.3). Every breath a tiny amount is released together with the more gross breath. The overall amount of life force wind contained in the middle channel determines the duration of one's lifespan: we die when this wind is consumed. *Soklung* can be understood as the body's consumable energy, much as a car's petrol is combusted to power its motor. In the human body, the fuel is derived from food essence (*dangma*) and oxygen. It is consumed in the brain to produce life-sustaining wind. Lifespan wind exits the mouth and nostrils imbued with various karmic imprints, which can be thought of as colored sand in a glass tube (see Figure 4.2). These colored bodily winds manifest fortune or misfortune according to their karmic quality. When a positive wind flows from the mouth and nose, it will bring success and happiness, whilst a negative wind will lead to suffering.

Tibetan medicine, Buddhist sources, and modern physiology all concur that a healthy person breathes around 21,600 times a day.[23] The breath is made of two components. Regular bodily breathing (*lé lung*) is the major part. It represents about 97% or 20,925 exhalations in a single day if calculated based on 15 breaths per minute. The second component is *soklung*, representing about 3% or 675 exhalations. Both parts flow together and have the same wind nature, but the latter is more subtle. In the tantric world, the breath is the main means by which to calculate the lifespan and to engage in spiritual practice. How many breaths are taken in 100 years? An adult man's normal breathing pattern is said to be 21,600 breaths per day, making approximately 7,776,000 breaths per year (with 360 days, based on Tibetan astrology). Multiplying this by 100 gives approximately 777,600,000 breaths in one lifetime. This amount contains 24,300,000 lifespan breaths.

The essence of the breath is also called *yéshé kyi lung* or transcendental wisdom wind. It is like honey from flowers, nectar from water, diamond from rock, and like the essence of fragrant plants. Therefore, another name is the quintessence of wind, *lung gi dangma*. This tiny subtle amount of the total *soklung* that flows with each breath forms one full breath every 32 general breaths.[24] This quintessence, over 100 years, will thus total 24,300,000 breaths. Controlling the transcendental wind through yogic techniques such as *lung bumpachen* reduces the consumption of this lifespan wind, thereby extending the lifespan. This calculation is part of the hidden rationale behind the Tibetan Buddhist retreat of three years and three days. If the practitioner is able to transform their winds into pure transcendental wind, they may be able to achieve enlightenment. Every day a small amount of lifespan wind is lost or used and consequently the total amount reduces daily, like a candle slowly being consumed by a flame.

The channels that wander like the *la*

The third group carries life energy which is able to move away from and come back to the body; it "wanders like the *la*." This topic is complex, requiring a great amount of time to understand it fully (see Section 18.1). Here, we should understand the *la* firstly as a life energy. The life force that wanders out like the *la* does not refer to the *la* body, but simply uses a likeness as illustration. It refers to an energy that is usually centered around the heart, generating a sense of self. Yet it also wanders in and around the body.

The wandering life energy exits and returns through the *la* channel of the ring finger, which connects to the heart-mind. The heart is the house of the *la* energy that flows through the two arms into the ulnar artery, until it reaches the tip of the ring finger. It exits via the ring finger, flowing out for a distance of 16 fingers and then returning, in synch with inhalation and exhalation. This repetitive cycle is called *la khyampa*. The channel involved is called *latsa*, the *la* pulse. Some *menpa* can read the pulse of this channel to make predictions on the lifespan and energetic situation of the patient.

---

21 Zur mkhar blo dros rgyal po, 1991, vol. 1, 166–173.

22 Oxygen and carbon dioxide correlate with the earth-water (*sachü lung*) and fire-wind breaths (*mé lung*) respectively.

23 Sde srid sangs rgyas rgya mtsho, 1994, vol. 1, 112.

---

24 The 32 breaths correspond to the 32 deities, winds, body natures, etc., as described in tantra.

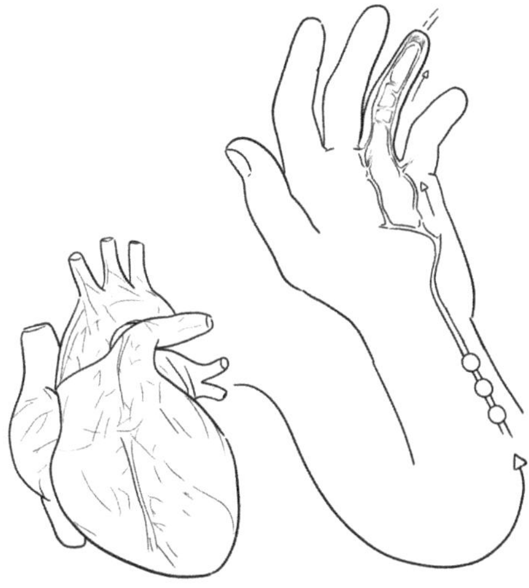

FIGURE 17.11 The *la* channel in the hand,
and where to read the *la* pulse

The heart is the main seat of consciousness (*künzhi*) and of the *la*. It also houses *dang*, which gives power to the mind and the *la*. The ring finger is called the gate of *la* energy. It is equally known as the entrance point for good and bad spirits. The *la* mostly detaches from the body and interacts with the outside world during sleep. In Tibetan societies, *la* is well-known because Tibetan astrology pays a lot of attention to it, as do healing rituals. People often wear a metallic ring on the ring finger to avoid the entry of negative forces.[25] In tantric yoga, during *lüjong* exercises for instance, practitioners close it with their thumbs.

---

25 An iron ring made from a warrior's sword is said to block
   negative forces. In many places, this ring is the sign of marriage.

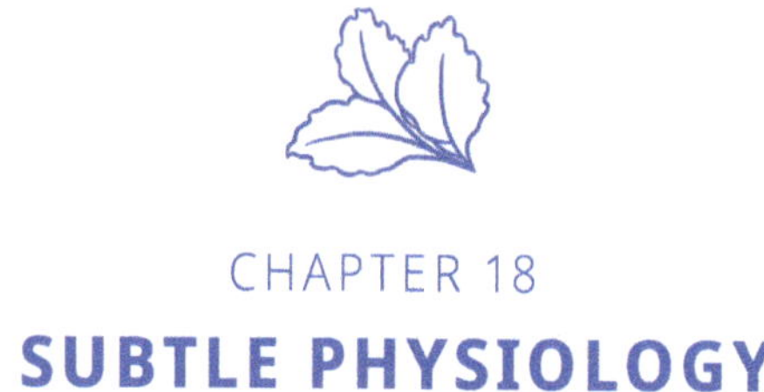

CHAPTER 18

SUBTLE PHYSIOLOGY

18.1 AN OVERVIEW OF THE *LA*

There are two different types of *la*. The first is the *la* body, which is referred to here as external *la*. It has a form similar to the material body. The second is the inner *la*, which is more subtle. The outer *la* is a reflection of the body, an energetic copy produced by the body-mind that is intricately connected to both the physical body and the mind. As long as we are fully aware, the outer *la* is joined with our body-mind. The connection between the outer *la* and the body is fostered by *dang*, but with increasing distance this link weakens. The *la* usually protrudes up to 16 fingers from the heart along with the breath and our thoughts. The heart, which holds the sense of self, is its seat.

The *la* can travel further away in a momentary loss of self-awareness, for instance when distracted or during sleep, like a kite soaring into the sky yet held by a thin wire. Sometimes it even naturally disconnects from the body for a while. To prevent sudden disconnection, it is advised not to suddenly disturb a sleeping person. It appears that the *la* body experiences feelings and sufferings as reflections of our own experiences. It can therefore suffer, get sick, and require healing as laid out in soul retrieval rituals.

Traumatic experiences can lead to more permanent separation. Most Tibetans know *la* as something related to vitality, and they have at least heard about "losing the *la*" (*la lakpa*)[26] and the need for a *la* retrieval ceremony (*laguk*, or *tséguk*). Causes of lost *la* are described in many folk tales, including being seduced by a nymph (*menmo*), or the *la* being stolen by evil spirits. Tibetan medicine, astrology, and popular sayings all offer examples of *la* leaving the body due to an accident, caused by sadness, depression or fear, due to shock or chronic trauma, or as a result of black

magic. *La* may more easily get lost in autumn and spring.

Outer *la* is not just linked to the physical body. It is also connected with sky and earth. At the moment a child is born, there is synchronicity with the local environment, creating a unique connection between the newborn and particular natural features of its birthplace. This forms the basis of the child's own inner-outer relationship with the world, which may include *la* stars, *la* trees, lakes, rocks, turquoise, animals (sheep especially), or other objects. It is difficult to discover which tree, for example, is connected to a particular person. But the energetic link exists, granting strength and stabilizing the *la* as well as the body-mind of the individual for the rest of their life. If all connections are good, *la* is stable, mind is tranquil, and the body is healthy. These ecological connections are studied in elemental astrology (*jungtsi*).

Symptoms of lost *la* include: unstable mind and emotions, discontentment, apathy, depression, fear, insecurity, feeling empty, panic attacks, increased anxiety, difficulty concentrating, diminishing memory, frequent nightmares, dreams of being naked, losing clothes or wearing ripped clothes, feeling strange in one's own body, pale face, sadness in the evenings, weak immune system, losing control over the mind, and even going insane. Generally, losing one's *la* brings about a weakening of the mental functions and feelings of alienation, of having a double personality. One loses the capacity to feel fully alive. Without *la*, a person is like an empty house or a car without an owner.

The author has spent decades trying to uncover the meaning of *la* across numerous medical, religious, and astrological texts, also investigating Bön and popular beliefs. All sources agree on the existence of *la*, and many provide explanations, yet none describe the specific appearance of *la* or its exact nature. Literally *la* signifies "higher" or "superior," as in lama (the guru or spiritual teacher) or as applied to masters, chiefs, and officials in general. The term *la* bears

---

26 Other variants of lost *la* include robbed, separated, sickened, stolen, and hidden *la*.

witness to their superior (subtle) bodies. Tibetans characterize a person who lacks intelligence and acts stupidly as "lacking higher life spirit" (*la sok*). A lama is said to guide people just as the *la* guides the body and mind. Based on this research, it appears that all humans and animals have three bodies:

1. A physical body: the product of the gross five elements

2. A mental body: the product of the afflictive mental consciousness and wind

3. And a *la* body: the subtle combined product of the physical and mental bodies, like a rainbow conjured by humidity and light; it is like a pseudo body-mind, an energetic body copy

The physical body remains on earth upon death and decays, whereas the mental body journeys towards the next reincarnation. Mind produces the mental body, whilst the subtle elements give rise to the gross elements, which then establish a new material body. The *la* body develops from the cooperation of these two bodies, like a flower growing when a seed and the earth are present as factors. Like a flower, *la* reflects both the current physical energy as well as the memory of the deceased person. *La* is not likely the very subtle mind. It is related to both subtle and gross mind. This is important to note because many psycho-emotional disorders are influenced by the *la*'s stability. A relation between *norlhagyel* minor wind (associated with body consciousness) and the existence of the *la* seems likely. *La* remains with the corpse until it is decomposed just like *norlhagyel*, especially with the bones. Both *norlhagyel* and *la* stick together with the remains of the body. Perhaps this is one reason why Tibetans prefer sky burial, as this burial method ensures that the *la* does not linger and therefore will not have to endure further suffering. The *la* of the deceased may in rare cases possess someone and express familial issues. Yet, it is difficult to distinguish here between spirits and *la*.

We will now approach the *la* from different perspectives.

Döl Bön

It is highly likely that *la* healing rituals originate from native shamanism, which is called Döl Bön. Over time, these were integrated into Tibetan Buddhist rites and healing practices. Döl Bön is still practiced widely in Siberia, Tibet, and along the Nepal-India border, and is related to animistic religions worldwide. Historically,

practitioners performed *la* rituals in a less organized fashion, which nowadays involves the use of printed texts. In soul retrieval rituals (*laguk*), evil spirits are given ransom in exchange for returning the patient's *la*.[1] In the author's experience, this type of ritual does give positive results. The following phrase sums up the Bön approach:

Propitiate the protector spirits,
subdue the harmful spirits.

Bönpos have profound knowledge of the natural environment, invisible positive and negative forces, and their relationship to human wellbeing, as indicated in the following event recounted by the author:

When I was student in Syabru Bensi (Rasuwa Jilla, Nepal) in the early 1970s, our old schoolhouse owner died. He was of the Tamang ethnicity. Nepali Tamang people follow the Nyingma Buddhist tradition with elements of local Bön shamanic practice. One day there was a feast for the deceased. I was curious, so I attended. Some Tamang lamas and one Tibetan lama were present. They made a small effigy of the deceased man and dressed it with his clothes. They offered the effigy the food, drinks, and even the type of cigarette that the deceased man had liked. Reciting religious texts and calling his name, the lamas summoned the deceased into the effigy. They then informed the man that he had died and convinced him to release any attachment he had to his family, house, property, and so on. Next, the effigy was sent off with a ransom ritual (*lü*), so that he would not remain attached to his past life.

Similar practices are also found in other Tibetan Buddhist schools that perform a ceremony for the deceased person involving their tutelary deity (*yidam*), to free the soul from negative karma. However, according to Milarépa's biography, *la* is not the consciousness or mind of the deceased person. It can however act like the person's mind, generating confusion with the deceased person's actual consciousness. Nevertheless, the person's consciousness has already journeyed towards a new life, driven by one's karma. But how long does the *la* spirit remain on earth? This is a question that has not been settled. In Tibetan astrology, specific necromancy rites are said to pacify the remaining *la*. One of Künkyen Jigmé Lingpa's (1730–1798) works contains the following words:[2]

---

1 "Soul" has been used frequently in translations of Tibetan Buddhist and Bon religious texts, but this does not mean that the *la* is equivalent to Christian understandings.

2 Tshul khrims gyal tshan, 1998, vol. 1, 513.

Life is terminated by evil spirits.
Consciousness follows karma,
and the *la* remains in the grave.

This statement makes clear that the external *la* is not mind itself. However, it is certainly a subtle energy body.

La in the *Gyüzhi*

Tibetan medical texts do not give much attention to the *la*, but the *Four Tantras* do contain a few scattered, rather superficial references. The section on the life channels (*tsé yi tsa*) in the *Explanatory Tantra* describes a channel that "wanders like the *la*" (see Section 17.6). The subtle *la* energy cycle (*la powa*) is also mentioned. The *Subsequent Tantra* mentions the following in the pulse chapter:[3]

When the mind is not liberated, it turns
downwards,
and is born into an ignorant samsaric body.
The wandering *la* pulse arises as the base of
the life force.
As long as this pulse remains, *la* and life
force will be stable.
If it changes, life will not be maintained.
If the *la* escapes, *la* and life force will be
exhausted.
Longevity and soul retrieval rites might
bring these back.

According to the *Gyüzhi*, the *la* energy flows through *la* channels. When faced with a patient's lost or separated *la*, an *amchi* may consult the Tibetan almanac and calculate the patient's *la* situation by determining whether they are in an obstacle year. Rituals, soul retrieval, or long-life initiations may then be advised. Sowa Rigpa thus recognizes *la* and considers it an important vital energy.

The inner flow of *la* energy according to the *Kālacakratantra*

The wandering *la* energy is not the same as the *la* body, which should not be confused with fluxes in the body such as hormonal cycles. The *la* body, however, does correspond to *dang*: the body's *tiklé* radiance.[4]

The location of the inner *la* changes day by day, which is known as *la powa*: the transference of *la* from one place to another within one month. The *la* cycle never stops unless the life force itself is finished.

It is a wandering, "superior" subtle life energy present in each being. The manner of its movement is termed *lané potsül*. The changing energy inside a person reflects the changing phases of the moon, which influences the mood and character of a person, their body and health. Similarly, the moon can be said to be the *la* of our planet. It is an energy that circles around and affects the Earth, acting like a synchronizing natural clock. The moon is a symbol of the *tiklé*, and an outer reflection of what also occurs inside our bodies.

The inner *la* is also used as a collective term for the essence of the material body, its subtle energy that consists of five components from a tantric perspective: *tsa* (channels), *lung* (wind), *drö* (psychic heat), and *tiklé* (essence drops), which are the physical basis for *namshé* (consciousness). In this context, *La* is also used as a synonym for evolving relative *bodhicitta* (*jangchup kyi sem gyégyur gyi rikchen*), which corresponds to the five-colored *tiklé*. This is why Ju Mipham Namgyel Gyatso writes in his commentary:[5]

The basis of lifespan and life force is
the quintessence of wind, *tiklé*, and
consciousness; this together is called the *la*.

Tsa refers to the 72,000 channels, where an equal number of *lung* energies flow. In the channels, wind transports the *tiklé*, which are burnt by heat, producing bliss and light. The perceiver of these sensations is consciousness itself, whereas the nature of consciousness is the light of awareness. This process takes place in countless major and minor channels throughout life. Through yogic methods, metabolic heat can be transformed into *tumo* fire that is utilized to burn the dualistic body-mind and its waste products, driving out ignorance. The ultimate result of this transformation is obtainment of a rainbow body.

Understanding this process, it is clear that the *la* is a quintessential energy that brightens the entire body-mind from the heart, the root of all channels and house of the *künzhi*. The vibrating waves of light of the inner *la* spread outwards, thus continuously reinforcing the outer *la* body which is usually described as *dang* in medical sources. The energies in this five-dimensional body-mind flow in accordance with the moon phases, increasing and decreasing in potency as the moon waxes and wanes. They are known as *kyangma* for men, and *roma* for women. These are basically the same but are governed by the moon and sun respectively. According to the author, the waxing moon stimulates the endocrine glands to produce more hormones, which takes place for women mainly from the lower abdomen upwards. The full moon corresponds to a state of maximum energy, which can easily lead to imbalance.

---

3 G.yu thog yon ta mgon po, 1993, 566.
4 For more details, see Sde srid sangs rgyas rgya mtsho, 1994, 112.

5 'Ju mi pham nnam rgyal rgya mtsho, 1988, 287–88.

The male cycle is usually given as an example. Women are opposite: the *la* is a lunar energy cycle in men, and a solar cycle in women. Men and women have contrasting bodies and feelings. This is related to their inner nature, which is referred to as relative *bodhicitta* or subtle *tiklé* energy.

The *la* cycle starts at new moon (first day of the Tibetan lunar month) and continues until full moon (15th day of the month). The *la* energy increases and then declines until the black or dark moon, when the cycle is complete (30th day). During the waxing moon the masculine lunar energy increases in men, starting from the first toe joints of the left foot (for women it is the opposite: the solar energy increases in the right first toe joints). The dark moon is the sign of minimum *la* energy (which is concentrated at the soles of the feet) for both men and women, while full moon is the maximum (at the crown point). These days the energies are polarized to the extreme, which is an imbalanced state of the body-mind from a medical point of view that may influence the mind and lead to increased emotional sensitivity and "lunatic" disturbances. The left channel (*kyangma*, Skt. *lalanā*) and right channel (*roma*, Skt. *rasanā*) are the inner lunar and solar systems of the body, which rule the body alternately. Eclipse then represents a neutral or balanced state, which corresponds to the central channel (*uma*, Skt. *āvadhūtī*). This balancing of the lunar and solar energies takes place during new and full moon. In-between day 30 and day 1, the whole body is charged with *bodhicitta* energy.

Buddhist practitioners reserve these special days for spiritual growth, but medical practitioners should equally be aware of their effect. To find out the *la* energy situation one should consult the Tibetan lunar calendar. Each day the *la* changes, being concentrated in a different area. The times at which the energy and location of the *la* change are at dawn and dusk, when it is (still) light enough to see the lines of the hands without artificial light.

TABLE 18.1 The male *la* cycle

Day	Moon	Energy letter	Phonetics	Location
1	New moon	ཨཿ	*aH*	First foot joints (left)
2	Waxing crescent	ཨི	*i*	Second foot joints
3	"	རྀ	*r-i*	Third foot joints
4	"	ཨུ	*u*	Ankle
5	"	ཨཱི	*I-i*	Knee
6	"	ཨ	*a*	Hip
7	"	ཨེ	*ei*	First finger joints (proximal phalanges)
8	First quarter	ཨར	*ar*	Second finger joints
9	Waxing gibbous	ཨོ	*o*	Third finger joints
10	"	ཨལ	*al*	Wrist
11	"	ཧ	*ha*	Elbow
12	"	ཡ	*ya*	Shoulder (left)
13	"	ར	*ra*	Throat
14	"	ཝ	*wa*	Fontanel
15	"	ལ	*la*	Forehead
15–16	Full moon	ཨོཾ	*oM*	Crown
16	Waning gibbous	ལཱ	*lA*	Occiput
17	"	ཝཱ	*wA*	Neck
18	"	རཱ	*rA*	Heart
19	"	ཡཱ	*yA*	Shoulder (right)
20	"	ཧཱ	*hA*	Elbow
21	"	ཨཱལ	*Al*	Wrist
22	"	ཨཽ	*au*	Third finger joints (distal phalanges)
23	Third quarter	ཨཱར	*Ar*	Second finger joints
24	Waning crescent	ཨཻ	*ei*	First finger joints
25	"	ཨཱ	*A*	Hip
26	"	ཨཱི	*lI*	Knee
27	"	ཨཱུ	*U*	Ankle
28	"	རཱྀ	*r-I*	Third toe joints
29	"	ཨཱྀ	*I*	Second toe joints
30	"	ཨཱ	*A*	First toe joints (right foot)

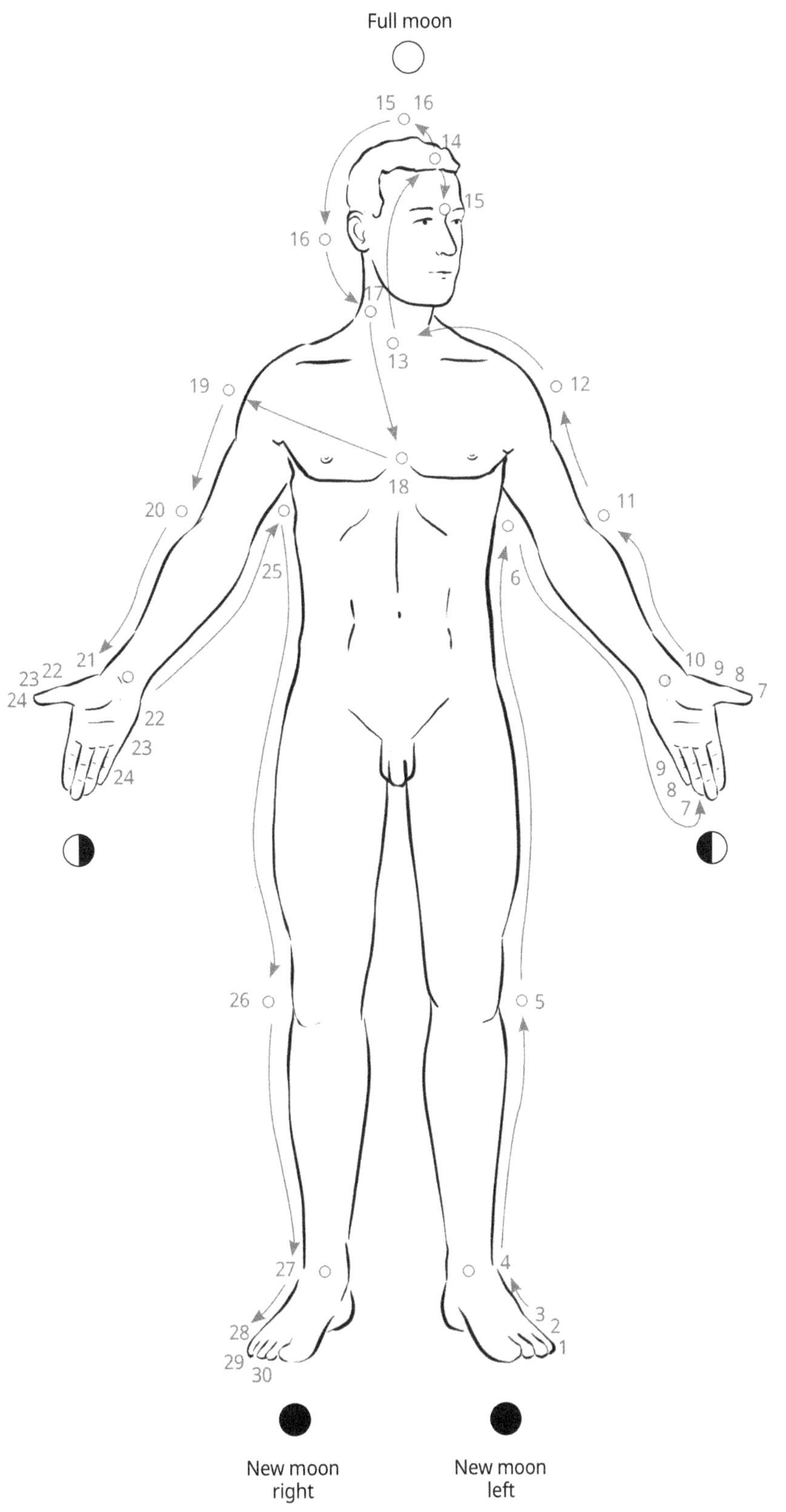

FIGURE 18.1 The lunar *la* cycle of men

TABLE 18.2 The female *la* cycle

Day	Moon	Energy letter	Phonetics	Location
1	New moon	ཨཿ	aH	First foot joints (right)
2	Waxing crescent	ཨི	i	Second foot joints
3	"	རི	r-i	Third foot joints
4	"	ཨུ	u	Ankle
5	"	ཨེ	I-i	Knee
6	"	ཨ	a	Hip
7	"	ཨེ	ei	First finger joints (proximal phalanges)
8	First quarter	ཨར	ar	Second finger joints
9	Waxing gibbous	ཨོ	o	Third finger joints
10	"	ཨལ	al	Wrist
11	"	ཧ	ha	Elbow
12	"	ཡ	ya	Shoulder (right)
13	"	ར	ra	Throat
14	"	ཝ	wa	Fontanel
15	"	ལ	la	Forehead
15–16	Full moon	ཨོཾ	oM	Crown
16	Waning gibbous	ལཱ	lA	Occiput
17	"	ཝཱ	wA	Neck
18	"	རཱ	rA	Heart
19	"	ཡཱ	yA	Shoulder (left)
20	"	ཧཱ	hA	Elbow
21	"	ཨླལ	Al	Wrist
22	"	ཨཽ	au	Third finger joints (distal phalanges)
23	Third quarter	ཨུར	Ar	Second finger joints
24	Waning crescent	ཨི	ei	First finger joints
25	"	ཨཱ	A	Hip
26	"	ཨླི	lI	Knee
27	"	ཨུ	U	Ankle
28	"	རི	r-I	Third toe joints
29	"	ཨླི	I	Second toe joints
30	"	ཨླ	A	First toe joints (left foot)

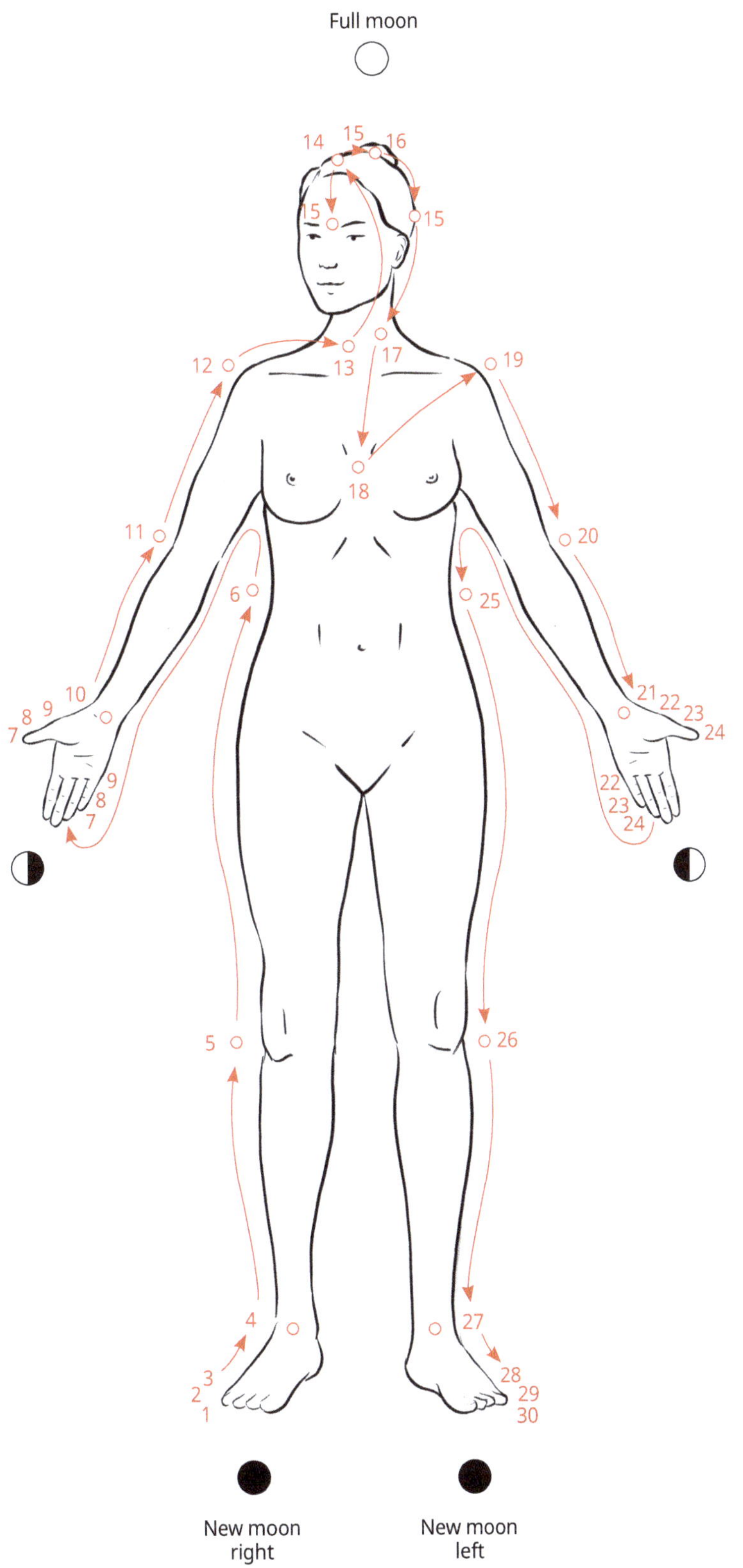

FIGURE 18.2 The solar *la* cycle of women

18.2 TANTRA-BASED CHANNELS

Channels (*tsa*), chakras (*khorlo*), gross and subtle *tiklé*, and especially wind (*lung*) and its functions are expounded in detail in *vajra* body teachings. Such teachings may use different terminologies, metaphorical names, and numbers of channels and chakras, so that a great deal of time is necessary to get an overall understanding. Oral transmission and empowerment as well as devotional practices are primary, rather than logic and rational knowledge. Tantric practice is squarely based on devotion to the guru and specific meditation deities. There could therefore be differences according to the master's tradition, personal vision, and experience. In tantra, the central wind channel is called *tsa uma*, the blood channel *roma*, and the phlegm or water channel *kyangma*.

Major and minor chakras are presented as inner body cities (*nang gi drongkhyer*), or alternatively as flowers with channels as petals. *Lung* transports the *tiklé* through the *tsa*, where these can be ignited by *drö* (heat), in turn producing bliss. This is experienced by the consciousness (*namshé*), which manifests feelings and emotions (*tsorwa*). Wind is the vehicle of consciousness. Consciousness is equated with the inhabiting male and female deities. Correctly practicing as instructed will affect all these body-mind aspects, allowing one to see and experience a reality based on the union of loving-kindness and emptiness. All of this is manifested by utilizing the channels, chakras, *tiklé*, *drö*, and consciousness, which are moved by the power of the winds.

Father Tantras mention 84,000 channels, and the Mother Tantras 72,000. Each channel circulates *lung* and houses the combustion of *tiklé* that produces the body and emotions. The channels are like a house, wind like a vehicle, *tumo* heat is power, the *tiklé* are a treasure, and consciousness is the owner of the body country. Unrealized beings live an illusory life, not knowing the inner and outer worlds, which leads to death and rebirth, aging and disease. They are absorbed in their daily lives like bees in a beehive, fish in a pond, or ants on an anthill, not seeing the bigger picture. The body is composed of numerous channels, winds, and consciousness, which produce emotions similarly to communities consisting of collectives of beings. The tantric way of practice is to understand and transform this collective body, liberating the mind from the world of illusion. Tantra relies on a different language and understanding of body, energy, and mind, which is generally forbidden to openly expose to others. We therefore refrain from explaining the *vajra* body in much detail here.

18.3 CHAKRAS (*KHORLO*)

Cakra is a Sanskrit word equivalent to *khorlo* in Tibetan, which means "wheel." Chakras are also called *tsakhor*, wheels of channels. They consist of major and minor channels and functions like city centers, directing the functioning of the body country and connecting to other centers through countless intersections. The central channel (*tsa uma*) is like a bamboo trunk with the chakras as its nodes, from which many branches grow. Teachings on the channels and chakras belong to the anatomy as well as subtle physiology of wind and mind in Tibetan medicine, and they belong to the *vajra* body in tantra. They are the seats of psychic and elemental forces, an important subject in higher medical study. The three major and the minor channels make the chakras that house the five emotions. The number of chakras described varies greatly. The *Kālachakratantra* describes six chakras, whereas *Nāropā's Six Dharmas* utilizes four, and the *Guhyasamāja* five. The tantric channels, their colors, numbers, and terms should be understood as part of the traditional language of instruction and practice without any external criticism. Some texts state that the middle channel is blue, and others say white, some say it is empty and others explain it is filled by lifespan wind. Here, we will introduce the chakras in an easy way from a medical point of view, without the need for spiritual restrictions.

The three chakras

What follows is based on the formation and existing channels sections of the *Explanatory Tantra's* fourth chapter.

1. The crown chakra (*chiwo déchen gyi khorlo*)

The crown chakra is white. It is the seat of the life-sustaining wind and the five minor winds. These winds function together with the sense consciousnesses and organs. Tibetan medicine explains that the crown chakra is the seat of the phlegm humor, which corresponds psychologically with ignorance, gross mind and its memory. The brain is heavy, watery and has a cold nature, but it also has the potential to awaken from ignorance. Tantra describes the crown chakra as the principal subject of practices aiming to consume dualistic thinking. It is also the seat of the *tiklé*, the subtle energy of the brain, which can be transformed into wisdom through meditation. It has the symbolic seed syllable *ŌṀ*, representing the body. Complete victory over duality is equal to enlightenment.

Therefore, this chakra is called *chiwo déchen gyi khorlo*: "the crown chakra of great bliss." It sits at the top of the body mandala, like a pagoda. The crown chakra is comprised of 500 channels: 200 *kyangma*, 200 *roma*, and 100 *uma* channels. These are the pathways that allow the mind to arise, and which transport the *tiklé*. They are responsible for the function of the sensory consciousnesses as well as controlling the whole body and its organs.

2. The heart chakra (*nying a chö kyi khorlo*)

The heart chakra is the capital city of the body-mind. It is red, facing down. It is the seat of pervasive wind and base of the *künzhi*. It is also the seat of accomplishing bile, and where the deep awakening memory channels reside. The heart chakra provides interest, the sense of "I" as well as the self-grasping mind. It functions as the basic source of the emotions of pride, ambition, anger, and aggressiveness, yet can also manifest love, compassion, and friendship, thus balancing the body-mind. In medicine, the heart chakra is the source of anger and bile, which is a destructive force. In tantra, it is called the dharma chakra, since it is here that the wisdom of discrimination can be developed, leading to realization. The enlightened knowledge of the self and of phenomenal existence has to be awakened from the *künzhi*. 500 channels, like those mentioned above for the crown chakra, provide the passageways to maintain its function, supporting the central channel.

3. The secret chakra (*sang ngé dékyong gi khorlo*)

The secret chakra is blue and faces upward. It is the seat of descending wind, of fear and jealousy, and manifests desire, anger, attachment, as well as joy. According to medical texts, it is the base of the wind humor, regulating the production of reproductive fluids, sexual activity, and conception. It is called the "bliss-guarding chakra of the secret place" in tantra. It is the engine that powers the manifestation of desire and attachment. This is why many psychological and emotional disorders manifest from this chakra.

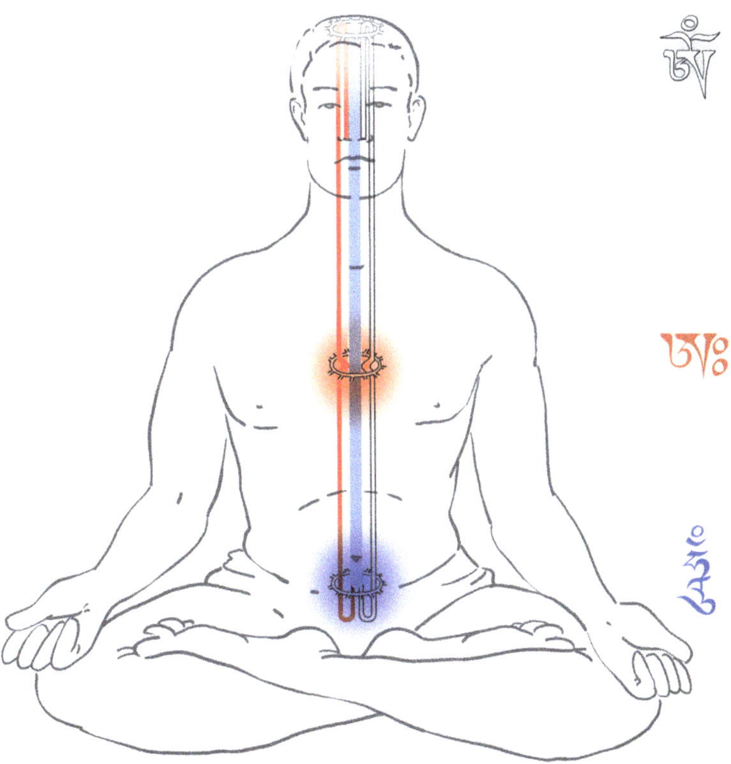

FIGURE 18.3 The three chakras

TABLE 18.3 The correspondences of the three chakras

Chakra	Appearance	Minor wind	Function	Humor (element)	Psychic base	Seed syllable
Crown	White downward-facing lotus	Life-sustaining wind	Material foundation, seat of *tiklé*, gross mind and memory, perception, thinking	Phlegm (water)	Ignorance and closed-mindedness, wisdom	*ŌṀ*
Heart	Red downward-facing lotus	Pervasive wind	Subtle mind and memory (*künzhi*), seat of "I"	Bile and blood (fire)	Anger and hatred, compassion	*AH*
Secret	Blue upward-facing lotus	Descending wind	Very subtle mind, arousal, reproduction	Wind (wind)	Jealousy, desire, fear, joy	*HUṀ*

500 channels also regulate the functions of the secret chakra throughout life.

The above three chakras correspond to the three dimensions of body, speech (energy), and mind, which are the products of the three mental poisons that materialize as the three humors. All body-mind manifestations can be explained through the operation of this triadic system.

The five chakras

The study of the five-chakra system focuses on the composition of the body-mind based on the five elements and the five mental poisons, and their spiritual transmutation into the Five Tathagatas (Rgyal ba rigs lnga). This system provides more systematic information on the relationship between mind and matter than the three chakras. Transmutation here refers to the spontaneous transformation of the samsaric body-mind using spiritual methods, much like iron is turned into gold through alchemy. The iron does not disappear but turns into another substance. Similarly, the ignorant mind transforms itself into Buddha-nature. The Five Tathagatas represent the enlightened body, speech, mind, qualities, and action of an individual buddha. Our emotions manifest from the function of the chakras and then run the business of samsara. But by penetrating the chakras using the techniques of spiritual yoga and meditation, one's mind can be purified much like gold can be rid of its oxidation. However, only a person with the right heart, strong determination, detachment

from samsara, and the proper guidance of the master will achieve this goal. The summary that follows is based on a combination of medical sources and the *Guhyasamāja Tantra*.

1. The crown chakra

The crown chakra, where life-sustaining wind is located, governs the general body-mind. It is ruled by the space element, is of white color, and it is the seat of ignorance. The crown chakra has 32 lotus petals that symbolize the 32 channels of the crown, which support the manifestation of ignorance. When ignorance is transformed through spiritual practice, it becomes the white Buddha Vairocana. The head is the aggregate (Skt. *skandha*) of form and corresponds to the enlightened buddha body. The seed syllable of this buddha and chakra is a white *ŌṀ*.

2. The throat chakra (*drinpa longchö kyi khorlo*)

The throat chakra, where ascending wind is located, governs speech and experiences taste. Because the mind enjoys these experiences, it is called the enjoyment chakra. It is associated with the fire and wind elements, and of red-greenish color. The throat chakra provides the condition for the manifestation of attachment and enjoyment. It has 16 lotus petals, symbolizing the 16 channels of the throat. When attachment is transmuted, it becomes the red Buddha Amitābha. It is associated with the feeling aggregate, which can be transformed into enlightened buddha speech. The seed syllable of this buddha and chakra is a red *AH*.

3. The heart chakra

The heart chakra is the seat of pervasive wind that governs the heart and chest area. It is ruled by the water (which predominates) and fire element. It is of blue color, with red inside. The heart chakra has eight petals, which are symbols of the eight consciousnesses (eyes, ear, nose, tongue, body, mind, mental affliction, and *künzhi* mind). These channels help manifest anger, aggression, and related emotions. On the other hand, they can also produce love, compassion, and wisdom, which leads to enlightenment. When anger is transmuted, the mind arises as the blue Buddha Akshobhya. Akshobya represents the enlightened buddha mind that is associated with the perception aggregate. The seed syllable of this buddha and chakra is a blue *HUṀ*.

4. The navel chakra (*téwa trulpé khorlo*)

The navel chakra is located in the lower abdomen, below the navel. It is the seat of fire-like wind, which governs the digestive fire (*médrö*). It is ruled by the earth element, of yellow color, and provides the conditions for pride, ambition, greed, and miserliness to arise. The navel emanation chakra is the place from where the embryo develops through the umbilical cord. It has 64 lotus petals which represent the 64 channels that help manifest the affliction mind of pride and egotism. However, it can also become the source of selflessness and generosity. When this mind is transmuted, it arises as the yellow Buddha Ratnasambhava, who corresponds to the formation aggregate and represents the enlightened buddha quality. The corresponding syllable is a yellow *SO*.

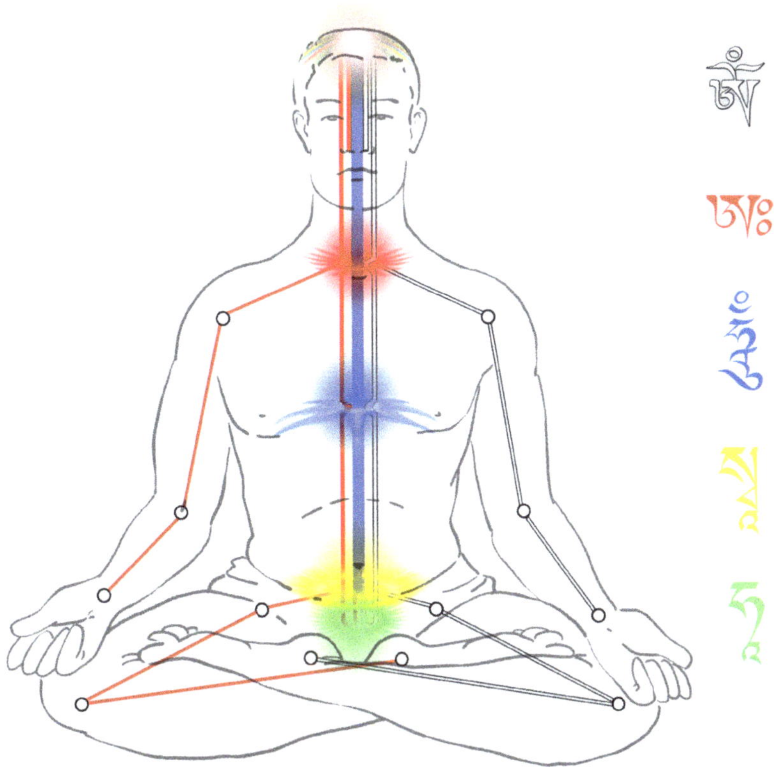

FIGURE 18.4 The five chakras

5. The secret chakra

The last chakra is located in the genital and coccyx area, and is governed by descending wind which rules the lower back and abdomen. It is wind element, green, and provides the condition for desire, jealousy, fear, and lust to arise. The bliss-guarding chakra of the secret place has 32 petals which symbolize the 32 channels that help manifest the above-mentioned mental afflictions. The secret chakra is the place of the discernment aggregate. When transmuted, the mind arises as the green Buddha Amoghasiddhi, enlightened buddha action. The buddha's and chakra seed syllable is a green *HA*.

There are many other minor chakras (*khorlo chungwa*) that are not described here. These include the forehead chakra, the 12 large body joints which correspond to the 12 zodiac signs, and the 360 body joints which correspond to the 360 days of the year. The minor chakras form bigger chakras, which then form the principal chakras just like smaller groups of stars form galaxies. All chakras, major or minor, gross or subtle, produce emotions and regulate the elements and mind functions. They preserve and transport *tiklé*, subtle wind energy, and consciousness. The body is like a universe and the chakras are its constellations. The *tiklé* are like planets that move in their orbits by means of wind energy.

TABLE 19.4 The correspondences of the five chakras

Chakra	Minor wind	Element	Color	Emotion	Aggregate	Wisdom	Buddha
Crown	Life-sustaining wind	Space	White	Ignorance	Form	Body	Vairocana
Throat	Ascending wind	Fire	Red	Attachment	Feeling	Speech	Amithāba
Heart	Pervasive wind	Water	Blue	Anger	Perception	Heart-Mind	Akshobhya
Navel	Fire-like wind	Earth	Yellow	Pride	Formation	Quality	Ratnasambhava
Secret	Descending wind	Wind	Green	Jealousy	Consciousness	Action	Amoghasiddhi

CHAPTER 19

DREAMS AND THE DYING PROCESS

When the time of youth is over, signs of aging begin to appear like autumn flowers. We get weaker, wrinkles appear, and memory declines. The body shrivels like an old fruit. White hairs grow like snowfall on trees in wintertime. In this stage of life, degeneration signs will naturally appear, letting us know that the elemental energies of earth, water, fire, air, and space are no longer capable of fully sustaining the body-mind. The digestive organs can no longer fully digest food and absorb nutritional essences. Therefore, body strength begins to decrease. This is called "aging disease" (*gé né*). As a result, the body house begins to deteriorate, and the mind suffers from feeling old. The intimate relationship of body and mind has endured over a long period of time, making it painful when they start to separate again.

The disease of old age receives ample attention in all systems of medicine, especially amongst religiously inclined traditions. The *Gyüzhi* dedicates a chapter to geriatrics, and another chapter to rejuvenation practices. The overall aim is to slow down the aging process and fortify the physical conditions that prolong life. Many Tibetan physicians have written works on these subjects, searching for possibilities to extend life, which is the fundamental idea of rejuvenation. Yet, the Buddhist view holds that all phenomena are governed by the law of impermanence. There is therefore no permanent cure to stop the aging and dying process. The body is seen as the karmic consequence of past lives. One should therefore accept and prepare for any result, whatever it may be. If one wants to be free from aging and death, one should avoid their causes, as expounded in the Four Noble Truths:

> Suffering exists.
> Because it has a cause,
> cessation is possible.
> This is the path.

The evolution of humans and all sentient beings is ruled by cause and effect. A person who knows the cause of suffering, who works hard on its prevention and purification, and who eradicates the roots of ignorance and delusions, will be led to liberation from the cycle of death and rebirth.

The search for immortality

In ancient times, people had great faith in religion, meditation, yogic methods, mantra recitation, and so on, hoping that these would ward off death. There are legends of yogis who lived hundreds of years, but they are relatively few, and eventually they still had to face the Lord of Death. Even the gods called "The Immortals" have to die. Medical research turned towards material methods to support and prolong life, yet the result has been rather limited. The interest then shifted to alchemy in medieval times. Various detoxified metals and minerals, especially mercury-sulfide and gold compounds, were used to substitute the bodily elements in order to slow down the aging process.[1] These techniques brought hope to many scholars, much more than other life-prolonging methods. Precious pills (*rinchen rilbu*) were made by physicians from transformed mercurial powder. On the benefit of *rinchen rilbu*, Gurupel says:[2]

> It is called *tiklé daryaken*.[3]
> Beings who taste the amount of a tiny
> sesame seed can reach the pure land of
> Khechara.

---

1 Tibetan alchemy is mostly based on translations from Sanskrit and on Nāgārjuna's works. Further research needs to be conducted on this subject and its history.

2 Sde dge'i drung yig gu ru 'phel, 1986, 372.

3 This is a Greek or Galenic medical term related to theriac, a panacea that cures snakebite. The corresponding Tibetan term is *tengchok*. *Daryaken* is believed to be a word of Zhangzhung origin.

Eventually, alchemical approaches declined. Tibetan alchemists appeared to have accepted that it is not possible to conquer impermanence and achieve freedom from disease and death through matter alone. Material energy is limited; it sustains the physical body, but it cannot increase the basic lifespan wind that is determined by past lives. Scholars also turned to Buddhist spiritual practice to find permanent freedom from suffering, integrating yogic exercises, alchemical preparations, non-dual or transcendental practices, and especially tantric transformation of the body-mind. The aim was to achieve a *vajra* body (*dorjé lü*), an indestructible state, and finally to attain the rainbow body (*ja lü*). Many succeeded, as confirmed by accounts that have been retold throughout history. However, this path is limited to certain practitioners only. The majority remains behind as ordinary mortals. In this manner, spiritual practice and self-transformation became the main instruments to end death (and rebirth) in Tibetan Buddhist culture.

The Mahayana Buddhist makes good use of the unfortunate situation of dying, turning it into an exceptional opportunity. The three stages of life related with death, bardo, and rebirth allow for highly sophisticated methods of mind transformation as a path towards liberation. At these stages, major emotions dissolve. The mind becomes very light, which makes it easier to experience ultimate reality. More detail can be found in the *Tibetan Book of the Dead*, and in *sādhanā* texts with different *yidam* deities that include the three *kāya* as paths (*kusum lamkhyer*). In the context of such practices, dreams are signs or messengers of the changing body-mind. We should therefore pay attention to our dreams and other omens for medical as well as spiritual purposes.

Prognosis of death

The *Gyüzhi* describes this subject with care, in parallel with the concepts and practices of tantric dissolution.[4] The text does not elaborate, however, on what happens after the physical body is dead. The process of dying and its prognosis is called *jikté*, which can be understood as "signs of destruction." The body's elemental functions collapse in reverse to their development during embryogenesis, with every moment taking us one step further. The elements which cooperate harmoniously at the beginning become enemies, and eventually start to fight each other. This elemental disharmony creates breakdown particles that block the life channel, which affect dreams, manifest omens, and influence the mind.

---

4   More detail on signs, dreams, and omens can be found in Pha khol, 1989, vol. 1, 296–303.

19.1 DISTANT SIGNS OF DEATH

A distant sign of death is a sign or warning that indicates that some changes are happening in the body-mind. There are three subdivisions: (1) observing the messenger, (2) dream prognostication, and (3) the patient's temperament.

Observing the messenger

Ponya signifies "messenger," the person who comes to invite or who goes to call the doctor or lama for help. The doctor or lama observes the messenger's clothing, mode of speaking, and emotions, and asks about what they have seen and experienced on the way. This information can act as a prognosis of the patient's recovery or decline.

The following signs are considered positive:

- An unusual messenger (wearing bizarre clothes), or a spiritual person of the same caste or area (as the physician) are signs that the patient can be cured

- The inviter encounters someone carrying grains, curd, etc. in full containers on their way

- The messenger perceives the following: ringing bells, lamps, flowers, roasted grains and food, sacred statues, people wearing white clothes or praying and practicing dharma, a standing banner, a burning fire, a horse, sheep, or a cow with their young, people eating and drinking with beautiful ornaments, people entering a house, or beautiful sounds

The following signs are negative signs, indicating there may be obstacles in healing the patient:

- The inviter arrives with fear, is impatient or anxious, rubs his hands (with a stone or other objects), calls the doctor from a distance, engages in negative activities, wears inauspicious ornaments (for instance, broken ones), and speaks with lamentations

- If the inviter visits when the doctor is in a bad mood, speaks inauspiciously, cuts objects or takes them apart, propitiates the ancestors, or performs a fire puja; these are signs that the patient may die

- If the inviter undertakes his journey to see the doctor on the Tibetan calendar days four, six, or nine, at solar or lunar eclipses, on negative days, and days ruled by negative constellations, or at midnight

- If during the journey, the inviter finds burnt or broken objects, hears cries or the sounds of killing

- If during the journey, the inviter is crossed by a cat, monkey, otter, snake, or by other inauspicious animals

- Seeing curd or milk taken out of a house by someone, or seeing an extinguishing lamp, or broken containers

These signs are also valid for the doctor who goes to visit a patient.

Dream prognostication

Dreams are the secret symbolic language of the mind. They are a common topic of interest in East and West. In the West, psychoanalysts such as Carl Jung (1875–1961) say an "important dream" speaks in a mysterious language. Western psychologists, however, often neglect religious and spiritual concepts related to dreaming, adopting a rather narrow scientific interpretation. Tibetan dream interpretation is colored by Tibetan cultural beliefs, and firmly influenced by the Buddhist philosophy of mind and phenomena. Some agreement does exist between Eastern and Western understandings of dreams, but there can also be considerable differences. According to Tibetan Buddhism, the all-ground of the mind (*künzhi*) is involved, which records all memories of past and present experiences.

There are several general dream types. The first derives directly from memories. It is like an imprinted film appearing in the mind triggered by thoughts and experiences that the person had during the day. The second type of dream comes from the consciousness that travels or wanders, investigating experiences in the form of a dream. Through dreams, the *künzhi* can reveal or communicate subtle information to the dreamer. Tibetan medicine lists six groups of dreams, from the time just after profound sleep until late morning. The duration of sleep is either six or eight hours, and can be divided into six sections:

1. Dreams of what was seen the day before, related with food and life influences

2. Dreams of what was heard the day before

3. Dreams of experiences of the day before

4. Dreams of prayers, the fulfilment of spiritual achievement

5. Dreams of fulfilling wishes

6. Dreams of bad omens or illness prognosis

Early night dreams are often forgotten and are usually not highly significant, while morning and late morning dreams could be good for interpretation, showing indications on health, business, spiritual progress, and the future.

During sleep or even when fainting, the sensory consciousness dissolves into the mental consciousness in the heart (see also Section 4.4). The mind goes into a deep sleep and momentarily goes into an unconscious state. After that, the mental affliction wind (*nyönmongpé lung*) arises and wakes up the heart memory. Driven by this wind, the mind then enters the two main channels of the right and left sides of the throat chakra. This allows the mind to dream. The consciousness is carried by *nyönmongpé lung* through the channels and the chakras of the upper, middle, and lower parts of the body. From there, movie-like dreams manifest which appear to the consciousness like reality. The brain might release chemical substances that make the mind hallucinate and see this different world. In any case, further research is needed on the subject. Based on the favorable and unfavorable experiences of the consciousness, a reflection, a film-like dream manifests. If the dreamer is ill or has a disease, he will dream of negative situations or will have nightmares. A healthy person will generally have dreams regarding normal and beautiful situations. There are three categories of dreams: (1) dreams of a healthy person, (2) of an unhealthy person, and (3) premonitory dreams, which has three subsections (general bad omens, predictive dreams, and spiritual visions).

Dreams of a healthy person

Healthy people dream of devas (*lha*, gods), kings and emperors, leaders, famous men and women, burning fires, beautiful lakes, upright religious banners and umbrellas, putting blood and feces on the body, wearing white, clean clothes, obtaining fruits, fruit trees, climbing up a mountain, entering into a palace, riding on a lion, elephant, horse or cow, crossing a lake or a river, climbing mountains or towers, travelling north and east, surviving difficult situations, defeating an enemy, worshipping protectors and parents, and so on. All these dreams are positive and are signs of long life, good health, and prosperity. Depending on their constitution, people are inclined to have particular dreams. These body nature signs are not considered to be negative.

- Wind nature dreams
  Blue and black colors predominate; about green meadows, flying birds, flowers, houses, clothes, flying, driving cars, riding horses, foxes, moving objects, blowing wind, agitation, anxiety, joy, a busy life, happy emotions, etc.

- Bile nature dreams
  Yellow and red colors predominate; about yellow earth, houses, clothes, flowers, gold, copper, a hot and burning fire, hot sun, bright colors, red or yellow animals, sweating, having a clear mind, fear, etc.

- Phlegm nature dreams
  White and grey colors predominate; about water, snow, white earth or surfaces, elephants, silver, pearls, clothes, an ocean, peaceful rivers, a calm and quiet body-mind, being stable and slow, feeling heavy, etc.

Dreams of an unhealthy person

Unhealthy dreams manifest from illness. Disease injures, blocks, or contaminates the life channels in which consciousness flows.

- Patients with a wind disorder have dreams with an excess of blue or dark colors. They have nightmares with fear or shock, see cruel people or cats chasing after them, and are running for their lives. Dreams can include falling from a high mountain or a house, or being squashed by a beam or a stone. They can be about living in cold and windy places, dangerous places, going into the darkness, or having difficulty being on time. Dreams of killing can occur, with blood, fighting, and torture. These are all signs of wind disorder. Wind disorder produces many dreams, and these are usually unstable and change rapidly.

- Bile disorder produces dreams including fire, burning, hot sun, volcanoes, deserts, sweating, heat, the color red, red fruits, red-colored animals like a bull, horse or tiger, blood, fear of fire, and visions of women and spirits.

- Phlegm disorder dreams often have water, wetness, cold, snow, raining, sleeping, lakes, swimming pools, oceans, waterfalls, bathrooms, the moon, and a heavy or slow quality.

- Fever manifests itself in dreams in the form of fire, burning, volcanoes, thorns, heat, and unpredictable events.

- Infection dreams are about dirtiness, falling in the mud, worms, insects, snakes, and receiving money or metals (gold).

- Heart disorders produce fearful dreams and nightmares such as animal attacks.

- Lung disorder dreams are about rocks, red colors, and suffocation.

- Liver disorders manifest as red-colored metals and rocks, fire, and the sun.

- Kidney disorder dreams are about water, rivers, dams and irrigation, meadows, gardens, and looking for a bathroom.

- Spleen disorder dreams are about a feeling of sinking in water or mud, or heaviness.

- Rheumatism and arthritis dreams are about hot springs, boiling water, rivers, and sunshine in a green garden.

- Serious diseases can produce negative dreams as signs of approaching death, such as losing one's clothes, hatred, fear, unhappy dreams, dreams of eclipses, shooting stars, comets, sunsets, being swallowed by a fish or other animals, lost battles or fights, and dreaming about danger to one's life.

- Lost *la* manifests as losing clothes, ugly or ripped clothes, losing one's skin, being naked, losing one's bag or ornaments or jewelry, empty houses, a ruined sanctuary, losing friends, family, job, shaving one's hair or moustache off, having one's name called by a dead person, seeing falling leaves, unhappy dreams, and forgetting one's own name or house.

Negative dreams

The following dreams are signs of being caught by the Lord of Death:

- Riding on a cat, monkey, tiger, wolf, or on a dead body

- Being naked and riding on a buffalo, horse, pig, donkey, or camel, and going toward the south

- Dreams such as a tree growing on one's head with a bird's nest, or a banana tree or a thorny tree growing from one's heart

- Taking out a lotus flower from one's heart, falling down from a steep hill, sleeping in a cemetery, seeing one's head broken, being surrounded by crows, dreaming of someone or of oneself being surrounded by *preta* beings (hungry ghosts, *yidak*) or reptiles

- The skin on one's legs or muscles falling off, returning back to one's mother's womb, being swept away by water, sinking in quicksand, being swallowed by a fish, finding iron or gold, losing one's business, and asking taxes from wandering peoples

- There are many other negative signs such as inviting a bride, drinking wine with dead individuals and/or being drugged by them, wearing red clothes and carrying a red rosary, or dancing with a dead person

When an ill person frequently has these dreams, it could be a sign of nearing death. However, it is not necessarily a sign of dying when such negative dreams appear once or twice to a healthy person. Pacification methods derived from Tibetan medicine, astrology, and religion are the basis for treating negative dreams. To pacify negative dreams, one should:

- Receive a long-life initiation

- Perform a special retreat related to the subject

- Recite longevity mantras

- Study and meditate on emptiness

- Practice dream yoga to recognize dreams as an illusory world

- Perform a soul retrieval ritual (*la guk, tsé guk*)

- Receive medical treatment

The patient's temperament

A sign of a disease which might be dangerous is when the psychology and temperament of the patient changes drastically, especially regarding their relationship with the physician or spiritual master:

- If the patient's mood changes and they become cruel to the doctor, spiritual master, or friends, and show dislike for medical treatment, this is a sign of negativity

- A complete change of character in a person from good to bad and vice-versa is a sign of dying

- If the patient becomes beautiful or prosperous, or the opposite in a short period of time, this also may be a sign of dying

- It is a negative sign when a patient always has a bad facial radiance, or is depressed, when crows do not eat the ritual cake dedicated to the patient, or if the chest (heart area) does not remain wet with water after having taken a bath; these are also signs of dying

- If the patient's fingers do not produce sound when snapped

- All the food they eat becomes waste products and the patient does not gain strength

- Lice and lice eggs are found on the body when before there were none, or the contrary, is also a sign of dying

- Seeing a cut head, or a missing head or limbs in the image left by the sun, a mirror, water, and the sky, are signs of dying

19.2 SIGNS OF NEAR DEATH

Signs of near death, which indicate that the patient could die soon, include:

- Bleeding from any of the nine orifices without particular cause

- Forgetting everything that has been said

- A limp or retracted penis

- Unusual sounds when sneezing and coughing

- Inability to smell an extinguished lamp

- No sensitivity whilst combing the hair

- A very oily scalp

- Hair and eyebrows forming a new line, inward-turning hairs

- The appearance of a moon-like shape with visible vein vessels in the forehead and lips

- False perceptions of the five sense organs

- Not being able to see one's arm from elbow to wrist when held in front of the middle of the two eyes

- Eyes staring like a rabbit

- Eyes retracting into their sockets or irises losing their brightness (liver dysfunction)

- Ears sticking to the sides of the head (kidney dysfunction)

- The loss of the natural inner ear sound (kidney dysfunction)

- No shadow, or steam rising from the head

- Flattening of the nostrils and a gathering of dry whitish mucus (lung dysfunction)

- The central part of the tongue becomes dark; the tongue is short, dry, and one cannot speak (heart dysfunction)

- Falling of the lower lip or shrinking of the upper lip (spleen dysfunction)

- Facial skin gathers dust, the breath is cold, and the teeth become dark

- Breath shortens and the body temperature diminishes

- The body is cold but with a high temperature inside

- A cold disease decreases the body heat or vice-versa, and a normal treatment does not give positive results, whilst the opposite treatment gives positive effects

Uncertain omens of death

There are also some uncertain or indefinite dreams and signs that may appear to the patients that are not fatal. These may disappear when the disease is cured or through spiritual healing methods.

Certain omens of death

However, if the disease shows signs of frequent relapse, it could be a sign of near death. A patient who has lost bodily strength, appetite, and wrist pulse will definitely die. Treatments can be performed but they will not give positive results. In short, the various signs of the dying process of the body aggregates are caused by the corruption and destruction of the elements' relationships with the humors, body constituents, and waste products. The elements and humors become enemies; they no longer cooperate with each other. This mirrors the external phenomena and processes that will take place during the destruction of the world, as the Medicine Buddha teaches us in his *sādhanā*.

19.3 SIGNS OF IMMINENT DEATH

The signs of dissolution of the body elements and sense consciousnesses will appear to all beings, whether they face a natural death, death by disease, or are spiritual practitioners. These are general signs of imminent death that are also described as dissolution or absorption signs in Buddhism. They manifest during the absorption of the five elements (earth, water, fire, air, and space) into the five sense consciousnesses (eyes, ears, nose, tongue, body, and mind). In the end, the elements dissolve into space and the other consciousnesses dissolves into the mind consciousness. Detailed explanations of this stepwise process and the accompanying meditations should be acquired from the spiritual practice of *kusum lamkhyer* and the Tibetan book of death (*Bar do thos grol, Liberation Through Hearing During the Intermediate State*).[5] Here, a brief synthesis of the dissolution process is presented. If possible, one should study the relevant texts and put them into practice during one's lifetime in preparation. If not, one should get help from a teacher who can instruct the dying person on the various stages with a clear voice. Various stages take place during dissolution. To begin with, the elements disintegrate and their functions cease. It starts with earth and is completed with ether. Consciousness starts with the eye and progresses to the body consciousness.

1. Earth element and eye consciousness absorption

The earth element of the body dissolves into the water element, and earth-related signs of losing weight, decreasing muscles, and so on, appear. At the same time, the consciousness of the eyes dissolves into the ear consciousness, resulting in the patient's inability to perceive form and color as well as visions that are like a mirage in a desert. Eyesight decreases, but the clarity and power of hearing increases.

Internal sign: the dying person begins to see visions which are like a mirage.

2. Water element and ear consciousness absorption

The water element of the body then dissolves into the fire element, and the body loses control of liquids and urination. The body does not produce water anymore; the mouth and tongue become dry. The person feels thirsty. The ear consciousness begins to dissolve into the nose consciousness. The patient gradually loses the ability to breathe, eventually seeing what seems to be smoke that rises and dissolves. Hearing power decreases, while the power of smell increases.

Internal sign: the dying person sees rising smoke in the atmosphere.

3. Fire element and nose consciousness absorption

The fire element then dissolves into the air element and the body loses temperature. Feet and hands become cold as heat concentrates in the heart. The nose consciousness dissolves into the tongue consciousness. One starts losing memory and feelings. The patient has no more sensitivity to smell, but the power of taste increases. The inner mind sees sparkles in the darkness.

Internal sign: the dying person sees visions of red sparkles in a dark environment.

4. Air element and tongue consciousness absorption

The air element of the body dissolves into the space element; the body gradually stops breathing. Exhalations become longer than inhalations, resulting in the slowing down of breathing. Physical movements and heartbeats stop. The body-mind loses control. The tongue consciousness dissolves into the tactile consciousness, resulting in the loss of taste. Gradually the body consciousness is absorbed into the mind consciousness, and then into the space element. All physical functions stop. The deeper, subtler mind sees darkness with a tiny light that is motionless. This is also called "the great contemplation stage" for tantric practitioners.

Internal sign: the dying person sees a vision of a tiny lamp in the darkness.

This is the state of death from the biomedical point of view. But according to Sowa Rigpa and Buddhism, this state is only external and referring to the body. The subtler mind has not yet completely perished. The completion and absorption of the mental consciousness lasts up to three days. Within three days (there are, however, some special cases), the consciousness wakes up and leaves the body and heart, entering the bardo state. Here, and from the beginning of dissolution, instructions on spiritual meditation and contemplation are advised. What follows below is explained in tantric sources.

Next, the subtle mind and emotion dissolution starts, which is marked by the appearance of the *tongpa zhi*: the four stages of emptiness. The mind becomes more and more subtle as the 80 gross emotions (*küntok gyéchu*) dissolve.

---

5 Karma gling pa, 1995.

1. The "white appearance," first stage of emptiness

The mind slowly wakes up from the state of darkness and perceives a whitish color, like moonlight on a clear autumn night. The 33 subtle emotions of attachment begin to dissolve. The paternal body-mind energy ceases to function and is absorbed into the middle channel.

2. The "red appearance," second stage of emptiness

The mind perceives a reddish color, like the sun reflected by the moon on a clear autumn night. The 33 subtle emotions of hatred begin to disappear. The maternal body-mind energy ceases to function and is absorbed into the middle channel.

3. The "dark appearance," third stage of emptiness

When the mind and subtle wind begin to dissolve into the very subtle mind, darkness like a late evening autumn sky is perceived. At this moment, the mind loses its awareness once again. The consciousness derived from the dying person's previous life ceases to function and is absorbed into space.

4. The "clear light appearance," the fourth emptiness

After a certain time, the mind recovers from the previous unconscious state, and perceives the clear light of an autumn morning sky. This is called the "mother light." It is primordial Buddha-nature (the Buddhadharma *dharmakāya* nature, *sangyé kyi chö kyi chökü rangzhin*). Simultaneously, the mind experiences the "son light" absorption stage, which is the light of the relative nature.

The most important goal for the departing consciousness is to recognize the mother light as the nature of their own mind. This light appears only briefly, but it is the one and only golden opportunity to benefit from the misfortune of dying. To know the mind, and to integrate this insight with *sādhanā* practice on one's *yidam*, is the way to travel to pure lands, to obtain liberation, or to choose one's rebirth.

PART 7

FRAMEWORKS

སློམ་གནི།

CHAPTER 20

MEDICINE TREES OF THE *ROOT TANTRA*

The medicine trees are diagrams that act as syntheses of the *Gyüzhi*. The general medical field of knowledge is symbolized by the root or ground. Trunks are the main subjects, branches and leaves are elaborating subsections. Flowers and fruits are the final results or goals. There are tree groups for each of the *Four Tantras*. Sowa Rigpa's unique medicine tree recitation practice is called *dong drem*. It is a powerful teaching and learning tool that helps to grasp the basics easily. In a few words, *dong drem* is the traditional way to study Sowa Rigpa. Students should ideally memorize the text beforehand and be able to identify the roots, trunks, branches and leaves, with their names and meanings. The presentation of the *Root* and *Explanatory Tantra* trees are considered compulsory material. When constructing the trees, the different parts are usually made from wood or bamboo, and colored according to the humors and body constituents (wind is blue, bile is yellow, blood is red, etc.).

The roots should first be displayed on the floor or a table, then the trunks should be added, then the branches, and finally the leaves. At the end, the flowers are displayed at the top of the tree of health. Because a healthy flower naturally produces fruits, these are placed above the flowers. To cover the *Root Tantra*, one should construct three roots, nine trunks, 49 branches, 224 leaves, two flowers, and three fruits. What follows is a summary of the accompanying text.[1]

20.1 THE FIRST ROOT: THE NATURAL STATE OF THE BODY

The *Root Tantra* consists of three roots:

1. The natural state of the body
2. The root of diagnosis
3. The root of treatment

The first root, the natural state of the body, has two trunks:

A. Healthy humor tree
B. Unhealthy humor tree

A. The trunk of health

The healthy humors tree, also known as the trunk of health, has three branches:

1. Three humors branch
2. Seven body constituents branch
3. Three waste products branch

A1. The three humors branch has 15 leaves

Each humoral subbranch has five leaves.

First, the five principal wind leaves:

1. (1) Life-sustaining wind (*lung sokdzin*) in the head
2. (2) Ascending wind (*lung gyengyu*) in the chest and throat
3. (3) Pervasive wind (*lung khyapjé*) in the heart
4. (4) Fire-like wind (*lung ményam*) in the abdomen

---

1 The exposition of the medicine trees provided below follows the *Gyüzhi* as well as Mkhyen rab nor bu, 1984 (1924), in particular.

5. (5) Descending wind (*lung tursel*) in the sigmoid colon

Second, the five principal bile leaves:

6. (1) Digestive bile (*tripa jujé*) in the stomach and small intestine
7. (2) Color-transforming bile (*tripa dangyur*) in the liver
8. (3) Accomplishing bile (*tripa drupjé*) in the heart
9. (4) Seeing bile (*tripa tongjé*) in the eyes
10. (5) Complexion-clearing bile (*tripa doksel*) in the skin

Third, the five principal phlegm leaves:

11. (1) Supporting phlegm (*béken tenjé*) in the chest
12. (2) Decomposing phlegm (*béken nyakjé*) in the stomach
13. (3) Experiencing phlegm (*béken nyongjé*) in the tongue
14. (4) Satisfying phlegm (*béken tsimjé*) in the head
15. (5) Joining phlegm (*béken jorjé*) in the joints

A2. The body constituents branch has seven leaves:

16. (1) Food essence or chyme (*dangma*)
17. (2) Blood (*trak*)
18. (3) Flesh (*sha*)
19. (4) Fat (*tsil*)
20. (5) Bone (*rüpa*)
21. (6) Bone marrow (*kang*)
22. (7) Reproductive fluids (*khuwa*)

A3. The waste products branch has three leaves:

23. (1) Feces (*shangwa*)
24. (2) Urine (*chin*)
25. (3) Sweat (*drima*, includes body dirt)

Summary: There are two trunks, three branches, and 25 leaves in total on the healthy tree.

B. The trunk of disease

The unhealthy humors tree trunk has nine branches:

1. (1) Distant causes of disease (*ring gyu*)
2. (2) Immediate causes (*nyé gyu*)
3. (3) Entrance gates (*juk go*)
4. (4) Locations (*né*)
5. (5) 15 pathways (*gyulam chonga*)
6. (6) Nine manifestation times (*dangdü gu*)
7. (7) Nine results of disease (*drébu gu*)
8. (8) 12 adverse reactions to treatment (*dokgyu chunyi*)

The unhealthy tree has 63 leaves.

B1. The distant and near causes branch has three leaves:

1. (1) Attachment (*döchak*) is the distant cause of the wind humor
2. (2) Hatred (*zhédang*) is the distant cause of the bile humor
3. (3) Closed-mindedness (*timuk*) is the distant cause of the phlegm humor

B2. The immediate causes (conditions) branch has four leaves:

4. (1) Wrong climate or unusual weather, which promotes disease
5. (2) *La* (subtle body) stolen by evil spirits
6. (3) Wrong nutrition, for example: drinking wine and eating meat on hot spring days increases bile; drinking too much strong coffee leads to wind disorder; and eating raw foods or overeating leads to phlegm disorder
7. (4) Wrong behavior, for example: wearing animal skins or warm clothes at midday in late spring could cause bile disorders; listening to loud music leads to wind disorder; resting or sleeping in cold and wet places produces phlegm imbalance

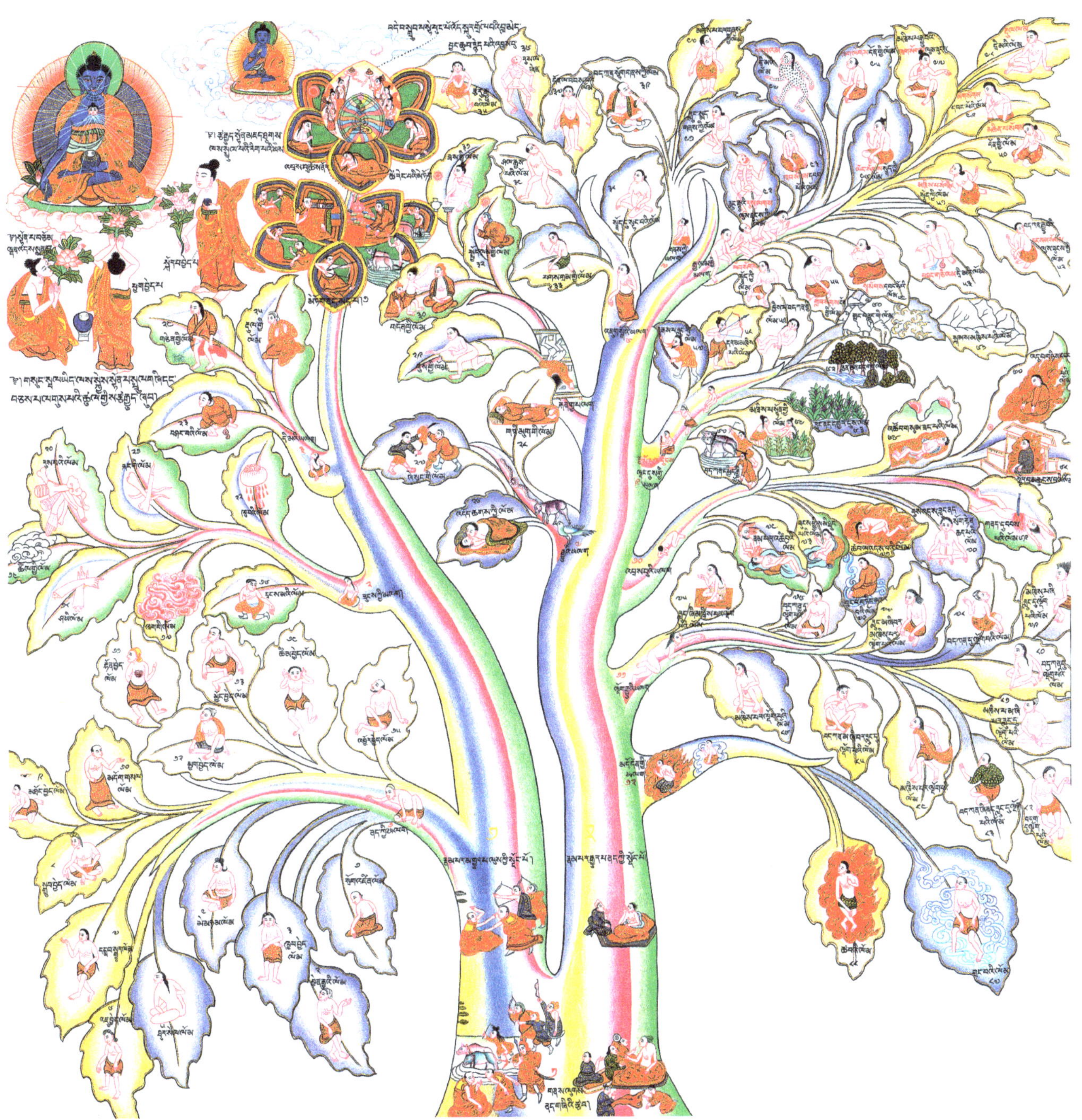

FIGURE 20.1 The tree of health and disease

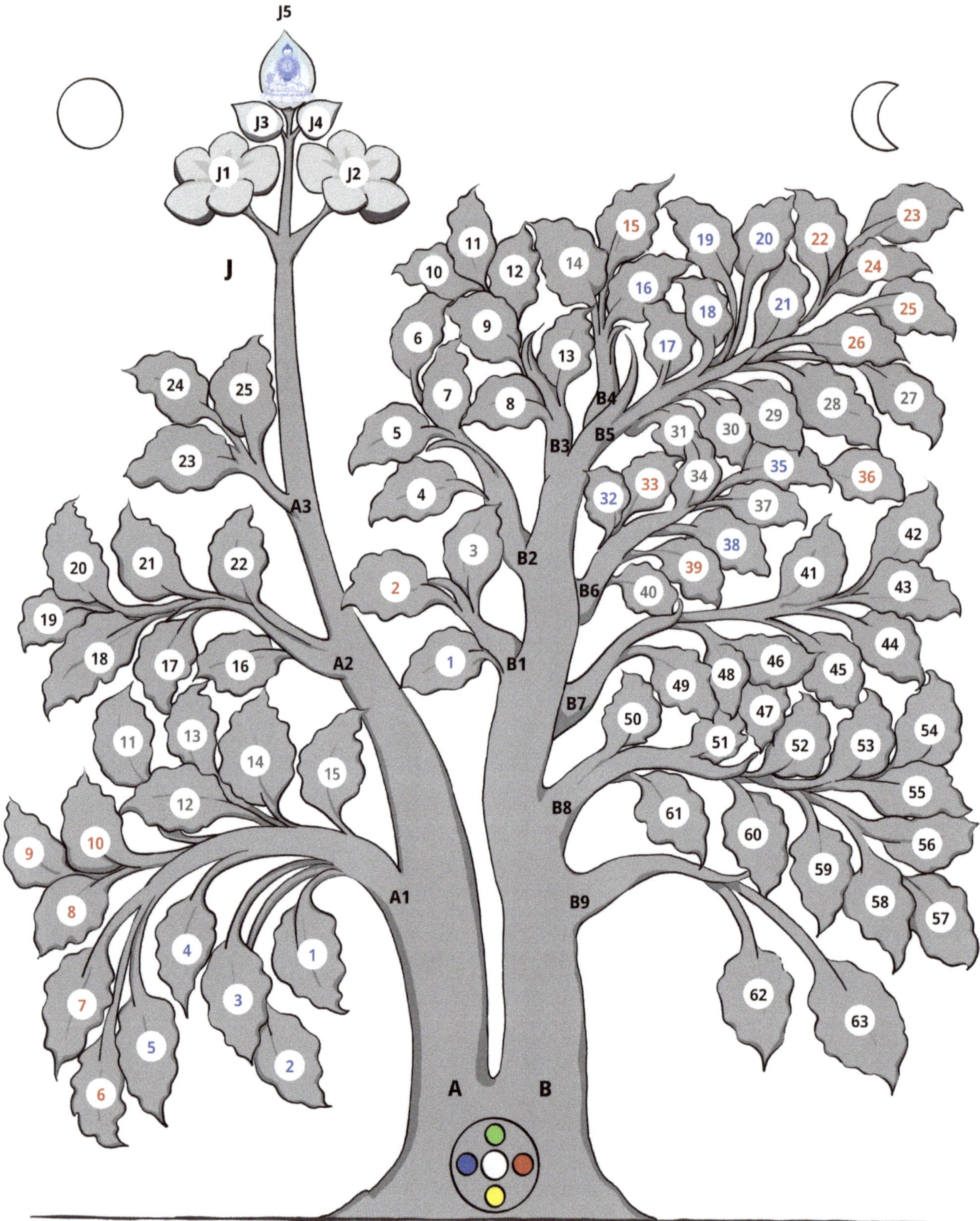

FIGURE 20.2 The sequential structure of the tree of health and disease

B3. The entrance gates branch has six leaves

The following example is based on a fever disorder in which fever-promoting factors first manifest in the skin:

8. (1) On the first day, the fever disease spreads to the skin; the skin becomes sensitive and shivery
9. (2) On the second day, it spreads into the flesh and manifests muscle pain
10. (3) On the third day, it flows into the blood, so the blood vessels feel tense
11. (4) On the fourth day, the disease spreads to the bones, making the bones ache
12. (5) On the fifth day, it attacks the solid organs and bronchitis, etc., could appear
13. (6) On the sixth day, the disease descends into the hollow organs, becoming a chronic fever that may bring diarrhea, colitis, and metabolic disorders

Generally, fever takes different times to reach the hollow organs depending on one's constitution and other factors. If the fever remains for more than 21 days in the body, it is considered to be a chronic fever.

B4. The locations of the humors branch has three leaves:

14. (1) Phlegm resides in the brain, which is its base, from where it flows down to all body parts like a river
15. (2) Bile resides in the middle part of the body (liver and gall bladder), which is its base, from where bile symptoms manifest and rise like fire
16. (3) Wind resides in the lower abdomen and sacral area, which is its base, from where wind symptoms manifest and move freely

After entering, diseases will accumulate in their locations as described above, becoming stronger and eventually manifesting symptoms.

B5. The 15 humoral pathways branch has 15 leaves

From the wind base, wind disorder goes to (attacks):

17. (1) The bones among the body constituents
18. (2) The ears among the sense organs
19. (3) The tactile function of the skin (and its subtle waste products)

20. (4) The heart and life channel among the vital organs
21. (5) The colon among the hollow organs

From the bile base, bile disorder goes to:

22. (1) The blood among the body constituents
23. (2) The eyes among the sense organs
24. (3) Sweat among the waste products
25. (4) The liver among the solid organs
26. (5) The small intestine and gallbladder among the hollow organs

From the phlegm base, phlegm disorder goes to:

27. (1) Flesh, fat, bone marrow, and reproductive fluids among the constituents
28. (2) The nose and tongue among the sense organs
29. (3) Feces and urine among the waste products
30. (4) The lungs, spleen, and kidneys among the solid organs
31. (5) The stomach, bladder, and reproductive organs among the hollow organs

B6. The manifestation times branch has nine leaves

Each humor has three leaves, in all there are nine leaves. Manifestation of humoral tendencies according to age:

32. (1) Aged people (*gépa*, above 60) become more and more wind-natured due to degeneration of the physical body. They acquire a natural tendency for wind disorders
33. (2) Adults (*darma*) are assertive and ambitious due to their bile nature. They are prone to bile disorders
34. (3) Children (*jipa*, until 12 years old for females, and 16 for males) are sleepy as they are of a phlegm nature. They have a tendency to develop phlegm disorders

Manifestation of humoral tendencies according to place of living:

35. (1) Cold and windy places increase wind
36. (2) Dry and hot places increase bile
37. (3) Wet and humid places increase phlegm

Manifestation of humoral tendencies according to time:

38.   (1) Wind disorders manifest in summer (rainy season), early evening and early morning, and when one is hungry
39.   (2) Bile disorders manifest in autumn, midday, midnight, and during digestion
40.   (3) Phlegm disorders manifest in spring, late evening and late morning, and immediately after meals

B7. The result of disease branch has nine leaves

Disease may eventually bring death, but not all causes of death are karmic; there are many other factors:

41.   (1) Consumption of the three pillars of life: lifeforce, karma, and fortune
42.   (2) Disease turning into an enemy, becoming fatal
43.   (3) Wrong treatment through diet, behavior, medicine, or therapy
44.   (4) Injury of the vital organs, such as the heart and brain
45.   (5) Consumption of lifespan wind (*soklung*) by delayed wind disorder treatment
46.   (6) Fever having crossed the mountain caused by delayed fever treatment
47.   (7) Deep stagnant coldness due to delayed phlegm disorder treatment
48.   (8) Allergy/intolerance (to foods, treatment, etc.)
49.   (9) *La* stolen by evil spirits

B8. The negative reactions branch has 12 leaves

Each humor has four leaves. Four wind treatment reactions:

50.   (1) The manifestation of a bile disorder after excessive wind disorder treatment
51.   (2) The manifestation of a phlegm disorder after excessive wind disorder treatment
52.   (3) The manifestation of a bile disorder after insufficient wind disorder treatment
53.   (4) The manifestation of a phlegm disorder after insufficient wind disorder treatment

Four bile treatment reactions:

54.   (1) The manifestation of a wind disorder after excessive bile disorder treatment
55.   (2) The manifestation of a phlegm disorder after excessive bile disorder treatment
56.   (3) The manifestation of a wind disorder after insufficient bile disorder treatment
57.   (4) The manifestation of a phlegm disorder after insufficient bile disorder treatment

Four phlegm treatment reactions:

58.   (1) The manifestation of a wind disorder after excessive phlegm disorder treatment
59.   (2) The manifestation of a bile disorder after excessive phlegm disorder treatment
60.   (3) The manifestation of a wind disorder after insufficient phlegm disorder treatment
61.   (4) The manifestation of a bile disorder after insufficient phlegm disorder treatment

B9. The conclusion branch has two leaves:

62.   (1) Wind and phlegm share the same cold nature
63.   (2) Bile and blood share the same hot nature

Sin (parasites and microorganisms) and *chuser* (plasma) can be either hot or cold.

Summary of the first root: There are two trunks, 12 branches, and 25 leaves in the healthy tree, and 63 leaves in the disease tree. In total, the healthy state of the body and humoral pathology are explained through 88 leaves.

20.2 THE SECOND ROOT: DIAGNOSIS

The tree of diagnosis has three trunks:

C.   (1) Visual diagnosis (*mik gi tawa*)
D.   (2) Palpation (*sormö rekpa*)
E.   (3) Questioning (*ngak gi triwa*)

C. The third trunk on visual diagnosis has two branches:

1.   (1) Tongue diagnosis
2.   (2) Urine analysis

D. The fourth trunk on pulse diagnosis has three branches:

3.   (1) Wind pulse
4.   (2) Bile pulse
5.   (3) Phlegm pulse

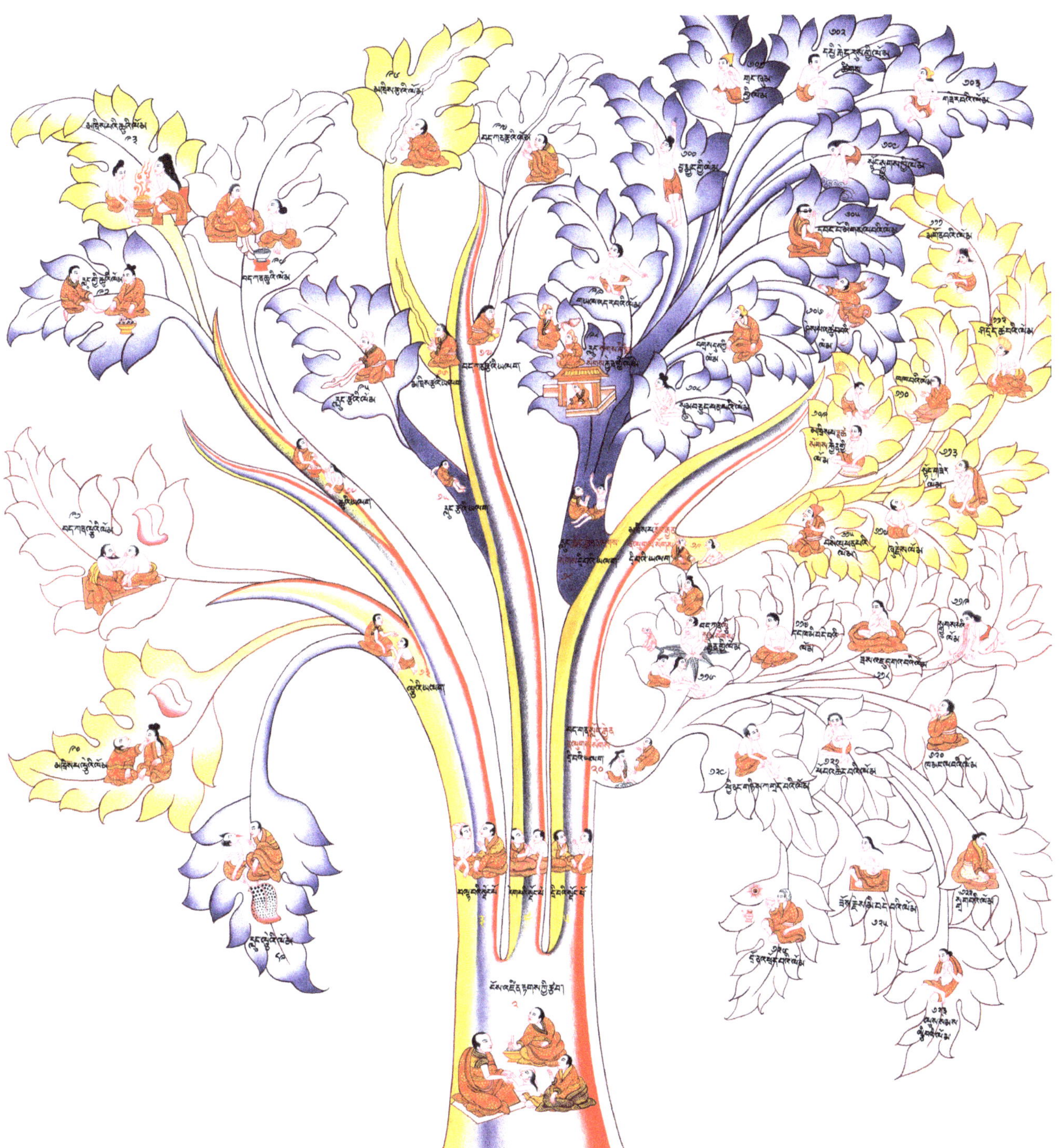

FIGURE 20.3 The tree of diagnosis

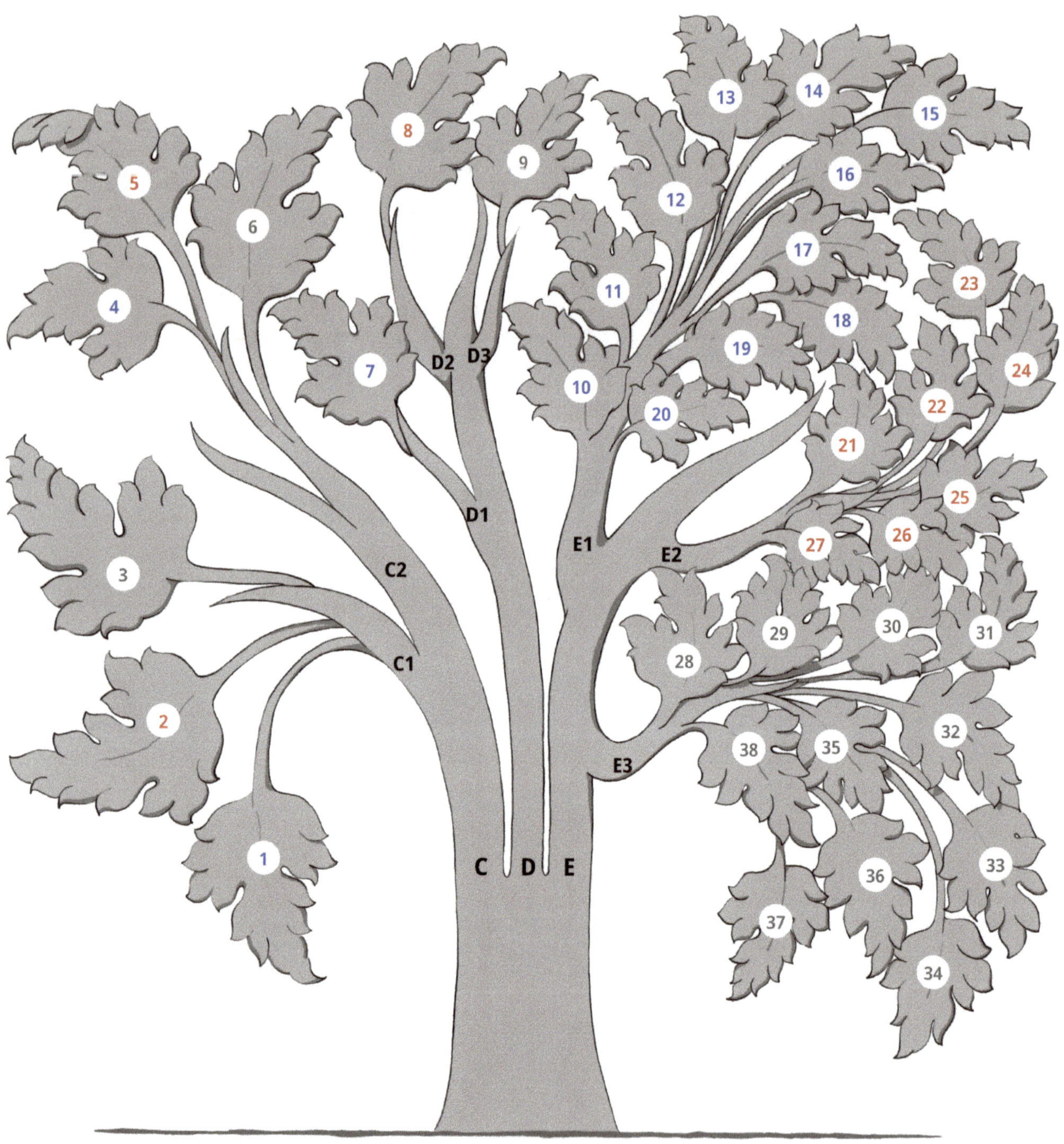

FIGURE 20.4 The sequential structure of the tree of diagnosis

E. The fifth trunk on questioning has three branches:

6.   (1) Wind questions
7.   (2) Bile questions
8.   (3) Phlegm questions

In total, the three diagnostic trunks have eight branches.

C. The trunk of visual diagnosis

There are nine leaves on the visual diagnostic branches.

C1. The tongue diagnosis branch has three leaves:

1.   (1) Wind disorder tongue is red, dry, and rough
2.   (2) Bile disorder tongue has a thick yellow-white coating
3.   (3) Phlegm disorder has a white coating, is pale, smooth, and wet (plenty of saliva)

C2. The urine analysis branch has three leaves:

4.   (1) Wind disorder urine is waterish and has large bubbles
5.   (2) Bile disorder urine is reddish yellow, with much steam, and is malodorous
6.   (3) Phlegm disorder urine is whitish, with little odor and steam

D. The pulse reading trunk

Each humor has one leaf, so there are three leaves:

7.   (1) Wind disorder pulse is floating, empty, and halting
8.   (2) Bile disorder pulse is rapid, full, and taut
9.   (3) Phlegm disorder pulse is sunken, weak, and slow

E. The questioning trunk

The questioning trunk has three branches and 29 leaves.

E1. The wind questions branch has 11 leaves

Causes:

10.   (1) Wind disorder is caused by the following conditions: light and rough quality food (e.g., excess consumption of strong tea, goat's meat, pork, and bitter and astringent foods in general), and wind-increasing behavior such as fasting

Symptoms:

11.   (2) Yawning and trembling
12.   (3) Needing to stretch often
13.   (4) Shivering (feeling cold)
14.   (5) Pain in the hips, waist, and all joints
15.   (6) Vague pains
16.   (7) Retching
17.   (8) Weakening of the senses
18.   (9) Mind becoming unstable
19.   (10) Pain manifesting when hungry

Diet test:

20.   (11) Oily and nutritious food are beneficial, reducing the symptoms

E2. The bile questions branch has seven leaves

Causes:

21.   (1) Bile disorder is caused by the following conditions: excess sharp and pungent food (too many spices), drinking strong alcohol, eating fatty meat, drinking milk, and behaviors such as staying in the sun, near to a fire or in hot places

Symptoms:

22.   (2) Bitter taste in the mouth
23.   (3) Headache
24.   (4) Body temperature increase
25.   (5) Pain in the shoulders and neck
26.   (6) Pain during digestion (feeling weak)

Diet test:

27.   (7) Food that is cooling is beneficial, reducing the symptoms

E3. The phlegm questions branch has 11 leaves

Causes:

28.   (1) Phlegm disorder is caused by the following conditions: excess heavy and oily foods, stale or raw vegetables, sweets, wheat products, and cooling behaviors such as staying in wet, humid, and cold places

Symptoms:

29.   (2) Poor appetite
30.   (3) Difficult digestion
31.   (4) Vomiting
32.   (5) Diminishing sense of taste
33.   (6) Bloating stomach
34.   (7) Belching
35.   (8) Heavy body and mind
36.   (9) Feeling cold externally and internally
37.   (10) Discomfort after eating

Diet test:

38.   (11) Warming foods are beneficial, reducing the symptoms

Summary: There are three trunks, eight branches, and six leaves in visual diagnosis, three leaves in pulse diagnosis, and 29 leaves on the questioning branch. In total, there are 38 leaves.

20.3 THE THIRD ROOT: TREATMENT

The treatment tree has four trunks:

F.   (1) Nutrition
G.   (2) Behavior
H.   (3) Medicine
I.   (4) Therapy

There are 27 branches on the treatment trunk.

F. The healing nutrition trunk has six branches:

1.   (1) Foods for wind
2.   (2) Beverages for wind
3.   (3) Foods for bile
4.   (4) Beverages for bile
5.   (5) Foods for phlegm
6.   (6) Beverages for phlegm

G. The healing behavior trunk has three branches:

1.   (1) Behaviors for wind
2.   (2) Behaviors for bile
3.   (3) Behaviors for phlegm

H. The remedies trunk has 15 branches.

Six materia medica branches:

1.   (1) Wind medicine compounded according to taste (*ro jor*)
2.   (2) Wind medicine compounded according to power (*nü jor*)
3.   (3) Bile medicine compounded according to taste
4.   (4) Bile medicine compounded according to power
5.   (5) Phlegm medicine compounded according to taste
6.   (6) Phlegm medicine compounded according to power

Six pacifying medicine branches:

7.   (1) Wind-pacifying medicinal broths (*khuwa*)
8.   (2) Wind-pacifying medicinal butters (*menmar*)
9.   (3) Bile-pacifying decoctions (*tang*)
10.   (4) Bile-pacifying powders (*churni* or *chéma*)
11.   (5) Phlegm-pacifying pills (*rilbu*)
12.   (6) Phlegm-pacifying calcinated ashes (*trésam*)

Three purifying medicine branches:

13.   (1) Wind-purifying enemas (*jamtsi*)
14.   (2) Bile-purifying purgatives (*shel*)
15.   (3) Phlegm-purifying emetics (*kyuk*)

I. The external therapy trunk has three branches

1.   (1) *Hormé*[2] for treating wind (*hor gyi métsa*)
2.   (2) Bloodletting for treating bile (*tarka*)
3.   (3) Moxibustion for treating phlegm (*métsa*)

In total, there are 27 branches and 98 leaves on the treatment trunk.

---

2 *Hormé* is a gentle warming therapy using herb bundles soaked in heated sesame oil.

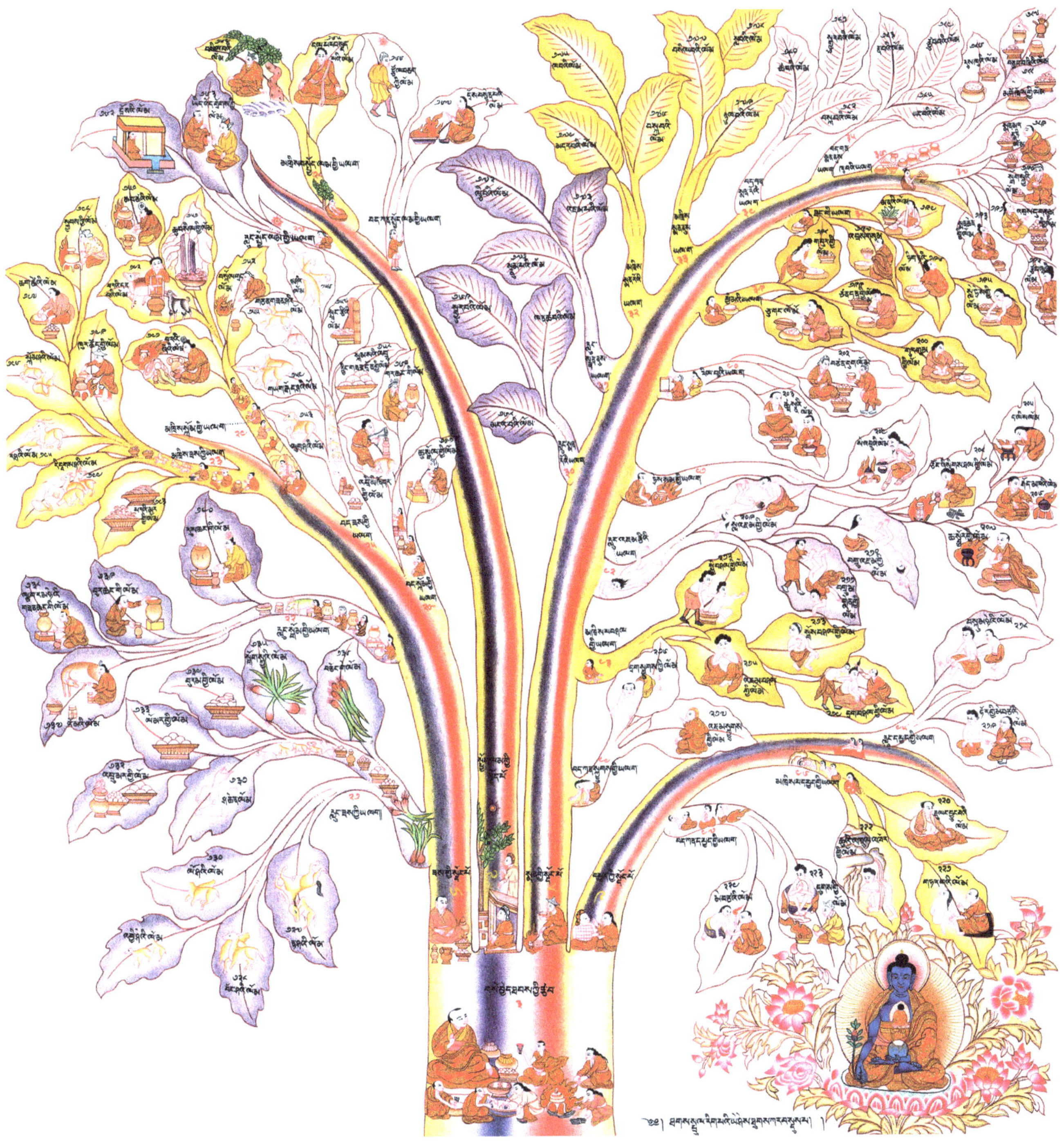

FIGURE 20.5 The tree of treatment

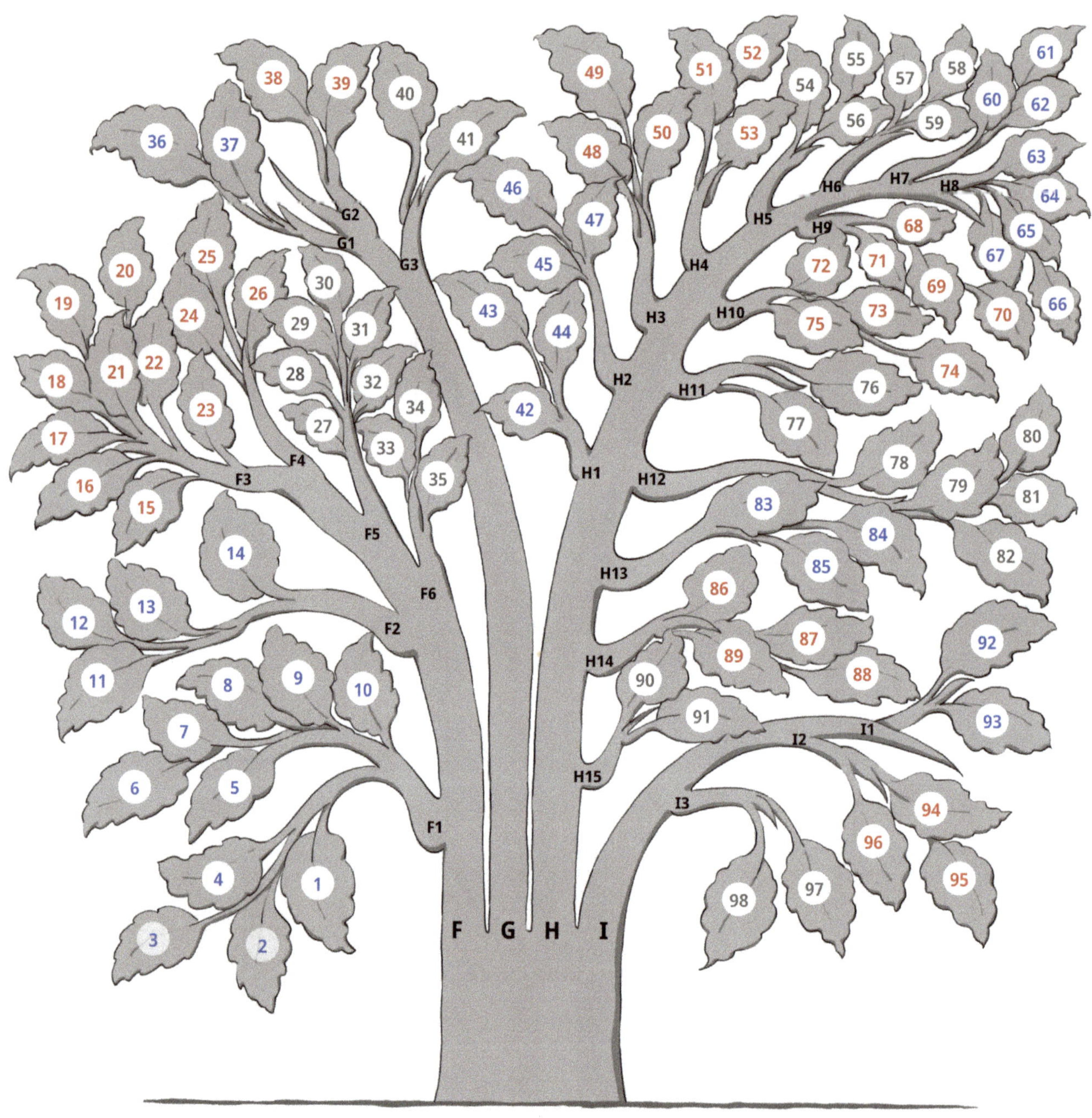

FIGURE 20.6 The sequential structure of the tree of treatment

F. The trunk of healing nutrition

There are 35 leaves on the healing nutrition trunk. The wind-curing foods and beverages branches together have 14 leaves.

F1. Wind-curing foods has 10 leaves:

1. (1) Horsemeat
2. (2) Donkey's meat
3. (3) Marmot's meat
4. (4) One-year old dried meat
5. (5) *Shachen*[3]
6. (6) Seed oils
7. (7) One-year old butter
8. (8) Molasses
9. (9) Garlic
10. (10) Onion

F2. Wind-curing beverages has four leaves:

11. (1) Warm milk
12. (2) *Chang*[4] made from angelica root (*chawa*) and *Polygonatum cirrifolium* (*ranyé*) powder.
13. (3) *Chang* mixed with unrefined sugar cane
14. (4) *Chang* mixed with bone soup

There are 12 leaves of bile-curing foods and beverages.

F3. Bile-curing foods has nine leaves:

15. (1) Curd from cow or goat milk
16. (2) Whey from cow or goat milk
17. (3) Fresh butter
18. (4) Game meat (e.g., deer)
19. (5) Goat meat
20. (6) Fresh *töl* meat[5]
21. (7) New barley porridge (without added salt or spices)
22. (8) Stew of a type of dandelion (cf. rocket salad)
23. (9) Dandelion stew

F4. Bile-curing beverages has three leaves:

24. (1) (Luke) warm water (without tea, butter, milk, or salt)
25. (2) Cold water (from snow-topped mountains and springs)
26. (3) Boiled cold water

There are nine leaves of phlegm-curing foods and beverages.

F5. Phlegm-curing foods has six leaves:

27. (1) Mutton
28. (2) Wild yak meat
29. (3) Carnivorous animal meat
30. (4) Fish
31. (5) Honey
32. (6) Warm polenta made from stored grain from dry areas

F6. Phlegm-curing beverages has three leaves:

33. (1) Curd and whey from she-yak milk
34. (2) Strong *chang*
35. (3) Boiled hot water

In total there are 35 leaves on the diet tree.

G. The trunk of behavior

Two leaves for each humor; in all six leaves for the behavioral tree.

G1. Wind healing behavior has two leaves:

36. (1) Wind patients should stay in a slightly dark room, in a warm house, and wear warm clothes
37. (2) Wind patients should be accompanied by pleasant friends

G2. Bile healing behavior has two leaves:

38. (1) Bile patients should stay nearby rivers, where there is a cool breeze, and stay in the shade
39. (2) Bile patients should take rest in a calm and quiet place

---

3 *Shachen* translates as "the great meat." It refers to human flesh, which has high potency to cure wind disorder. However, it is mostly substituted with dried wild yak's heart or rabbit heart.

4 *Chang* is an alcoholic Tibetan beer drink. It is possible to use Japanese sake or red wine instead.

5 The animal born from the she-yak crossed with an ox, a yak-cow hybrid.

G3. Phlegm healing behavior has two leaves:

40. (1) Phlegm patients should do physical work and exercise
41. (2) Phlegm patients should stay in dry and warm places

There is a total of six healing behavior leaves.

H. The trunk of medicine

The medicine tree has 50 leaves. There are 18 taste and power medicines that cure disorders of the three humors. The first six leaves are for wind disorder.

H1. Three leaves with taste-based medicines for wind disorder:

42. (1) Sweet medicine such as *buram* (unrefined cane sugar)
43. (2) Sour medicine such as old *chang* (old wine, sake)
44. (3) Salty medicine such as *gyamtsa* (rock salt)

H2. Three leaves with power-based medicines for wind disorder:

45. (1) Oily medicine such as *agaru* (*Aquilaria agallocha*)
46. (2) Heavy medicine such as *kharutsa* (black salt)
47. (3) Smooth medicine such as *kandakari* (*Rubus niveus* / *Solanum surratense*)

The second group of six leaves of taste and power medicines are for bile disorder.

H3. Three leaves with taste-based medicines for bile disorder:

48. (1) Sweet medicine such as *gündrum* (*Vitis vinifera*)
49. (2) Bitter taste medicine such as *ser gyi métok* (*Herpetospermum pendunculosum*)
50. (3) Astringent medicine such as *tsenden karpo* (*Santalum album*)

H4. Three leaves with power-based medicines for bile disorder:

51. (1) Cooling medicine such as *gabur* (*Cinnamomum camphora*)
52. (2) Thinning medicine such as *dong ga* (*Cassia fistula*)
53. (3) Blunt medicine such as *chugang* (*Bambusa textilis* / kaolin)

The third set of six leaves of taste and power medicines are for phlegm disorder.

H5. Three leaves with taste-based medicines for phlegm disorder:

54. (1) Pungent medicine such as *nalésham* (*Piper nigrum*)
55. (2) Sour medicine such as *sendru* (*Punica granatum*)
56. (3) Astringent medicine such as *baru* (*Terminalia bellerica*)

H6. Three leaves with power-based medicines for phlegm disorder:

57. (1) Sharp medicine such as *gyatsa* (sal ammoniac)
58. (2) Coarse medicine such as *tarbu* (*Hippophae rhamnoides*)
59. (3) Light medicine such as *tsitraka* (*Plumbago zeylanica*)

There is a total of 18 leaves on the medicine branch.

There are 23 pacifying formulas for the three humors, of which eight are pacifying formulas for wind disorder.

H7. Three leaves with medicinal broth formulas for wind disorder:

60. (1) Bone broth made from sheep's anklebone
61. (2) Four essence broth made from meat, butter, sugarcane, and *chang* combined
62. (3) Dried sheep head broth

H8. Five leaves with medicinal butter formulas for wind disorder:

63. (1) Medicinal butter made with *dzati* (*Myristica fragrans*)

64. (2) Medicinal butter made with *gokpa* (*Allium sativum*)
65. (3) Medicinal butter made from the three fruits (*drébu sum*): *arura* (*Terminalia chebula*), *barura* (*Terminalia bellirica*), and *kyurura* (*Emblica officinalis*)
66. (4) Medicinal butter made from the five roots (*tsawa nga*): *chawa* (*Angelica sinensis*), *batru* (*Mirabilis himalaica*), *lagang* (*Polygonatum cirrhifolium*), *zéma* (*Tribulus terrestris*) and *nyéshing* (*Asparagus racemosus*)
67. (5) Medicinal butter made with *tsenduk* (*Aconitum richardsonianum* var. *crispulum*)

Next, eight pacifying formulas for bile disorder.

H9. Four leaves with decoction formulas for bile disorder:

68. (1) Decoctions made with *manu* (*Inula racemosa*) as principal ingredient
69. (2) Decoctions made with *létré* (*Tinospora cordifolia* / *T. sinensis*) as principal ingredient
70. (3) Decoctions made with *tikta* (*Swertia chirayita*) as principal ingredient
71. (4) Decoctions made with the three fruits as principal ingredients

H10. Four leaves with powder formulas for bile disorder:

72. (1) Powder medicine made from *gabur* (*Cinnamomum camphora*)
73. (2) Powder medicine made from *tsenden karpo* (*Santalum album*)
74. (3) Powder medicine made from *gurgum* (*Carthamus tinctorius*)
75. (4) Powder medicine made from *chugang* (*Bambusa textilis* / kaolin)

Next, seven pacifying formulas for phlegm disorder.

H11. Two leaves with pill formulas for phlegm disorder:

76. (1) Pills made with *tsenduk* (*Aconitum richardsonianum* var. *crispulum*)
77. (2) Pills made with various salts

H12. Five leaves with calcinated ash medicines for phlegm disorder:

78. (1) Calcinated ash made from *sendru* (*Punica granatum*)
79. (2) Calcinated ash made from *dali* (*Rhododendrum primulaeflorum*)
80. (3) The Gömakha formula (a formula described in the *Subsequent Tantra*'s pharmacy chapter)[6]
81. (4) Toasted salts
82. (5) Burnt calcite stone powder

There is a total of 23 leaves on the pacifying medicine branch. Subsequently, there are nine leaves on the internal purification medicine branch.

H13. Three leaves with wind-purifying enemas:

83. (1) *Léjam* for wind disorder
84. (2) *Trujam* for wind-bile disorder
85. (3) *Trumalen* for wind-phlegm disorder

H14. Four leaves for bile-purifying purgation:

86. (1) General purgative practice: preliminary test preparation
87. (2) Specific practice: cleaning the mouth after administering purgative medicine
88. (3) Avoiding vomiting caused by using a strong purgative
89. (4) Fomentation on the abdomen for smooth purgative therapy

H15. Two leaves for phlegm-purifying emesis:

90. (1) Squatting while pulling up the knees for strong emetic therapy
91. (2) Squatting while covering the body with a blanket for mild emetic therapy

There are nine leaves on the purification branch. In total, there are 50 leaves on the medicine tree.

---

6   G.yu thog yon tan mgon po, 1993, 585.

I. The trunk of external therapies

The external therapies tree has seven leaves.

I1. Two leaves on the wind external therapy branch:

92. (1) Using mustard oil or one-year-old butter to massage the wind points (*ku nyé*)
93. (2) *Hormé* on the wind points, with bundles made from powdered *gonyö* (*Carum carvi*), *dzati* (*Myristica fragrans*), and melted butter

I2. Three leaves on the bile external therapy branch:

94. (1) Sweating (*ngül dön*)
95. (2) Bloodletting (*trak tarwa*)
96. (3) Cold showers (*chü trülkhor*)

I3. Two leaves on the phlegm external therapy branch:

97. (1) Hot salt pack fomentation on the abdomen (*tsa duk*)
98. (2) Moxibustion on the joints (*métsa*)

There are seven leaves on the external therapy trunk. In total, 98 leaves—comprised of 35 leaves on the nutritional trunk, six on the behavioral trunk, 50 on the medicinal trunk, and seven on the therapy trunk—relate to treatment.

Altogether, there are 224 leaves: 25 leaves on the healthy tree, 63 leaves on the unhealthy tree, 38 leaves on the diagnostic tree, and 98 on the treatment tree.

20.4 THE GOALS

The flowers and fruits of health

After having completed the construction of the roots, trunks, branches, and leaves, one should place two fresh, colorful flowers that blossom on the top of the healthy tree.

J1. The flower of good health

The first flower is a symbol of the achievement of a healthy life after having followed the right diet and behavioral regimens, etc., which give health and the ability to perform physical tasks, as well as education, arts, and sports.

J2. The flower of long life

The second flower represents longevity, the result of good health, and is symbolized by an old person carrying a walking stick but possessing a clear mind.

J3–5. Three fruits

After the flowers, one should add three fruits on top. They are the symbol of the ideal state of body, mind, and speech, which is achieved through positive health, wealth, and the practice of dharma, leading to freedom from suffering in this life and beyond.

J3. The first fruit is the symbol of one who knows all the spiritual and worldly dharmas in this life.

J4. The second fruit is the symbol of one who is able to collect wealth[7] through positive health, as well as enjoyment in life.

J5. The third fruit is the symbol of the achievement of complete liberation from suffering, the accumulation of permanent happiness, and enlightenment by means of a rainbow body. The latter is called the "fruit of the fruit," the essence of life. To achieve such flowers and fruits is the final goal for both patients and physicians, the liberation from samsara and the fulfillment of all desires and wishes.

---

7 This wealth is described by means of the seven noble riches: faith, generosity, discipline, learning, modesty, sense of shame, and insight.

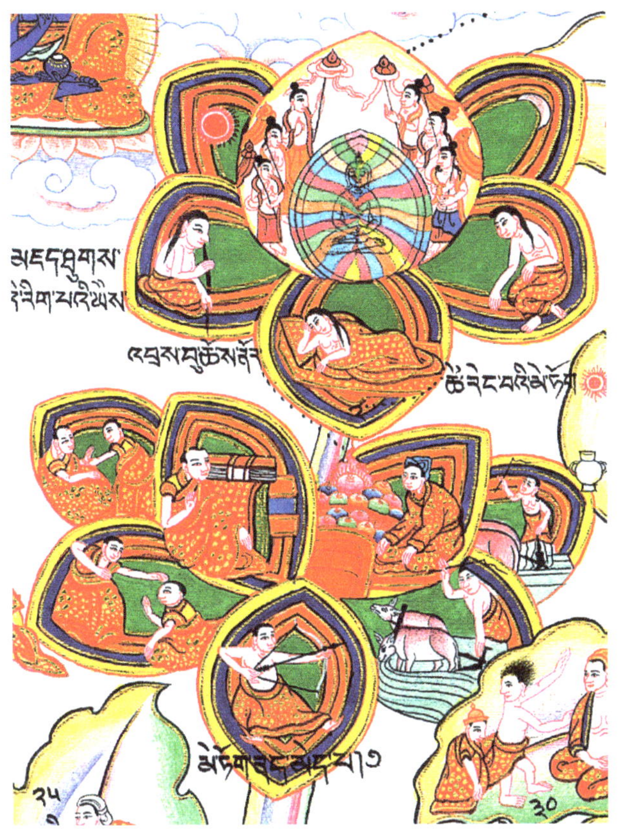

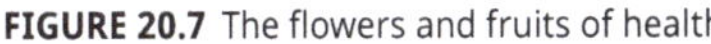

FIGURE 20.7 The flowers and fruits of health

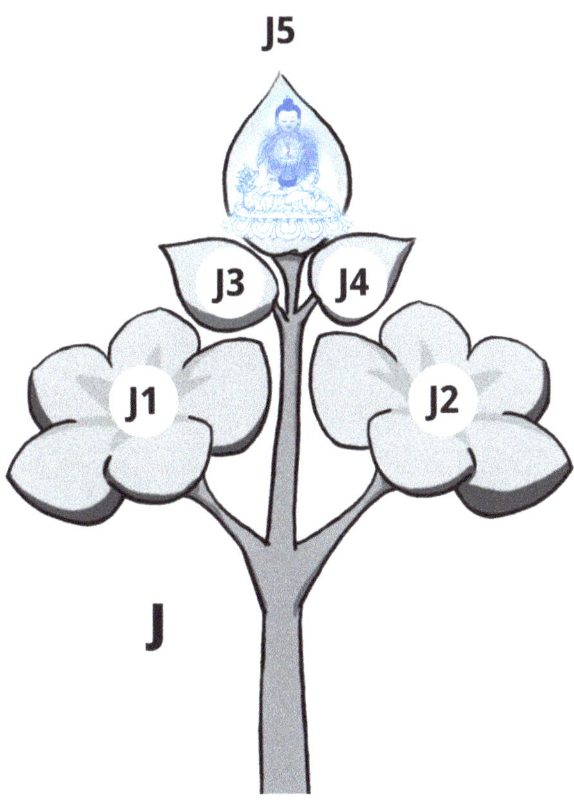

FIGURE 20.8 The sequential structure
of the flowers and fruits of health

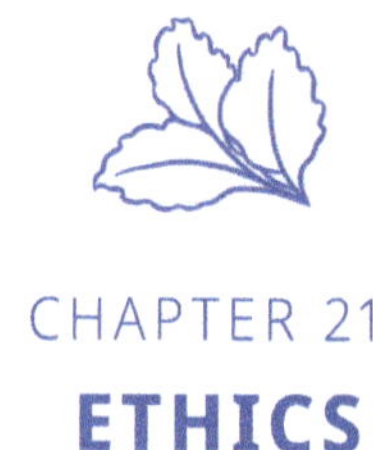

CHAPTER 21

ETHICS

21.1 THE IMPERIAL CODE OF CONDUCT

This chapter introduces Tibetan medical ethics, focusing on the physician's code of conduct. Medical ethics has two aspects, relating to different historical developments: (1) the imperial code, which is largely secular, and (2) the *Gyüzhi*'s Buddhist educational framework.

Medical ethics developed along with societal changes and through cultural exchange with neighboring countries. A first ethical code seems to have been established under the patronage of the Tibetan emperors Songtsen Gampo and Trisong Detsen between the seventh and eight centuries CE. At that time, the Asian medical traditions were much less systematized. The establishment of this ethical framework coincides with the dawn of Sowa Rigpa, as well as with significant social, legal, and moral changes in the Land of Snow. Songtsen Gampo (605–649) was the first emperor who promoted a medical system in Tibet. He was very pleased to have gathered three great physicians coming from India, China, and Persia. He praised them and declared the following words:[1]

> Not studying the ways of the three great traditions,
> you cannot be counted amongst great physicians.
> Because you will be of no benefit to yourself or others,
> like attempting to grasp thin air.
> Great Sage Bharadvaja,
> Galéno, the Ambassador,
> Hanwen Hangte, authorized by the king,
> you, the three miraculous ones,
> are to be praised as vases of immortality.

Songtsen Gampo thus promoted Indian, Greco-Arabic, and Chinese medicine as necessary contributors to the health of his subjects. All physicians were obliged to study the three traditions, and practitioners of each of these were recognized and permitted to practice. Emperor Trisong Detsen (742–798) continued this legacy by inviting renowned physicians from seven nations to Samyé Monastery in Central Tibet, aiming to further improve the science of healing. He even pretended to be ill, testing the skill of the visiting physicians.[2] The emperor was impressed by their knowledge and diagnostic accuracy. He then apologized to the physicians for disrespecting them with his tests, presenting many gifts. He also drafted the following 13 codes of conduct (*latsik chusum*) which regulate the doctor-patient relationship:[3]

1. Physicians must be honored by the black-haired Tibetans because they give life

2. The king is respected by all black-haired ones, physicians honored by him are granted the title "Lord of Lords" (*lharjé*)

3. They are protectors of wandering beings, so offer them the highest seat

4. Place a carpet, tiger and leopard skin, and silk brocade on their seats

5. See them off and receive them by horse, and pay their fees in gold

6. Obey their advice and do not go against their word

---

1 Sde srid sangs rgyas rgya mtsho, 1982, 150–51.

2 Sde srid sangs rgyas rgya mtsho, 1982, 170–71.

3 There are no Tibetan historical records concerning the ancient medical ethics of Hippocrates, nor from Chinese or Indian traditions.

7. Even my kingdom, I offer without regret as the price for my life

8. Do not ask for a thousand coins in case of death caused by wrong treatment, but be ready to pay gold even for receiving dust as medicine

9. Offer beverages and a quarter of sheep meat

10. To be able to see them continuously, avoid complaining and talk behind their backs

11. Offer them clothes, crude silk, and *gyamtak* (*rgyam thag*)[4]

12. The duty of all is to greet them and pay respect

13. In this life, forever remember and repay their great kindness

These are the 13 highly important rules. Whosoever transgresses them will be punished.

He concluded with the following advice to both physicians and patients:[5]

Physicians are like fathers,
they should treat the patient with compassion.
Patients are like sons,
do not declare their faults.

Such ethical foundations were laid between the seventh and ninth centuries CE. Unfortunately, Buddhism and medicine subsequently went into decline with the fall of centralized Tibetan rule. In 842, Langdharma assassinated his brother King Tri Relpachen, and three years later Langdharma himself was also killed. With warring princes and warlords struggling for power, the mighty Tibetan empire disintegrated into many small princedoms, and a dark period ensued for more than two centuries. Dharma, medicine, and all other sciences and their institutions nearly vanished.

21.2 THE *GYÜZHI'S* BUDDHIST EDUCATIONAL FRAMEWORK

When this long dark night finally passed, the new dawn shed a light of renaissance through the windows of the house of Tibet. Thanks to the Gugé kings Lha Lama Yéshé Ö and Jangchup Ö, Lotsawa Rinchen Zangpo, Atisha Dipankara Shrijnana, Marpa Lotsawa, and so on, Dharma and medical science were reintroduced into Tibet from India in the 11th century. Nevertheless, the most influential text concerning the medical profession and its overarching framework is certainly *Bdud rtsi snying po yan lag brgyad pa gsang ba man ngag gi rgyud*: the *Gyüzhi*.

Lama Yutok Yönten Gönpo the Younger composed the *Gyüzhi* in the 12th century based on Buddha's teachings, Vāgbhaṭa's *Aṣṭāṅga*, and several other sources. He made the *Medicine Buddha Sutra* and Five Buddhas the heart of medico-spiritual practice. He also laid down Tibetan medical ethics for physicians in a designated chapter, focusing on mind training and how to eventually become a truly altruistic bodhisattva-physician—a medical saint—and to achieve Buddhahood. It was Yutok the Younger who provided a complete guide for the physician's life and philosophy. He clearly defined what it means to be a good doctor, warning against malpractice. The ethical code of physicians is the subject of chapter 31 of the *Explanatory Tantra*. Chapter 31 covers the doctor's actions of body, speech, and mind in relation with patients, their responsibilities, and the potential fruits of medical practice. What follows is a synthesis of this chapter.

In short, aspiring doctors should abide by the following three sets of guidelines:

1. The required qualities to become a good physician

2. Medical education and training

3. The results of being a good physician

---

4 This is an ancient word of which the exact meaning has not yet been found.

5 Ibid., 174. There is quite a lot of variation within the 13 codes of conduct, comparing for instance the Dési's historical account with Drangti Penden Tsojé's 13th-century work (Brang ti dpal ldan 'tsho byed, 2005, 77–82). For more details, see Byams pa 'phrin las, 1990, 34.

The key method to learn medicine quickly is to search for the right master and to win their heart. This is the secret of learning Sowa Rigpa the fastest way. According to the tradition, the master-disciple relationship is the key for a complete education in all the sciences, including learning about the body-mind through philosophy and medicine. In this sense, learning medicine is not just learning the art of healing. It also entails acquiring a deep understanding of self and environment. In Vajrayana Buddhism, the lama or guru is regarded as the Buddha's representative or embodiment when it comes to personal practice. The entirety of the Buddhadharma is transmitted from the master, the lineage holder, to the students. Therefore, the ethical code says:[6]

> Find a teacher endowed with vast knowledge and rich experience, good-natured, not greedy, and kind.
>
> Students should perform all works without hypocrisy, and all deeds in accordance with their wishes.
> Continue to remember their kindness.
> As a result, you will learn fast and become skilled.

When the master truly opens their heart to the disciple, the moon-like nectar that pacifies the heat of delusions can be transmitted. For this to occur, the disciple should have the capacity and qualities to receive and digest it; to be mentally prepared for the teaching. The disciple should be of high quality, sincere and genuine. To maintain a good relationship with the master, the disciple should pay respect and serve the master from the beginning to the end, with loyalty and without deceit. A perfect disciple needs to cut through ego-clinging and pride, offering actions of body, speech, and mind without prior conditions. These qualities will help the student win the teacher's heart and to unite with the master's consciousness, allowing for true knowledge to be transferred.

Definition of a physician

A qualified medical doctor has studied and put into practice the 156 chapters of the *Four Tantras*, has graduated, and received a certificate. A doctor of medicine or healer-physician (*tsojé menpa*) knows mind and emotions, the body and humoral function, etiology, pathology, treatment, materia medica, and pharmacy, and applies this knowledge skillfully.

Physicians and surgeons are designated by four titles:

1. *Menpa*: "healer," who cures disease and benefits the patient's body-mind

2. *Pawo*: "hero(ine), warrior;" physicians are brave and treat without fear

3. *Menpha*: "medicine father," who protects patients like his own children

4. *Lharjé*: "Lord of Lords," because even kings obey the words of a physician; Emperor Trisong Detsen granted this title to physicians in the eighth century, as mentioned above.

Physicians are furthermore classified into four categories:

1. Supreme physician
2. Extraordinary physician
3. Ordinary physician
4. Nurse

1. Supreme physician

A supreme or unsurpassed physician is indistinguishable from the Medicine Buddha and all other buddhas, who are victorious over the four demons and the three mental poisons. The supreme healer-physician subdues all diseases resulting from wind, bile, and phlegm.

2. Extraordinary physician

An extraordinary physician is a bodhisattva, a fully altruistic being that aids others through their power of clairvoyance. They are able to know the mind and desires of others, and to provide suitable aid. Bodhisattvas possess great love and compassion, and treat all sentient beings with equanimity. As such, extraordinary bodhisattva physicians balance the body-mind and liberate from suffering.

3. Ordinary physician

An ordinary physician is a normal human being trained in medical science, putting this knowledge into practice. All medical schools and physicians of this world generally belong to this group. This category is described in detail in the ethics (and nursing) chapter of the *Explanatory Tantra*, and consists of two sections:

---

6   G.yu thog yon tan mgon po, 1993, 98.

- Good physicians: the friend of patients

- Quacks, bad, and wicked doctors: the enemy of patients

Good physicians: the friend of patients

Good physicians are protectors of human life. They are good-hearted by nature and have a nourished mind, having received proper education in medicine and Dharma. There are three subcategories:

- Royally sanctioned physicians
  This group of physicians, called *nangrik*, contains practitioners who are descendants of physicians who were originally recognized by the Tibetan kings. They are the first family lineages, including the Nine Expert Physicians tradition and Yutokpa's lineage. These still command great respect and trust in Tibetan and Himalayan societies up to this day, even though the royal courts have disappeared. In contemporary times, the personal physicians of high lama's or VIPs also attract large amounts of patients. Trust based on name seems to function in all times.

- Trained under expert physician
  This type is called *jéjang*. It includes practitioners who themselves do not belong to a family tradition, but who have trained under the above-mentioned royally sanctioned or prominent physicians.

- *Légom* physician
  This type of physician did not learn from renowned physicians, but gained experience as an assistant (also in pharmacy works) and through long-term service.

All three groups are friends of patients. Qualified physicians also have the following 13 characteristics:

1. Born to a noble or physician's family,[7] or learned through the pure teachings of the lineage of medicine

2. Diligence in medical works

3. Intelligence to discriminate right and wrong

4. Keeps the six physician's commitments (*damtsik druk*)[8]

5. Knows the traditional medical literature, theories, and their profound meanings

6. Rich in practical experience in treatment

7. Familiarity and skillfulness in all medical practices

8. Gives up the eight mundane dharmas (*jikten chö gyé*),[9] and engages with patients with the compassion of the holy Buddhadharma

9. The physician's nature is restrained and gentle

10. Skill in the art of healing with body, speech, and mind

11. Is loving towards all sentient beings

12. Is altruistic

13. Has realized all medical sciences in theory and practice

The ancient medical treatise *Somaradza* (*Sman dpyad zla ba'i rgyal po*) also gives the following advice to physicians:[10]

A physician who possesses such qualities is a good doctor, a protector of beings, a descendant of lineage-holding medical saints, and considered a living emanation of Buddha Bédurya, the King of Medicine.

---

7   There seems to be a contradiction here. Emperor Songtsen Gampo discouraged descendants from noble families to learn medicine to prevent discrimination of poor people. Yutokpa's *Gyüzhi*, however, praised nobility as a positive quality. Still, he also encouraged caring for the poor through the altruism of Dharma.

8   This corresponds to the six bullet-points under the third beneficial quality required of medical students, as laid out above.

9   Gain, loss, pleasure, misery, praise, degradation, reputation, and infamy.

10   *Sman dpyad zla ba'i rgyal po*, 1985, 55.

Quacks, bad and wicked doctors: the enemy of patients

Quacks have not studied medicine properly. They act as doctors to earn fame and money. Quack doctors are enemies of longevity. People seeking health should keep away from them. There are four types:

1. Old patient doctors
   Patients with long treatment histories have accumulated a lot of personal experience on medicines and therapies, and they advise others on treatment; this could helpful for similar cases but not for others, which may be very risky

2. Book doctors
   Some study with a teacher for a short period, copy some formulas, and proclaim that they are now able to treat disease; such person is not able to diagnose and treat without referring to books, there is no confidence that comes with experience

3. Self-study doctors
   Without having received proper medical education, this type of quack collects medical literature, steals doctor's notes, and uses stolen or purchased medicines; without oral teachings and transmission from a master, the treatment will not be helpful and will be a danger to the patient's health

4. Drug seller doctors
   Sellers of herbs and spices or merchants know what single ingredients are good for what; without deeper knowledge on pharmacognosy and compounding methods, this could lead to health scandals

Secondly, bad doctors are physicians, who lack knowlegde and experience. They are characterized by 12 faulty qualities:[11]

1. A doctor who lacks a noble family background or lineage is like a fox on a king's throne, who will not gain the respect of others

2. A doctor who is ignorant on medicine is like a person blind from birth; consulting them is like showing an object to a blind person who cannot distinguish what to treat

3. A doctor who has neither studied the texts properly nor has practical experience is like meeting a stranger on the road; patients will doubt their diagnosis

4. A doctor without knowledge of diagnostic methods is like a person wandering in foreign lands without relatives; they will not detect a single disease

5. A doctor without knowledge of pulse and urine analysis is like a spy who is not able to send messages; they will not get information on the hot or cold nature of disorders

6. A doctor who is not able to make predictions based on diagnosis is like a leader who is uncapable of addressing their people; this will lead to disgrace and a poor reputation

7. A doctor who has no experience in the treatment of disease is like shooting an arrow at a target in a dark room; the antidote will not strike the disease

8. A doctor who has no knowledge on diet and behavior is like a ruler whose country turned against him; diseases will gain strength and will ruin the body constituents

9. A doctor with no knowledge on pacifying medicines and their preparation is like a farmer without knowledge on agriculture; the preparation and dose will be excessive or insufficient, promoting imbalance

10. A doctor without knowledge on purgation and purification is like pouring water on a sand hill; it will disturb the functioning of the humors and constituents

11. A doctor without medicine, surgical and therapy instruments is like a warrior without weapons; they cannot subdue the disease enemy

12. A doctor uninformed on venesection and moxibustion is like a burglar who lacks information on the vault

Bad doctors will misdiagnose and provide the wrong treatment. They endanger life like demons in human form holding the noose of the Lord of Death.

Doctors with the following 15 negative behaviors are wicked or poor and should be actively avoided.

---

11 Sum ston ye shes gzung described 13 faults in his *Explanatory Tantra* commentary *'Grel pa 'bum chung gsal sgron*, 1999a, 241–45.

Three crazy physicians:

1. Collecting wealth by means of negative actions, generating negative karma for the next life
2. Being jealous of colleagues with superior knowledge, not accepting their superiority but instead pretending to be a great scholar
3. A doctor who treats patients, but loses their fee and name to other physicians

Three immoral physicians:

1. Trying to get more attention by employing magic or tricks to remove gallstones, cataract, or tumors
2. Not keeping promises to patients
3. Being lazy and addicted to alcohol

Three foolish physicians:

1. Hunting for fame without proper knowledge
2. Pretending to be rich
3. Contempt for professional colleagues

Three moron physicians:

1. Not being able to earn a living, but still refusing fees from patients
2. Not having an analytical mind to make clear observations
3. Not understanding the situation of terminal patients and continuing treatment

Three weak physicians:

1. Losing patients to colleagues
2. Borrowing medicines and medical instruments from others
3. Needing to consult books while treating patients

The nurse

The nurse (*menzhap*) is a physician's assistant, while *néyok* is the term used for assistants or helpers of patients. As mentioned in the *Explanatory Tantra*, nursing is a very important aspect of treating patients.[12] Ethics is especially relevant for nurses because they are in close contact with patients. Nursing requires a good heart and great patience. Mentally preparing as well as consoling the patient is often more the responsibility of the nurse than of physicians. A good nurse must possess the following four qualities:

1. A nurse must be capable and skilled in nursing, and in assisting doctor and patient

2. A good heart and strong love and compassion are essential

3. Hygiene: to be able to keep the patient's room and house (or hospital) tidy, clean and healthy; washing the patient and their bedding and clothing regularly

4. Intelligence: to be able to give proper guidelines on diet, lifestyle, and prevention at the right moment; assess the patient's situation and communicate well with physicians; know how to best care for patients physically and mentally

Wicked nurses

Nurses who are unskilled, selfish, and unkind during treatment and who use harsh words, who are unhygienic or unqualified are not advised as supports for healing.

The physician's work and responsibilities

After laying out the qualities of a good physician and the classification into good and bad practitioners, we have now arrived at the fundamentals of the work and ethics of Sowa Rigpa physicians, which consists of two sections: (1) the physician's ordinary works, and (2) the physician's particular works.

The physician's ordinary works are threefold: physical, verbal, and mental. Firstly, physicians should obtain a variety of medicines and therapeutic instruments, and apply these with diligence.

Secondly, speech is a crucial instrument to communicate with the patient: to gather a complete case history, and to be able to explain treatment and prevention measures. In some sensitive cases, skillful words are especially important. Three ways are given to diagnose wisely:

1. If physician and patient both agree on the signs and symptoms of disease, the physician should explain the nature of the disease, its causes, conditions, and treatment like blowing a conch in the marketplace.

---

12 Nursing is not mentioned in chapter 31 on ethics. The section here is based on chapter 26 of the *Explanatory Tantra*.

The physician may accept the patient if he is able to restore health or, decline terminal cases.

2. Be wise in reading the patient's mind. Some patients have a fixed mind, for instance a strong conviction that their disease is caused by poisoning. If the physician has a different interpretation, he should first agree with the patient while treating the actual disease according to their own findings.

3. In case accurate predictions cannot be made: It is extremely difficult to accurately predict if a patient is going to survive or die, or to what extent life is in danger. This depends on the individual's invisible life energy, fortune (*lungta*), and karma. Patients whose live is at risk should be given hope. If an accurate diagnosis cannot be made and the patient cannot remain under further observation, it may be necessary to be ambiguous, to speak with a forked tongue. All predictions and decisions should be made with attention to mundane dharma and social mores.

Thirdly, mental work involves observation, study of patient cases, researching medical literature, and continual effort to learn and improve.

The physician's particular works

This is the soul of the ethical code, consisting of three sections: (1) right view, (2) practice, and (3) conduct.

On a religious and philosophical level, *amchi* are generally followers of Mahayana Buddhism. More specifically, the superior view for doctors is Master Nāgārjuna's Middle Way (*Umapa*, Sanskrit: Madhyamaka). The Middle Way approaches all phenomena as having no independent reality apart from the causes and conditions from which they arise. Correspondingly, disease and symptoms all arise from causes and conditions; there is no permanent cause, no indestructible self or creator. One should avoid philosophical wrong views such as "neither existence, nor non-existence," eternalism (everything is permanent), or nihilism (nothing exists). Applied in medical practice, physicians should always avoid extreme ideas in both diagnosis and treatment.

With the right view in mind, physicians should familiarize themselves with the Four Immeasurables through meditation and put them into practice. This has two aspects:

1. Meditation and practice of the Four Immeasurables

2. Paying attention to avoid the Four Downfalls

The Four Immeasurables are:

*   When seeing suffering patients, open your heart and generate loving-kindness towards them; pray that all sentient beings may have happiness and its causes

*   During medical practice: treat the patient with great compassion, considering them like your own child; pray that all sentient beings may be free from suffering and its causes

*   After treatment: rejoice about your work, and pay thanks to the art of healing and the lineage masters; pray that all sentient beings may never be separated from great joy

*   At the end of the day: dedicate the merit gained through your work, that it may become the cause of the liberation of all beings from suffering and diseases of body, speech, and mind, and lead to permanent happiness and enlightenment; pray that all sentient beings may dwell in equanimity, unaffected by attraction to dear ones and aversion to others

Meditation and practice of these Four Immeasurables develops the practitioner's *bodhichitta*, and eventually leads to rebirth in Medicine Buddha's pure land.

Our minds are corrupted by delusions that often favor wrong thoughts and actions. This is the very nature of samsara, the cycle of suffering into which we were born. Concerning to the physician's life and profession, this implies that it is hard to be a good doctor. It requires great effort to gain a high reputation. But amassing wealth, fame, and power naturally increases one's ego as long as the mind is not tamed by the Dharma. The egoistic mind easily turns to the Four Downfalls, which prevent excellence like stones tied to the feet. They are the opposite of the Four Immeasurables:[13]

1. Running after fame: this is called the downfall of wrong happiness.

2. Treating patients as property: this is the downfall of unloving-kindness

---

13 This version of the four downfalls is quoted from Sum ston ye she gzung, 1999a, 292–97. There are several explanations of these downfalls or "wrong turning points" in different *Gyüzhi* commentaries.

3. Torture and experimentation: the performance of strong treatment and violent surgery (such as removing organs) without real need for it, aiming to gain fame and wealth; this is the downfall of being uncompassionate

4. Discrimination: caring more for rich and important patients, accepting easy cases while avoiding and declining others; this is the downfall of non-equanimity

Physicians should pay great attention to not fall for wrong thoughts and actions. These are like thieves and spies of demons that steal merit and contaminate the heart. They rob us of genuine altruistic life and spiritual development, instead throwing us into the boundless ocean of samsara.

The conduct of physicians is twofold: positive or negative. Firstly, the 10 negative actions should be avoided. Instead, one should engage in their positive opposites:

1. Do not kill, even for the sake of the patient's life or family. Never give up: a good heart and sustained effort may even cure difficult cases

2. Do not steal from patients, or indirectly take their belongings

3. Abstain from sexual misconduct with patients and their relatives[14]

4. Do not lie to or deceive patients, and do not prescribe harsh treatments to lose patients one does not want to treat

5. Do not slander or speak divisive words to patients or their helpers, family, and doctors

6. Do not utter idle speech

7. Do not use harsh words when communicating with patients

8. Avoid covetousness: do not crave for or seek to obtain a patient's valuables

9. Do not intentionally harm the patient by applying strong and violent therapies

10. Avoid wrong views: do not rejoice when hearing a patient has died; be compassionate and share your condolences

Shakyamuni Buddha declared that accumulating merit by working with patients is the same as serving the Buddha. Physicians in particular should act ethically, since they hold precious human bodies and lives in their hands. In this case, treating patients becomes a great source of merit and spiritual progress incomparable to any of the other sciences.

Positive conduct is characterized by altruism. Physicians should abide by the six perfections (Skt. *pāramitā*), which ought to be integrated into daily medical practice.

1. Generosity (*jinpa*)

- Give free treatment to the poor, to animals, and to patients in need without hesitance; this is material generosity

- Offer freedom from the fear that comes with suffering and dying to patients and animals; this is the gift of fearlessness

- Offer consolation and moral support that heals the patient's heart; this is the generosity of the Dharma

2. Moral discipline (*tsultrim*)

- The physician should practice self-discipline, and strive towards a body, speech, and mind uncontaminated by delusions; mindfully balancing the humors and disorders of others is controlling immorality

- Strengthen the six causes for being a good physician by developing the mind; this is the collection of positive morals

- Make the patient a priority and work hard to help; this is the moral discipline of helping others

3. Patience or tolerance (*zöpa*)

- Be of maximum benefit even to enemies, without any doubt; this is called the tolerance of equanimity

---

14 Even great physicians can succumb to negative actions. Méla Chakdum—one of Yutok's previous reincarnations—was appointed as court physician in Oḍḍiyāna. A love affair developed while treating the queen. The king spared him from death, but had his hands cut off, banishing the physician from the kingdom. Méla Chakdum then came to Tibet, where he got many disciples and became a legendary physician. His teachings were later collected as part of the well-known text titled *Bum khu tshur* (Phyag sman rin rgyal, 2004).

- Trust the Triple Gem as a support and guide throughout the ups and downs of your life; this is the tolerance of hardship

- Face difficulties without fear, and take on all the challenges that arise when learning the art of medicine; this is fearless tolerance

4. Effort (*tsöndrü*)

- Respect spiritual masters and teachers, and abide by their words; this is respectful effort

- Spare no effort in treating patients; this is continuous effort

- Remember your motivation to liberate all sentient beings from samsara; this is spiritual effort

5. Concentration (*samten*)

- Focus the mind through meditation on positive actions, which brings physical and mental bliss; this is called special blissfulness

- Work with the direct experience of meditative concentration; this is bestowing peace

- Generate clairvoyance through contemplation; this is helping others by meditative power

6. Wisdom (*shérap*)
This is discerning awareness that understands what is to be cultivated and what is to be abandoned.

- Acquire wisdom through hearing

- Acquire wisdom through contemplation

- Acquire wisdom through meditation

21.5 THE RESULTS OF BEING A GOOD PHYSICIAN

Well-trained and nourished by the teacher's knowledge and the Dharma, the student grows their tree of knowledge. Without losing track, practicing correctly, and dedicating one's life to helping patients, the physician is considered an emanation of the Medicine Buddha who drives out disease and misfortune. Good practitioners who abide by the six positive qualities will achieve both the temporal and ultimate results.

The temporal results of good practice will arise in this life in the form of happiness, respect by others, and power, prosperity, and a joyful and peaceful life. All these results are due to the art of healing, by sharing your talent with others. Treat even your enemies like brothers and sisters. Apply the diagnostic tests and treat according to the disease nature. This treatment method will increase your merit and soon your reputation. Famous physicians should be skillful, gentle, with little desires, morally disciplined, and focused on helping others. When you are in high demand, charge reasonable fees at the right time, but do not take advantage. Do not forget to charge your fee when appropriate. Even long-time patients may forget your kindness, and might not repay you later. If the patient is poor, give free medication. But for others, free service can create malevolence. Psychologically, it is not beneficial for patients to be cured at no cost. This could even lead to a lesser effect of the treatment. From the physician's side, the mind also clings to not having received anything in return, which contaminates consciousness and the patient-physician relationship.

The ultimate result of being a good physician who has abandoned deceit and desire, and who is dedicated to healing and leading an altruistic life, is the unsurpassed state of enlightenment. This, the Medicine Buddha has proclaimed.

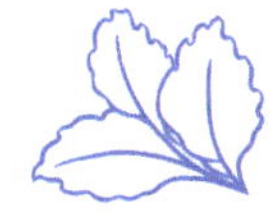

CONCLUSION

The *New Light* textbook series is meant to provide all the basic materials required to study and practice Sowa Rigpa, as well as leads for further research. For health professionals in particular, these teachings introduce an alternative view on the body-mind and its humoral energetics. Although directly based on the *Four Tantras* (*Gyüzhi*), several new chapters and topics have been added in *New Light on Tibetan Medicine: Volume I - Foundations* in order to present a contextualized overview that is suitable for contemporary purposes. We encourage the reader to consult *New Light* alongside (a translation of) the *Gyüzhi*, allowing for deeper insight into the often concise verses of this text.

The foundational framework of the *Gyüzhi*, with its four treatises and 156 chapters, however, is important to retain here as well. The oral lineage (*nyengyü*) instructions that accompany this scripture state that it is structured in a way that reflects the nature of the mind as well as the resulting formation of the body—from embryonic development up until death and the dissolution process. This sequence, which is kept as much as possible in the *New Light* series, is a skillful means that simultaneously guides students and practitioners in the somatic study of medicine and in mind training. The *nyengyü* transmission further explains that the *Four Tantras* can be taught in accordance with both sutra and tantra. Yutok the Younger himself declared that it is a hidden tantra, in the form of medicine, that is not different from the highest tantras. It was expounded by manifestations of the Five Tathagatas (often called "Dhyani Buddhas" in the West), for instance, each of which heals one of the five mental poisons. Therefore, studying and practicing the *Gyüzhi* is equal to studying the *vajra* body and practicing tantric *sādhanā* complete with generation and completion stages. This profound stepwise healing of the body-mind is what sets Sowa Rigpa apart from secular medical sciences.

A synopsis of *Volume I - Foundations*

To remember and show respect to the ancient masters in whose footsteps we follow, *New Light*'s *Foundations* begins with chapters on the history of Sowa Rigpa. Describing the diverse origins of the science of healing from a traditional lineage-based perspective, special attention is given to the *Vinaya Sutra on Medicine* and the *Golden Light Sutra*—Buddha Śākyamuni's direct medical teaching. The essence of these foundational source texts of Buddhist medicine has been transmitted via Jīvaka and many other lineage holders, eventually contributing to the glory of the *Four Tantras*. Jīvaka, Śākyamuni's personal physician, was later identified as an emanation of the Medicine Buddha, Master of Medicine and King of Aquamarine Light (*Bhaiṣajyaguruvaiḍūrya-prabhārāja*). His later emanations include Nāgārjuna and Vāgbhaṭa, the latter of whom composed the *Ashtāngahridayasaṃhitā*. The Medicine Buddha's principal reincarnation in Tibet was Yutok Yönten Gönpo, who compiled the *Gyüzhi* relying partly on the *Ashtānga*. Through the integration of Buddhist philosophy and ethics, it has remained the foundation of Sowa Rigpa up to this day. Based on his teachings, numerous Tibetan medical schools and lineages have flourished over the centuries.

After laying out the historical and religious context, *Foundations* commences with the actual elucidation of the *Gyüzhi* by starting with the first word of its title: ambrosia or nectar, which is a translation of *amṛta* (from the Sanskrit title) and *dütsi* (Tibetan). The term *dütsi* literally means "(anti-)demon essence," which refers to the mythical origins of poison and disease as well as medicine and healing. Next, the Medicine Buddha, his emanations, and the palace-city of Tanaduk are described with its four mountains. Tanaduk can be interpreted on external, internal, and secret levels, the former including an introduction to Tibetan materia medica and the latter corresponding to one's own body-mind.

Having gone through the abovementioned preliminaries, the content of the *Four Tantras* is enumerated as a list of 156 chapters. This covers its main practice, with the three humors (*nyépa sum*) acting as its backbone. The humors originate from ignorance and the three mental poisons, which implies that the entire medical system revolves around what could be called psychology for lack of a better word: how consciousness generates a physical body endowed with senses and emotions. Nevertheless, the *Gyüzhi* itself has no separate chapter on the mind and its functions, a topic that is scattered across distant verses. It is important to note here again that Tibetan medical psychology aligns more closely to tantra rather than sutra explanations of mental activity, and that Sowa Rigpa looks at the mind through the prism of bodily physiology instead of directly speaking about emptiness. Although the ultimate goal is the same, this makes a big difference in terms of approach. Tantric instructions assert that if one is able to control the winds (*lung*), one can control the mind. The winds, together with the channels, represent the physical body. So, through the body, we can work with consciousness in a more concrete manner. To gain a deeper understanding of these connections and especially the transformation of mind into matter, Chapter 4 was added to this book.

Following this, the book dives into humoral physiology, which is the largest part by far. Starting off in general, the causes (sources), conditions (physical locations), and resulting functions of the *nyépa sum* are first covered systematically. Secondly, the distinguishing characteristics of wind (*lung*), bile (*tripa*), and phlegm (*béken*), and their specific principal branches are treated one by one. Once more, extra information was added by the author, including potential symptoms of congenital humoral malfunction, and illustrations that highlight links between the *nyépa* and tantric channels, body areas, organs, and biomedical systems. The five minor winds (*yenlak gi lung nga*) have been brought to the center stage to better understand the workings of the brain and sense organs. The body is indeed formed in line with the mind as its karmic result, and is preconditioned by the morphology of the elemental forces initially obtained from the parents (including genes). The product is one's individual body constitution or type. The *Explanatory Tantra* lays out the three basic body types clearly. Building on these, the three dual constitutions that can be observed more regularly have been elaborated along with several newly added subcategories.

Once the humoral system is established, life depends on the metabolism of the digestive fire (*médrö*). For the purpose of clarity, digestion is subdivided into two parts: the general stages taking place in the digestive tract, which can be understood through the metaphor of cooking, and the specific chain of processes that gives rise to the body constituents and major as well as minor waste products. Under the name of metabolism, many classes of tiny beings (*sinbu*)—including microorganisms such as bacteria—contribute to overall health as well as the decomposition of food. Therefore, *sinbu* are the often-unacknowledged working population of the body country. The male and female reproductive fluids are the final body constituent; they are understood as "essence drops" (*tiklé*) that nourish the tissues and organs, their refined product being radiance (*dang*). Hormones (*kham kyi dangma*), reinterpreted here as subtle fluids closely related to the *tiklé* and *dang*, sustain the seat of the all-ground (*künzhi*) in the heart while also being involved in sexual differentiation and the menstrual cycle. Altogether, the body-mind system depends on the equilibrium of its 25 components: the humors (three times five branches), seven body constituents (*lüzung dün*), and three waste products (*drima sum*). This is the concept of health through balance (*ta mel né mé*), through which a harmonious mindset and even deep awareness can be naturally achieved.

The significance of female physiology for the science of medicine can hardly be underestimated as the actual development and growth of a human body commences in the uterus. Chapter 12 was added for this reason, introducing the six stages of a woman's life in relation to fertility and further exploring the role of hormones—and female sex hormones (*motsi*) in particular—from an integrated perspective. Next, the embryology chapter details the causes for body formation, the factors and mode of conception, as well as presenting an outline of the 38 weeks of fetal development. Immediately following conception, the five gross elemental energies obtained from the parents encircle the bardo consciousness, eventually producing the five extremities (head, arms, and legs), five vital, hollow (not counting the reproductive organs, which are associated with all elements combined) and sense organs, five fingers, and so on, which all relate to the five chakras. To come to a more profound understanding of the channels and winds, which are explained in parallel, one should read more and meditate on the mind and its first reflections when awakening from sleep. In short, the five elements create all the fivefold bodily components as well as the five minds/emotions. Nevertheless, the interactions of karma and the elements inside the mother's womb remain a miracle. When the body is built, it acts like a fully furnished abode of the mind and organs, like a king's palace. Such metaphorical comparisons, although simple, carry hidden meanings pertaining to all the body's main functions.

The *Explanatory Tantra* does not cover the organs in detail, whereas the *Oral Instruction Tantra*'s pathological perspective is helpful if interpreted from the contrary standpoint of normal healthy physiology. Even though luminaries such as Taktsang Lotsawa Shérap Rinchen (1405–1477) have written about the organs,[1] there is a need for more empirical and anatomically precise description. Organs are the fruits and bases of the five elements and the five mental poisons, which contact the external world through the windows of the senses. Their relationships with both positive and negative mental states have been elucidated further based on the author's clinical experience. On a spiritual level, the organs are the centers of the Five Tathagatas and their healing powers.

The channels (*tsa*) and chakras (*khorlo*) are a complicated subject, especially if one attempts to search for a single fixed system with representative colors that correspond closely to anatomical structures. Lacking the insight of tantric training, the many differences between different traditions easily lead to confusion. This notwithstanding, more profound research on *Gyüzhi* literature reveals that medical explanations on the channels draw on tantric sources. Texts such as Künkhyen Péma Karpo's commentary on Nāropā's yogic techniques clarify many of these contradictions by distinguishing between visualized meditative channels, the *vajra* body, and somatic channels.[2] Still, topics such as the identification of the life channel (*tsé yi tsa*) remain inconclusive. Largely adhering to the *Explanatory Tantra*, four overarching categories are covered: channels of formation, existence, connection, and of the life force. One should understand here that it is the same three main channels and their branches that are approached from different viewpoints, namely (1) embryology, (2) the four or five chakras as nodes of activity, (3) the medically more relevant blood, lymphatic, and nervous systems, and (4) the pervasiveness of life force (*sok*) and breath.

The just-mentioned final category leads us into subtle physiology. The phenomenon of separated or lost *la* is not prominent in the *Four Tantras*, but knowledge can be gleaned from astrology and rites such as "soul retrieval" (*laguk*). By evaluating the healing efficacy of such rituals, it becomes clear that the *la* is in fact an important contributor to the strength and stability of the body-mind. The *la* body is a usually invisible energetic interface that is produced from and acts in-between the physical and mentally projected bodies, a kind of body-mind copy or hologram. This third bodily dimension generally has the same structure as the gross body of the person to which it belongs, but it does not depart with consciousness after death, instead dwelling around the corpse until the bones have decayed. This might be one reason why Tibetans prefer sky burial; to sever attachment and thus lessen the sufferings of those who stay behind. Besides the *la*, more tantric notions of channels were also briefly introduced under the heading of subtle physiology. The aim in this context is to utilize the secret structure underlying the body-mind to induce radical transformation. Because these techniques are strongly based on faith and devotion, however, it is better not to publicly reveal too much. The exposition of the channels and chakras corresponds to the completion stage, working with the *vajra* body. In the *Gyüzhi*, four chakras are indirectly described under the four great channels of existence (*sipé tsa chen zhi*). Three- and five-chakra systems also each have their validity. In reality, however, our bodies our composed of countless major and minor nodes and networks.

Throughout development, completion, and use, the body ages and obstacles may appear. Signs of decline manifest like falling leaves in autumn. As time passes, inner changes reflect in the outer world as misfortune or success. Demons or evil spirits are all reflections of the body-mind. This is why due attention is given to the patient's dreams as well as other omens in diagnosis. Eventually, signs of decline, near and immanent death are bound to appear. On a medical level, we can infer the dissolution process of the elements and sense consciousnesses through the dying process. In terms of spiritual practice, we witness the dissolution of the subtle mind. During this process, the gross and subtle winds will come to flow in the opposite directions as in embryonic development. In the end, the mind once again enters into the space/emptiness from where it arose. Since dying and falling asleep share similarities, practitioners have the opportunity to familiarize themselves with this crucial life passage through dream yoga.

The medicine trees (*dong drem*) parallel the closing part of *sādhanā* practice. When students have successfully memorized the *Root* and *Explanatory Tantras*, the construction and recitation of the corresponding allegorical tree diagrams summarizes and concludes the formal study of these treatises. The ground, roots, trunks, branches, leaves, flowers, and fruits are color-matched and laid out sequentially following the illustrations included in the set of medical *tangka* paintings created under the auspices of Dési Sangyé Gyatso (1653–1705).

The last chapter of the *Explanatory Tantra* concerns professional ethics. After briefly introducing the much older imperial code of conduct, the penultimate chapter of this volume therefore details the required qualities to become a good physician and different ways to train ourselves. This moral framework aims to integrate Mahayana Buddhist compassion into every step of the doctor-patient interaction, which can be achieved by applying the Four Immeasurables.

---

1   See Byams pa 'phrin las, 1990, 197.

2   'Brug chen bzhi pa padma dkar po, 1983.

This pragmatic path towards body-mind transformation eventually leads to enlightenment as avowed by the Medicine Buddha. Acting like a healing buddha day and night is the ideal post-meditative state of Sowa Rigpa practitioners.

Finally, a concise Medicine Buddha *sādhanā* for daily practice is provided in the Appendix, composed by the author based mainly on the *Medicine Buddha Sutra of 800 Verses* and *Gyüzhi*'s medicine blessing passage.

Outlook

With the synopsis presented above in mind, we can conclude this volume by reflecting once more on the oral lineage teachings which frame the content of the *Four Tantras* along three major axes: medical knowledge on the material body, insight into the nature of mind, and the stages of tantric transformation. Embryology represents the generation stage (*kyé rim*) as it involves the visualization of the body mandala. This mandala is ultimately no other than the *nirmāṇakāya*, the physical manifestation of Buddha-nature that is adorned by the organs. When form has fully manifested, one enters into *tsalung* meditation to work with the subtle channels and chakras, thus practicing the techniques of the illusory body (*saṃbhogakāya*). Next, one reaches the completion stage (*dzok rim*), which involves the dissolution of the body-mind (*dharmakāya*) in a process similar to dying. In this way, the *Four Tantras* cure the three or five mental poisons as the worldly body is transmuted by means of true love and compassion. As the Medicine Buddha expounded, one needs to look no further for other spiritual means: caring for the sick is a stepping-stone towards complete liberation.

In the subsequent textbooks of the *New Light on Tibetan Medicine* series, we strive to continue to guide readers along this path to a modest degree by sharing contemporary explanations on diagnosis, treatment, and pathologies.

APPENDIX

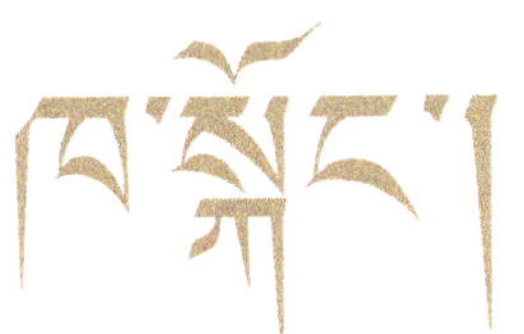

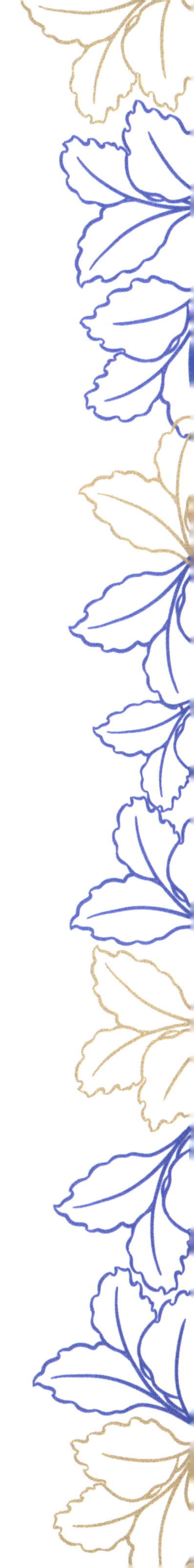

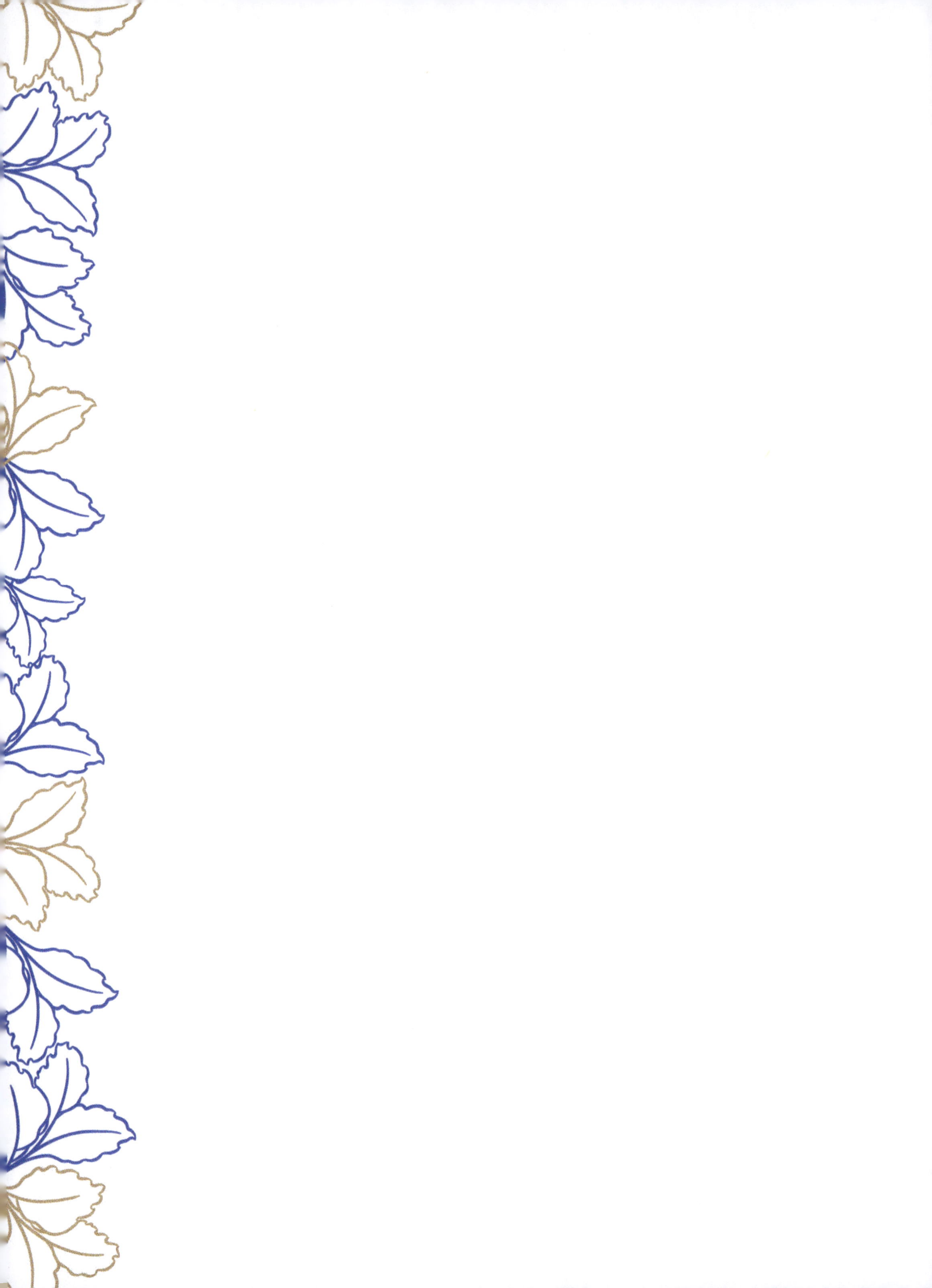

CONCISE DAILY
MEDICINE BUDDHA PRACTICE

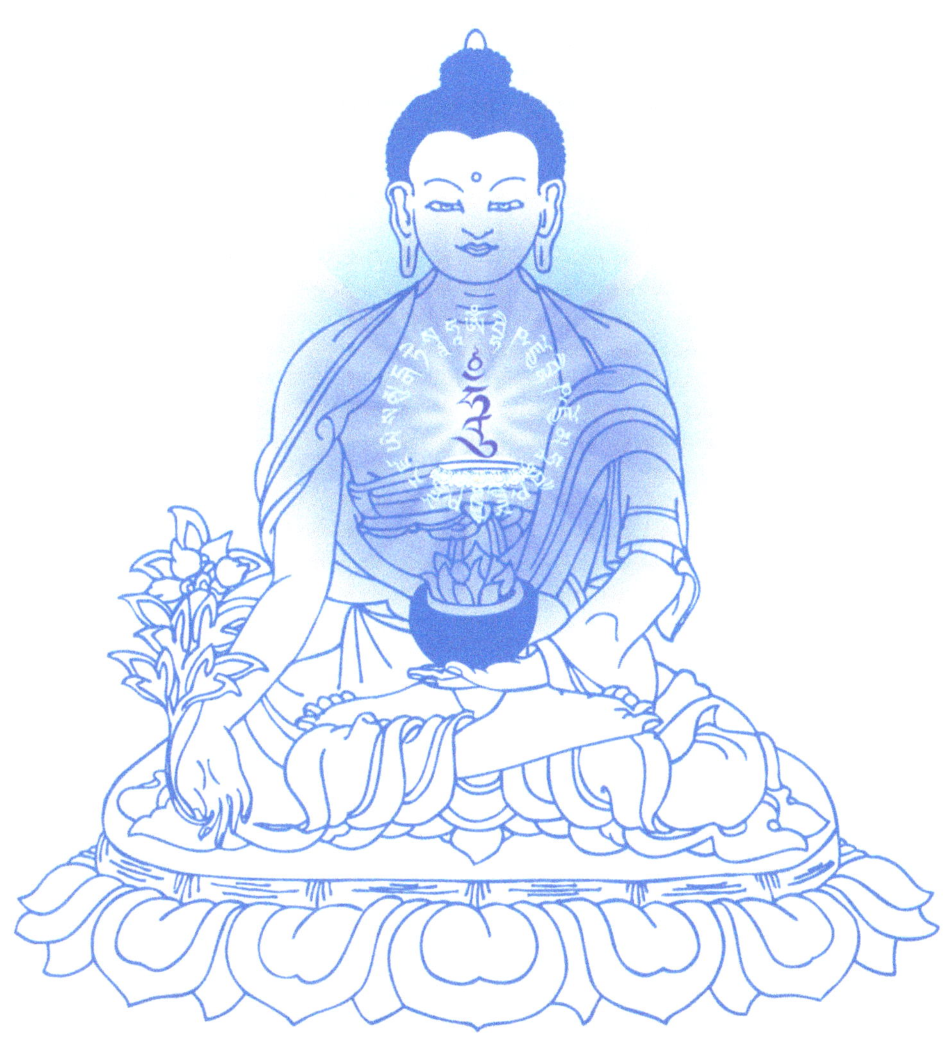

FIGURE A.1 Sangyé Menla with seed syllable and mantra at the heart

Taking refuge

Recite three times:

Sang gyé chö dang tsok kyi chok nam la
Jang chup bar du dak ni kyap su chi
Dak gi jin sok gyi pé sö nam kyi
Dro la pen chir sang gyé drup par shok

I go for refuge until I am enlightened,
to Buddha, Dharma, and Sangha, the supreme
assembly.
Through the virtues I collect by giving and
other perfections,
may I become a buddha for the benefit of all
beings.

Generating *bodhicitta*: the Four Immeasurables

Recite three times:

Sem chen tam ché dé wa dang dé wé gyu dang
mi drel war gyur chik
Sem chen tam ché duk ngel dang duk ngel gyi
gyu dang drel war gyur chik
Sem chen tam ché duk ngel mé pé dé wa dang
mi drel war gyur chik
Sem chen tam ché nyé ring chak dang nyi dang
drel wé tang nyom la né par gyur chik

May all sentient beings have happiness and
its causes.
May all sentient beings be free from suffering
and its causes.
May all sentient beings never be separated
from great joy.
May all sentient beings always dwell in
equanimity, unaffected by attraction to dear
ones and aversion to others.

Praise to the Supreme Healer, Medicine Buddha Bédurya

Tuk jé dro wé dön dzé chom den dé
Tsen tsam tö pé ngang drö duk ngel kyop
Duk sum né sel sang gyé men gyi la
Bé durya yi ö la chak tsel lo

I prostrate to the King of Aquamarine Light,
Buddha Bédurya Ökyi Gyelpo,
the Master of Medicine and Awakened One,
who acts to benefit beings,

protects them from the miseries of inferior
realms,
and dispels the three mental poisons and their
resulting ailments,
merely by hearing his name.

Invocation of the Medicine Buddha and his disciples[1]

Dün gyi nam khar seng tri pé dé teng
Sang gyé men gyi la ma ku dok ngo
Dak lo dé pé sö nam zhing chok tu
Sé dang ché pa né dir shek su söl

In the space before me, I invite the blue-
colored Medicine Buddha,
seated upon a lion throne, lotus and moon
cushions.
O Medicine Buddha Bédurya and your
disciples, please come!
You are the supreme field for my faithful
mind's collection of merit.

Self-generation as the Medicine Buddha[2]

Rang nyi bé durya ö men gyi gyel
Men gyi nö ni dü tsi lhung zé sam
Men la drang song nam kyi shi pa jö
Tso dzé men pé gyel po chom den dé
Duk sum né sel sang gyé men gyi la
Ku dok ting ga bé durya yi ö
Trül pé ku la tsen dang pé jé den
Lung tri bé ken né kyi dung pa la
Né kyi nyen po chak yé a ru ra
Chak yön dü tsi lhung zé par pu nam
Bé durya yi ö la chak tsel lo

Medicine Buddha is pleased by your request. He dissolves into aquamarine light, which enters your body,
speech, and mind.

Instantly, I become Buddha Bédurya
Ökyi Gyelpo,
and visualize the medicine container
as a nectar vase.
O Supreme healer, King of Physicians,
Blessed One!

---

1 This invocation can also serve as the front generation.

2 Only for those who received the empowerment. Others
may visualize the Medicine Buddha on top of their crown.

You are victorious from the three mental poisons.
Your serene aquamarine body is adorned with the 32 major and 80 minor good marks, and is full of healing light.
You are holding in your right hand a stem of chebulic myrobalan, which represents the physical ailments' antidote.
And in your left hand a bowl of nectar, to purify the ignorant mind and increase awareness.
The rays coming from your body go to all directions of samsara to bless and cure all beings' physical and mental disorders, and negative karma.

Praise to the lineage gurus

Rik pé né chok cho gyé tuk su chü
Tsé la wang wé chü len ngö drup nyé
Ngön shé nying jé dro chok du wa nyom
Drang song rik dzin nam la chak tsel lo

To you, holy sages, who have realized the art of the 18 sciences,
attained miracle power,
and immortality by extracting the essence,
who have achieved the power of clairvoyance and compassion,
which heals the imbalance of the various ailments, I offer prostrations.

The assembly is encircled by the lineage gurus.

Mandala offering

Sa zhi pö kyi juk shing mé tok tram
Ri rap ling zhi nyi dé gyen pa yi
Sang gyé zhing du mik té bül wa yi
Dro kün nam dak zhing du chö par shok

The land is sprinkled by perfume and fresh flowers are displayed.
Mount Méru is decorated by the sun, moon, and the four continents.
I offer this mandala to the Medicine Buddha, the Supreme Healer.
May all beings be reborn in his pure land and become realized.

IDAM GURU RATNA MANDALAKAM NIRYATAYAMI

Aditionally, recite the Vajrasattva mantra and confess.

Blessing by the power of words of truth

Lha nam kyi ni dü tsi ta bu dang
Lu nam kyi ni tsuk nor ta bu dang
Drang song nam kyi chü len ta bu ni
Kün la men ché nyé war né gyur chik

To the gods, medicine is like nectar.
And in the naga realm, it is like the crown jewel.
For the sages, it is like *chülen.*
May potent medicines and therapies always be at our disposal.

Pacifying disease by medicines, therapies, and other methods

Lung tri bé ken zhi gya tsa zhi né
Tsé la bar du chö pa zhi wa dang
Nö pé gek rik tong trak gyé chu dang
Yé drok sum gya druk chu la sok pa
Sam pé bar du chö pa zhi war dzö

May these subdue the 404 diseases caused by wind, bile, and phlegm, which threaten life, and also subdue the 1,080 types of harmful interferences,
and the 360 inborn spirits which provoke mental obstacles.

Visualization of blessing

At the heart appears a lotus and moon disc. Standing at the center of the moon disc is the blue seed-syllable *HŪṂ*, surrounded by the syllables of the mantra. As you recite the mantra, visualize rays of light radiating in all directions from the heart. The rays go to all parts of your body and drive out all physical, energetic, and mental disorders in the form of black smoke, fire or water, insects, and so on. The light also travels to all directions, pervading the six realms of existence. Through your great love, wishing all beings to have happiness, and through your great compassion—wishing them to be free from all suffering—all their afflictions and diseases are purified as they reach the state of Medicine Buddhahood. Recite the mantra at least 21 times.

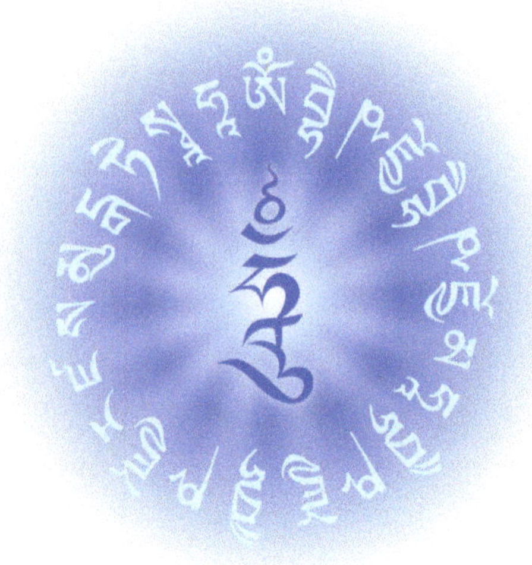

FIGURE A.2 The seed-syllable *HŪṂ* surrounded by the short mantra

Short Medicine Buddha *dhāraṇī*

TÉ YA THA OM BÉ KHA DZÉ BÉ KHA DZÉ MA
HA BÉ KHA DZÉ BÉ KHA DZÉ [BÉ KHA DZÉ]
RA DZA YA SA MUNG GA TÉ SO HA

Long Medicine Buddha *dhāraṇī*

OM NA MO BHA GA WA TÉ BÉ KHA DZÉ GU
RU BÉ DURYA PRA BHA RA DZA YA TA THA GA
THA YA AR HA TÉ SAM YAK SAM BU DHA YA
TÉ YA THA OM BÉ KHA DZÉ BÉ KHA DZÉ MA
HA BÉ KHA DZÉ BÉ KHA DZÉ [BÉ KHA DZÉ]
RA DZA YA SA MUNG GA TÉ SO HA

Absorption and dissolution

After the proper visualization and transformation of your body-mind, the protectors, lineage gurus, and the two bodhisattvas dissolve into the Medicine Buddha. The buddha then dissolves into the mantra, and the mantra into the *HŪṂ* syllable. At the end, the *HŪṂ* gradually dissolves into blue-white light, and into emptiness.[3] Meditate beyond thoughts and words as much as you can.

After this meditation, reappear as Medicine Buddha like sunrise, holding on to this vision as long as possible, day and night.

Dedication prayer

Chok chu jik ten tam ché du
Men dang men pa dak dang ni
Né yok tün pé za tung sok
Yo jé kün tu jung war shok

Dro wa né pa ji nyé pa
Né sö gyur gyi bar du ni
Men dang men pa nyi dang ni
Dé yi né yok jé par shok

Men nam tu dang den pa dang
Sang ngak dé jö drup par shok
Kha dro sin po la sok pa
Nying jé sem dang den gyur chik

Gé wa di yi nyur du dak
Sang gyé men la drup gyur né
Dro wa chik kyang ma lü pa
Dé yi sa la kyé war shok

May all 10 directions of the samsaric world provide medicines,
physicians, nurses, and full facilities of food and shelter for poor and sick people.
May I be reborn as medicine, physician, and nurse,
and perform healing and service until all sick people are cured.

May all medicines become powerful against disease.
May spiritual practitioners achieve their *siddhi*.
May all *ḍāka*, *ḍākinī*, evil spirits, and so on gain love and compassion in their hearts.

By the power of this merit, may all beings attain the enlightenment of Medicine Buddha, without leaving any behind.
May all achieve the reign of Buddha-nature.

Tashi Gého! Sarva maṅgalam!

---

3   For advanced practitioners, more detailed instructions on the final dissolution stages are required.

༼༢༡༽ སངས་རྒྱས་སྨན་གྱི་བླ་མའི་རྣལ་འབྱོར་
རྒྱུན་ཁྱེར་མདོར་བསྡུས་བཞུགས་སོ།

༈ སྐྱབས་འགྲོ།

།སངས་རྒྱས་ཆོས་དང་ཚོགས་ཀྱི་མཆོག་རྣམས་ལ། །བྱང་ཆུབ་
བར་དུ་བདག་ནི་སྐྱབས་སུ་མཆི། །བདག་གི་སྦྱིན་སོགས་
བགྱིས་པའི་བསོད་ནམས་ཀྱིས། །འགྲོ་ལ་ཕན་ཕྱིར་སངས་
རྒྱས་འགྲུབ་པར་ཤོག

ལན་གསུམ་འདོན།

༈ རྒྱུན་གྱི་སེམས་སྐྱེ་ཕྱིར་ཚད་མེད་བཞི་སྒོམ་པ།

།སེམས་ཅན་ཐམས་ཅད་བདེ་བ་དང་བདེ་བའི་རྒྱུ་དང་མི་འབྲལ་
བར་གྱུར་ཅིག །སེམས་ཅན་ཐམས་ཅད་སྡུག་བསྔལ་དང་སྡུག་
བསྔལ་གྱི་རྒྱུ་དང་བྲལ་བར་གྱུར་ཅིག །སེམས་ཅན་ཐམས་
ཅད་སྡུག་བསྔལ་མེད་པའི་བདེ་བ་དང་མི་འབྲལ་བར་གྱུར་ཅིག
།སེམས་ཅན་ཐམས་ཅད་ཉེ་རིང་ཆགས་སྡང་གཉིས་དང་བྲལ་
བའི་བཏང་སྙོམས་ལ་གནས་པར་གྱུར་ཅིག

ལན་གསུམ་འདོན།

༈ སངས་རྒྱས་སྨན་བླ་ནི་ཧྲཱིཿ ཡི་འོད་ལ་བསྒོད་པ།

།ཕྱགས་རྗེས་འགྲོ་བའི་དོན་མཛད་བཅོམ་ལྡན་འདས། །མཚན་
ཙམ་མཐོས་པས་དང་འགྲོའི་སྡུག་བསྔལ་སྐྱོབ། །དུག་གསུམ་
ནད་སེལ་སངས་རྒྱས་སྨན་གྱི་བླ། །བཻ་ཌཱུརྻ་ཡི་འོད་ལ་ཕྱག་
འཚལ་ལོ།

༈ སངས་རྒྱས་སྨན་གྱི་བླ་མ་སྤྱན་འདྲེན།

།མདུན་གྱི་ནམ་མཁར་སེང་ཁྲི་པད་ཟླའི་སྟེང་། །སངས་རྒྱས་
སྨན་གྱི་བླ་མ་སྐུ་མདོག་སྔོ། །བདག་བློ་དང་པའི་བསོད་ནམས་

ཞིང་མཆོག་ཏུ། །ཁྱེས་དང་བཅས་པ་གནས་འདིར་གཤེགས་
སུ་གསོལ།

༈ སྨན་བླ་སྐོམ་པ།

།རང་ཉིད་ནི་ཐུགས་འོད་སྨན་གྱི་རྒྱལ། །སྨན་གྱི་སྤྱོན་ནི་བདུད་ཚེ
སྲུང་བཟེད་བསམ། །སྨན་བླ་དང་སྟོང་རྣམས་ཀྱིས་ཤེས་པ
བཞེད། །འཚོ་མཛད་སྨན་པའི་རྒྱལ་པོ་བཅོམ་ལྡན་འདས།
།དུག་གསུམ་ནད་སེལ་སངས་རྒྱས་སྨན་གྱི་བླ། །སྐུ་མདོག
མཐིང་ག་བཻ་ཌཱུརྻ་ཡི་འོད། །སྤྱལ་པའི་སྐུ་ལ་མཚན་དང་དཔེ
བྱད་སྤྲས། །རྒྱུད་མཐིས་བད་ཀན་ནད་ཀྱིས་གདུངས་པ་ལ།
།ནད་ཀྱི་གཉེན་པོ་ཕྱག་གཡས་ཨ་རུ་ར། །ཕྱག་གཡོན་བདུད
ཚེ་སྲུང་བཞེད་པར་ཕུ་བསྐྱམས། །བཻ་ཌཱུརྻ་ཡི་འོད་ལ་ཕྱག
འཚལ་ལོ།

༈ སྨན་གྱི་རིག་འཛིན་ཆོས་སྐྱོང་རྣམས་ཀྱིས་བསྐོར་བ་ནི།

།རིག་པའི་གནས་མཆོག་བཅུ་བཅུད་ཕྱགས་སུ་ཆུད། །ཚེ་ལ་
དབང་བའི་བཅུད་ལེན་དངོས་གྲུབ་བརྙེས། །མདོན་ཞེས་སྦྱིང་
རྗེས་འགྲོ་མཆོག་འདུ་བ་སྙོམས། །དང་སྙོང་རིག་འཛིན་རྣམས
ལ་ཕྱག་འཚལ་ལོ།

༈ མཐའ་རྒྱས་པ་དང་མ་བྱུང་ན་བསྡུས་པ་འབུལ་ནི།

།ས་གཞི་སྤོས་ཀྱིས་བྱུགས་ཞིང་མེ་ཏོག་བཀྲམ། །རི་རབ་སྤྱིང་
བཞི་ཉི་ཟླས་བརྒྱན་པ་ཡིས། །སངས་རྒྱས་ཞིང་དུ་དམིགས་ཏེ
འབུལ་བ་ཡིས། །འགྲོ་ཀུན་རྣམ་དག་ཞིང་དུ་སྤྱོད་པར་ཤོག

༈ སྨོན་ལམ་བཅོས་ཀྱི་ནུས་པ་བྱིན་གྱིས་བརླབ་པ་ནི། བགྱིས། དགེའོ། སཪྦ་མངྒ་ལཾ།

།ལྷ་རྣམས་ཀྱི་ནི་བདུད་རྩི་ལྟ་བུ་དང་། །ཀླུ་རྣམས་ཀྱི་ནི་གཙུག་ནོར་ལྟ་བུ་དང་། །དྲང་སྲོང་རྣམས་ཀྱི་བཅུད་ལེན་ལྟ་བུ་ནི། །ཀུན་ལ་སྨན་དཔྱད་ཉེ་བར་གནས་གྱུར་ཅིག

སྨོན་རྣམས་པ་ཨ་ཏུ་པ་སངས་ཡོན་ཏན་ནས་སྨོན་མདོ་བརྒྱུད་བཅུ་པ། རྒྱུད་བཞིའི་སྨོན་བྱིན་རླབས་དང་རྒྱལ་བ་ལྷ་པའི་སྨོན་ལྨ་མདོ་ཚོག་སོགས་ནས་བཏུས་ཏེ་ཕྱོགས་སྒྲིག་བགྱིས་པའོ།

༈ ནད་གདོན་ཞི་བའི་སྨན་བླའི་གཟུངས་སྔགས་བཀླ་བ།

།ཀྲུང་མཐྲིས་བད་ཀན་བཞི་བརྒྱུ་རྩ་བཞིའི་ནད། །ཚེ་ལ་བར་དུ་གཅོད་པ་ཞི་བ་དང་། །གནོད་པའི་བགེགས་རིགས་སྟོང་ཕྲག་བརྒྱུད་བྱུ་དང་། །ཡེ་འདྲོག་སུམ་བརྒྱུ་དྲུག་ཅུ་ལ་སོགས་པ། །བསམ་པའི་བར་དུ་གཅོད་པ་ཞི་བར་མཛོད།

གཟུངས་སྔགས་ ༢༡ འདོན།

༈ གཟུངས་ཐུང་།

ཏདྱ་ཐཱ། ཨོཾ་བྷཻ་ཥེ་ཛྱེ་བྷཻ་ཥེ་ཛྱེ། མ་ཧཱ་བྷཻ་ཥེ་ཛྱེ་བྷཻ་ཥེ་ཛྱེ། རཱ་ཛཱ་ཡ་ས་མུངྒ་ཏེ་སྭཱ་ཧཱ།

༈ གཟུངས་རིང་།

ཨོཾ་ན་མོ་བྷ་ག་ཝ་ཏེ། བྷཻ་ཥ་ཛྱེ་གུ་རུ་བཻ་ཌཱུརྱ་པྲ་བྷ་རཱ་ཛཱ་ཡ། ཏ་ཐཱ་ག་ཏཱ་ཡ། ཨ་ཧྟེ་ཏེ་སམྱཀྶཾ་བུདྡྷཱ་ཡ། ཏདྱ་ཐཱ། ཨོཾ་བྷཻ་ཥེ་ཛྱེ་བྷཻ་ཥེ་ཛྱེ། མ་ཧཱ་བྷཻ་ཥེ་ཛྱེ་བྷཻ་ཥེ་ཛྱེ། རཱ་ཛཱ་ཡ་ས་མུངྒ་ཏེ་སྭཱ་ཧཱ།

༈ བསྔོ་བ་སྨོན་ལམ།

།ཕྱོགས་བཅུ་འཇིག་རྟེན་ཐམས་ཅད་དུ། །སྨོན་དང་སྨན་པ་དགའ་དང་ནི། །ནད་ག་ཡོག་མཐུན་པའི་ཟ་བཅུད་སོགས། །ཡི་བྱད་ཀུན་ཏུ་འབྱུང་བར་ཤོག །འགྲོ་བ་ནད་པ་ཇི་སྙེད་པ། །ནད་གསོས་འགྱུར་གྱི་བར་དུ་ནི། །སྨན་དང་སྨན་པ་ཉིད་དང་། །དེ་ཡི་ནད་ག་ཡོག་བྱེད་པར་ཤོག །སྨན་རྣམས་མཐུ་དང་། །གསང་སྔགས་བཀླ་བརྗོད་འགྱུལ་བར་ཤོག །མཁའ་འགྲོ་སྲིན་པོ་ལ་སོགས་པ། །སྙིང་རྗེའི་སེམས་དང་ལྡན་གྱུར་ཅིག །དཀོ་བ་འདི་ཡི་སྒྱུར་དུ་བདག །སངས་རྒྱས་སྨན་བླ་འགྲུབ་འགྱུར་ནས། །འགྲོ་བ་གཅིག་ཀྱང་མ་ལུས་པ། །དེ་ཡི་ས་ལ་སྐྱེ་བར་ཤོག །

GLOSSARY OF TIBETAN TERMS

A

amchi (am chi)
Practitioner of Sowa Rigpa, Tibetan medical physician (syn.: *menpa*)

aso (a so)
One of the two types of uterine *sinbu* (cf. *ngel sin*)

B

bakchak (bag chags)
Mental predispositions, latent karmic residues

bardo (bar do)
Intermediate state, usually refers to period in-between death and rebirth

bardö namshé (bar do'i rnam shes)
Bardo consciousness

bawa (lba ba)
Goiter

béken (bad kan)
Phlegm

béken chi (bad kan spyi)
General phlegm (humor)

béken gyi tsenyi dün (bad kan gyi mtshan nyid bdun)
The seven characteristics of phlegm

béken jorjé (bad kan 'byor byed)
Joining phlegm, one of the five phlegm branches

béken mukpo (bad kan smug po)
Brown phlegm

béken nyakjé (bad kan myag byed)
Decomposing phlegm, one of the five phlegm branches

béken nyongjé (bad kan myong byed)
Experiencing phlegm, one of the five phlegm branches

béken rangzhin (bad kan rang bzhin)
Phlegm constitution

béken tenjé (bad kan rten byed)
Supportive phlegm, one of the five phlegm branches

béken tsimjé (bad kan tshim byed)
Satisfying phlegm, one of the five phlegm branches

belgö chutsa (sbal mgo'i chu rtsa)
Thigh channels, lit. "frog head water channels"

bélung rangzhin (bad rlung rang bzhin)
Phlegm-wind constitution

bépé tsa (sbas pa'i rtsa)
Internal nerves, lit. "hidden channels" (cf. *dar gyi changtak chusum*)

bépé tsé yi kawa sum (sbas pa'i tshe yi ka ba gsum)
The three hidden pillars of life

bésin (bad srin)
Phlegm microorganisms and parasites, mainly located in the stomach

bétri (bad mkhris)
Béken and *tripa* combined (cf. *drangtri*)

bétri rangzhin (bad mkhris rang bzhin)
Phlegm-bile constitution

bönpö tö (bon po'i thod)
One of the three main skull bone channels, lit. "Bönpo's knot" (cf. *trényel*)

buga nangwa (bu ga snang ba)
"Openings-appearing" wind, branch of *soklung a* during week 11 of fetal development

buguchen (bu gu can)
Tubular phlegm nerve channel group

bümé tselwa (bud med brtsal ba)
Searching for a suitable (female) partner, part of eight branches of medicine (cf. *rotsawa*)

bur gyüpa (bur rgyus pa)
"Passage insertion" wind, branch of *soklung a* during week 13 of fetal development

butak (bu thag)
Umbilical cord, lit. "fetal thread" (syn.: *tétak*)

C

chak kyi go (lcags kyi sgo)
"Iron door" wind branching from *soklung a* during week 30 of fetal development

chakpé gyu (chags pa'i rgyu)
Conception factor(s)

chakpé tsa (chags pa'i rtsa)
Formation channel(s)

chaktsül rikpa (chags tshul rig pa)
Embryology (syn.: *ngelchak rikpa*)

champa (cham pa)
Flu, common cold, influenza

chang (chang)
Fermented beer-like, alcoholic drink

ché (lce)
Tongue

chéma (phye ma)
Medicine in powder form (syn.: *churni*)

chépé dün so gyé (gces pa'i mdun so brgyad)
The incisors, lit. "the eight precious front teeth"

cherpa (mcher pa)
Spleen

chi yi buga gu (phyi yi bu ga dgu)
The nine external orifices

chi yi tsakar (phyi yi rtsa dkar)
External or peripheral nerve(s)

chin (gcin)
Urine, one of the *drima sum*

chindri nakpo (mchin dri nag po)
Lower "black diaphragm," pancreas (?)

chingak (gchin 'gags)
Dysuria

chinpa (mchin pa)
Liver

chinyi (gchin snyi)
Frequent urination disorder

chitsa (phyi rtsa)
Peripheral nerves, lit. "outer channels" (ant.: *nangtsa*)

chitsuk (spyi gtsug)
The crown of the head, the central crown point (ZH1)

chiwa (lci ba)
Heavy, *béken* characteristic

chiwo déchen gyi khorlo (spyi bo bde chen gyi 'khor lo)
The great blissfulness crown chakra

chöjé kyi dram so gyé (gcod byed kyi 'gram so brgyad)
Molars, lit. "eight cutting and grinding teeth"

chong né (gcong nad)
Chronic metabolic disease(s)

chongchen zéjé (gcong chen zad byed)
Consumption disease

chongzhi rik nga (cong zhi rigs lnga)
The five types of calcite

chu (chu)
Water, water element

chu (mchu)
Lip(s)

chü kham nyingpo (chu'i khams snying po)
Essence of water (cf. *tiklé*)

chü trülkhor (chu yi khrul 'khor)
Cold showers, an external therapy indicated for excess bile

chülen (bcud len)
Rejuvenation practice, lit. "essence extraction" (Skt.: *rasāyana*)

churni (chur ni)
Medicine in powder form (syn.: *chéma*)

chuser (chu ser)
Blood plasma, lit. "yellow fluid"

chutsa (chu rtsa)
Water (energy) channels (cf. *tsa kyangma*)

chutsa trengbu chudruk (chu rtsa phreng bu bcu drug)
The 16 minor nerve channels

chutsen (chu tshan)
Hot spring(s)

chutsen rik nga (chu tshan rigs lnga)
The five hot spring waters, types of hot spring

chuwa chugu (chu ba bcu dgu)
The 19 ligaments

D

dakdzin (bdag 'dzin)
Self-grasping, an aspect of mind located in the heart, ego

damtsik druk (dam tshig drug)
The six commitments or *samaya* vows of physicians

dang (mdangs)
Body radiance, complexion, the final refinement of *dangma*

dangdü gu (ldang dus dgu)
Nine disease manifestation times, one of the nine branches of the unhealthy humors tree

dangma (dwangs ma)
(Liquid) food essence present in stomach and intestines, chyle; one of the *lüzung dün*

dangma lenpé tsagu (mdang ma len pa'i rtsa dgu)
The hepatic portal vein system, lit. "the nine nutrition-absorbing channels"

dar gyi changtak chusum (dar gyi dpyang thag bcu gsum)
The 13 inner (involuntary) nerves, lit. "the 13 hanging threads"

darma (dar ma)
Adulthood

daryaken (dar ya kan)
Theriac, panacea (syn.: *tengchok*)

datsen (zla mtshan)
Menstruation, the "monthly sign"

denpé rangzhin (ldan pa'i rang bzhin)
Combined constitution of two dominant *nyépa*

déwé kham gyuwé tsa (bde ba'i khams rgyu ba'i rtsa)
The "entering the realm of bliss channel" (syn.: *düpé tsa*)

döchak ('dod chags)
Attachment, the distant cause of the wind humor

dokching gyurwa (zlog cing bsgyur ba)
"Reversed transformation" wind, a branch of *soklung a* during week 8 of fetal development

dokgyu chunyi (ldog rgyu bcu gnyis)
12 adverse reactions to wrong treatment, eighth branch of the unhealthy humors tree

domen (rdo sman)
Stone medicine, *Gyüzhi* materia medica category

dön (gdon)
Evil spirits; psychiatry, one of the eight branches of medicine

dön nga (don lnga)
The five vital or solid organs, lit. "the five functionaries"

dön nö (don snod)
The (five solid and six hollow) organs

dong (gdong)
Face

dong drem (sdong 'grems)
The medicine tree (construction) practice

dorjé lü (rdo rje lus)
Vajra body, the tantric subtle body or an indestructible state

dötsa (bdsod rtsa)
Veins, stable blood channels (cf. *soktsa nakpo*)

dra ché (dgra lce)
One of the four son lungs

drakzhün rik nga (brag zhun rigs lnga)
The five types of mineral pitch

dramtsé ('grams tshad)
Spread fever

dranglung (grang rlung)
Cold wind

drangtri (grang mkhris)
Cold bile (cf. *bétri*)

drangtri rangzhin (grang mkhris rang bzhin)
Cold bile constitution

drangwa (grang ba)
Cold, *lung* characteristic; general term for cold abdominal diseases

dré ('bras)
Malignant tumor (as opposed to *tren*); fruit

dré né ('bras nad)
Malignant tumor disease

drébu gu ('bras bu dgu)
The nine results of disease, one of the nine branches of the unhealthy humors tree

drébu sum ('bras bu gsum)
The three myrobalan fruits: *arura*, *barura*, and *kyurura*

drek (dreg)
Gout

drelwé tsa ('brel ba'i rtsa)
Connecting channels

drenpa (dran pa)
(Gross) memory, recollection

drenpé wangpo selwé tsa (dran pa'i dbang po gsal ba'i rtsa)
Memory-clearing channels

drenshé (dran shes)
Memory consciousness, recollecting mind

drenshé tramo (dran shes phra mo)
Subtle mind memory

drésher menbu (gre sher rmen bu)
Thyroid gland

dréwa (gre ba)
Throat

drichen (dri chen)
Feces (syn.: *shangwa*)

dridong ('bri gdong)
"Wild female yak's face" wind, branch of *soklung a* during week 17 of fetal development

drima (dri ma)
Sweat and body dirt, one of the *drima sum*

drima mépa (dri ma med pa)
Stainless wind, branch of *soklung a* during week 18 of fetal development

drima sum (dri ma gsum)
The three principal waste products

drinam (dri snams)
Malodorous, *tripa* characteristic

drinpa longchö kyi khorlo (mgrin pa long spyod kyi 'khor lo)
The throat enjoyment chakra

drö (drod)
Heat

drongkhyer dzinpa (grong khyer 'dzin pa)
"City ruler," a subtle wind branching from *soklung a* during week 25 of fetal development

drülgo dengdré menbu nyi (sbrul mgo ldeng 'dra'i rmen bu gnyis)
Lit. "the two cobra-headed lymph glands"

drumbu (grum bu)
Rheumatism, arthritis

drumö chutsa (gru mo'i chu rtsa)
Elbow channels

drumpa ('brum pa)
Smallpox

drupa lü (grub pa lus)
Embryonic bodily development

düdé rangzhin ('dus sde'i rang bzhin)
Collective community constitution

dujé kyi lé (du byed kyi las)
Volitional formations, formative actions (cf. *lé*, *tendrel yenlak chunyi*)

duk (dug)
Poisons or toxicology, one of the eight branches of medicine

duk sum rakpa (dug gsum rags pa)
The three gross mental poisons

dül (rdul)
Natural psychic energy carrying fire in embryonic form (cf. *sem kyi rangzhin gyi nüpa sum*)

dungtsuk (mdung tshugs)
One of the three main skull bone channel groups, lit. "piercing spear"

düpé soktsa chik ('dus pa'i srog rtsa gcig)
The combined channel of all organs, involved in hormonal and reproductive functions

düpé rangzhin ('dus pa'i rang bzhin)
Combined constitution

düso sum ('dus so gsum)
Point where the blood channels come together at the fontanel

dütsi (bdud rtsi)
Nectar, ambrosia, lit. "(anti-)demon essence"

dütsi drowa (bdud rtsi 'gro ba)
"Nectar passage" wind, branch of *soklung a* during week 16 of fetal development

dütsik druk (dus tshigs drug)
Six medical seasons or "joints of time," consisting of two months

duwa nam zhi ('du ba rnam bzhi)
Four humor bloods

dzéjé kyi chéwa zhi (mdzes byed kyi mche ba bzhi)
Canines, lit. "the four beautiful fanged teeth"

dzo na (mdzo sna)
Son lung located above the heart, lit. "nose of a yak-cow crossbred"

dzöka (mdzod ka)
Alpha treasury wind, branch of *soklung a*

dzok rim (rdzogs rim)
Completion stage in tantric ritual practice (cf. *kyé rim*)

dzupmo (mdzub mo)
Fingers, digits including toes

G

ga shi (rga shi)
Ageing and death (cf. *tendrel yenlak chunyi*)

gakpa (gag pu)
Diphteria

gangpa (lgang pa)
Urinary bladder, one of the *nö druk*

gangtö gangmé (sgang stod sgang smad)
One of the five mother lungs, consisting of two parts lateral to the spinal cord

gaptsé (gab tshad)
Hidden fever, a chronic fever which hides in the (phlegm) organs

gé né (rgas nad)
Aging disease

gek rik (bgegs rigs)
Obstacles, obstacle-creating evil spirits, obstacle makers

gépa (rgas pa)
Eldery (older than 60); geriatry, one of the eight branches of medicine

géwa nga (dge ba lnga)
The five virtuous factors of excellent teachings

go (mgo)
Head

gogü buga (sgo dgu'i bu ga)
The orifices of the nine doorways of the body

gya chenpo (rgya chen po)
Exalted subtle wind, branch of *soklung a* during week 6 of fetal development

gya dar (rgya dar)
The meninges, lit. "Chinese silk" (syn.: *lépé gyadar*)

gyangjé ser gyi drönmé (rgyang byed gser gyi sgron me)
The light of the liver and gallbladder that shines from the eyes, lit. "the golden light seen from a distance"

gyelwa rik nga (rgyal ba rigs lnga)
The five Tathagatas or "Victors" representing the Five Buddha Families

gyétsé (rgyas tshad)
High fever

gyulam buga (rgyu lam bu ga)
Nutritional passages, lit. "hollow pathways"

gyulam chonga (rgyu lam bco lnga)
15 pathways of humoral circulation (one of the nine branches of the unhealthy humors tree)

gyuma (rgyu ma)
Small intestine, one of the *nö druk*

gyumé pu (rgyu ma'i spu)
Gastro-intestinal villi, lit. "intestine hair" (syn.: *powé pu*)

gyüpa (rgyus pa)
Tendon

gyusor chunyi (rgyu sor bcu gnyis)
Duodenum (syn.: *zangtsak lugu go*)

gyuzer (rgyu gzer)
Gastro-enteritis

H

hor gyi métsa (hor gyi me btsa)
Hormé, a gently warming external therapy for the treatment of wind imbalance

J

ja gap (bya sgab)
Son lungs named after the front shoulder blade muscle

ja lü ('ja' lus)
Rainbow body

ja tsön na nga ('ja' mtshon sna lnga)
Elemental energies encircling the *künzhi* mind, lit. "the five kinds of rainbow reflections"

jajé ('ja' byed)
"Paralysis-causing" bile nerve channel group

jampa ('jam pa)
Smooth, *béken* characteristic

jamtsi ('jam rtsi)
Mild enema

jangchup kyi sem gyégyur gyi rikchen (byang chub kyi sems rgyas 'gyur gyi rigs can)
Evolving relative *bodhicitta* energy

jangsem kar mar (byang sems dkar dmar)
White and red *bodhicitta*, referring to semen and menstruation (including ovum)

jarbak (byar bag)
Sticky/slimy, *béken* characteristic

jéjang (rjes sbyang)
A type of physician who trained under a prominent family lineage holder

jéjé (rjed rjed)
Amnesia, a type of psychiatric disease

jikté ('jig ltas)
The process of dying and its prognosis, lit. "signs of destruction"

jikten chö gyé ('jig rten chos rgyad)
The eight worldly dharmas: gain, loss, pleasure, misery, praise, degradation, reputation, and infamy

jinlap kyi ka (byin rlabs kyi bka')
Blessed teachings (cf. *kama*)

jinpa (sbyin pa)
Generosity, one of the six perfections

jipa (byis pa)
Children (younger than 12 for males and 16 for females); pediatrics, one of the eight branches of medicine

jipa nyerchö (byis pa nyer spyod)
Child care

juk go ('jug sgo)
Entrance gates, one of the nine branches of the unhealthy humors tree

jungpö dön ('byung po'i gdon)
Wandering (evil) spirits (cf. *dön*)

jungtsek ('byung brtsegs)
The tiers in which the elements arise and are positioned in the body

jungtsi ('byung rtsis)
Elemental astrology

jungwa chenpo nga ('byung ba chen po lnga)
The five basic/gross elements

jungwa ngé dangma ('byung ba lnga'i dang ma)
Essence energy of the five elements

jungwé dül ('byung ba'i rdul)
Subatomic elemental particle

jungwé dültren ('byung ba'i rdul phran)
Nucleus of an elemental particle

K

kama (bka' ma)
Buddha Word, direct oral transmission

kang (rkang)
Bone marrow, one of the *lüzung dün*

kangbam (rkang bam)
A serious leg inflammation caused by poor blood circulation, sometimes translated as scurvy or elephantiasis

kartika (karti ka)
Crystal-like white channel at the center of the heart chakra (cf. *yi zangma*)

ké (ske)
Neck

kézer né (skad 'zer nad)
Hoarseness

kha (kha)
Mouth

kham déshek nyingpo (khams bde gshegs snying po)
Essence of Buddha-nature (cf. *sem*)

kham kar (khams dkar)
Semen

kham kar gonga (khams dkar sgo nga)
Ovum, lit. "white essence egg"

kham kar mar (khams dkar dmar)
The white and red essential natures, semen and menstruation (including ovum, cf. *khuwa kar mar*)

kham kyi dangma (khams kyi dang ma)
Hormone, a biomedically derived term, lit. "natural essence of the body"

kham marpo (khams dmar po)
Menstrual blood, red nature reproductive fluid

khelma (mkhal ma)
Kidney(s)

khendra (khan dra)
Concentrated solid extract

khorlo ('khor lo)
Chakra, lit. "wheel"

khorlo chungwa ('khor lo chung ba)
Minor chakra(s)

khu chu (khu chu)
Seminal fluid

khuwa (khu ba)
Semen, one of the *lüzung dün* (cf. *kham kar mar*); medicinal broth

khuwa kar mar (khu ba dkar dmar)
White and red fluids, semen and menstruation (including ovum, cf. *kham kar mar*)

khuwé bu (khu ba'i 'bu)
Spermatozoa

khyampo ('khyam po)
One of the three main skull bone channel groups, lit. "wandering"

khyilwa ('khyil ba)
Winding subtle wind, branch of *soklung a* during week 7 of fetal development

khyilwé tsa ('khyil ba'i rtsa)
The lymbic system of the brain, lit. "coiled channel"

kom né (skom nad)
Thirst disease

küntok gyéchu (kun rtog brgyad cu)
The 80 gross emotions

küntu chöwa (kun tu 'phyo ba)
"Floating in all direction," a subtle wind branching from *soklung a* during week 24 of fetal development

küntu düpa (kun tu sdud pa)
Assembling subtle wind, a branch of *soklung a*

küntu gyelwa (kun tu rgyal ba)
All-victorious wind, branch of *soklung a* during week 22 of fetal development

kunyé (bsku mnye)
Body massage, generally indicated for wind disorder

künzhi (kun gzhi)
All-ground, the storehouse and base of all experience, an aspect of subtle mind

künzhi yi kyi namshé (kun gzhi yid kyi rnam shes)
Subtle mental consciousness

küpé go (skup pa'i sgo)
"Thread entrance" wind, branch of *soklung a* during week 14 of fetal development (syn.: *kupé kha*)

küpé kha (skud pa'i kha)
"Thread opening" wind, branch of *soklung a* during week 14 of fetal development (syn.: *kupé go*)

kusum lamkhyer (sku gsum lam 'khyer)
Taking the three bodies or *kaya* of a buddha as paths

kyabap (skya rbab)
Body swelling, the first stage of edema, lit. "whitish wave"

kyéché (skye mched)
Source, sensory field (cf. *tendrel yenlak chunyi*)

kyéché chunyi (skye mched bcu gnyis)
The 12 sources or bases of perception

kyéché druk (skye mched drug)
The six sensory fields or sources

kyépel wangpo (skye 'phel dbang po)
Reproductive organs, one of the *nö druk*

kyé rim (bskyed rim)
Generation stage in tantric ritual practice (cf. *dzok rim*)

kyéwa (skye ba)
Birth (cf. *tendrel yenlak chunyi*)

kyéwa ngönpar drupa (skye ba mngon par grub pa)
"Remembering past lives," a subtle wind branching from *soklung a* during week 26 of fetal development

kyikbu (skyigs bu)
Hiccups

kyuk né (skyugs nad)
Vomiting disorder

kyukpa (skyugs pa)
Emesis, vomiting

L

la guk (bla 'gugs)
Rites to summon or retrieve *la*

la khyampa (bla 'khyams pa)
Wandering *la*

la lakpa (bla brlags pa)
Lost *la*

la phowa (bla 'pho ba)
The transference of *la* from one place to another over the course of the month (cf. *lané potsül*); astral body

la yi chutsa (rla yi chu rtsa)
Buguchen nerve branches of the thigh channels (cf. *belgö chutsa*)

lama (bla ma)
Guru, master, spiritual teacher

lané potsül (bla gnas 'pho tshul)
The mode of operation of the *la* cycle (cf. *la powa*)

langtap (glang thabs)
Colic

latsa (bla rtsa)
La pulse, felt at the ulnar artery of the wrist; *la* channel

latsik chusum (bla gtsigs bcu gsum)
13 codes of conduct of physicians, laid down by Trisong Detsen

lé (las)
Karma

lé kyi lung (las kyi rlung)
Karmic body wind, a product of *lung dzinpa*

lé drel (las 'brel)
Karmic connection

lé kyi lung ngönpar düpa (las kyi rlung mngon par sdud pa)
"Manifest karmic assembly" wind, branch of *soklung a*

légom (las goms)
A type of physician who gained expertise through long-term assistantship and service

léjam (sle 'jam)
A type of enema suitable for single wind disorder

lélung (las rlung)
Bodily or karmic breath, the major part of each breath

lenpa (len pa)
Grasping (cf. *tendrel yenlak chunyi*)

lépa (klad pa)
Brain

lépé gyadar (klad pa'i rgya dar)
Meninges, lit. "Chinese silk cover of the brain" (syn.: *gyadar*)

lha (lha)
Divinity, celestial beings inhabiting the higher realms of samsara, "white" spirit

lhajin gyi lung (lha sbyin gyi rlung)
Tongue minor wind

lharjé (lha rje)
"Lord of Lords," honorary title given to physicians by Trisong Detsen

lhenkyé ma (lhan skyes rma)
Co-emergent lesions, being born with a wound; may correspond to congenital disease

lhenkyé né (lhan skyes nad)
Hereditary or congenital disease, may correspond to genetic disease

likluk (rlig rlugs)
(chronic) hydrocele

lo (blo)
Intellect (cf. *sem*)

long ga (long ga)
Colon, large intestine, one of the *nö druk*

lotsawa (lo tsa ba)
Honorary title for Tibetan translator of canonical texts

lowa (glo ba)
Lung(s)

lowa bu nga (glo ba bu lnga)
The five son lungs, the anterior lobes of the lungs

lowa ma nga (glo ba ma lnga)
The five mother lungs, the posterior part of the lungs

lu (klu)
Naga, underworld spirit associated with snakes and reptiles; the minor wind of vision

lü (lus)
Body; general internal medicine, one of the eight branches of medicine

lü (klud)
Ransom ritual

lu dön (klu gdon)
Malignant *lu* spirit, characteristically causing skin disorders

lü kyi drapé (lus kyi 'dra dpe)
Body similes

lü kyi namshé (lus kyi rnam shes)
Body consciousness

lü kyi rangzhin (lus kyi rang bzhin)
Body constitution

lü kyi trasin (lus kyi phra srin)
Bodily microorganisms (cf. *sinbu*)

lü kyi yéwa (lus kyi dbye ba)
Body classification

lü lung (klu'i rlung)
Naga (minor) wind

lü peltsül (lus 'phel tshul)
Fetal development

lüjong (lus sbyong)
Physical exercises that are part of Tibetan tantric yoga, lit. "body training"

luk khel tsek dra (lug mkhal rtsegs 'dra)
Temporal muscles "like piled sheep's kidneys"

lung (rlung)
Wind (element), wind (humor); oral transmission

lung bumpachen (rlung bum pa chen)
Vase breathing (Skt.: *kumbhaka*), a type of yogic breath retention

lung chi (rlung spyi)
General wind

lung dzinpa (rlung 'dzin pa)
Life-retaining wind

lung gi dangma (rlung gi dang ma)
The quintessence of wind (cf. *yéshé kyi lung*)

lung gi rangzhin (rlung gi rang bzhin)
Wind constitution

lung gi tsenyi druk (rlung gi mtshan nyid drug)
The six characteristics of wind

lung gyengyu (rlung gyen rgyu)
Ascending wind, one of the five wind branches

lung khyapjé (rlung khyab byed)
Pervading wind, one of the five wind branches

lung ményam (rlung me mnyam)
Fire-like wind, one of the five wind branches

lung rakpa (rlung rags pa)
Gross wind

lung sem yer mé (rlung sems dbyer med)
The inseparability of wind and mind

lung sokdzin (rlung srog 'dzin)
Life-sustaining wind, one of the five wind branches

lung trawa (rlung phra ba)
Subtle wind

lung tursel (rlung thur sel)
Descending wind, one of the five wind branches

lung uma (rlung dbu ma)
Central wind of the central life channel

lungta (klung rta)
Fortune of a person

lungtri rangzhin (rlung mkhris rang bzhin)
Wind-bile constitution

lungtsa (rlung rtsa)
Wind channel

lungtsap (rlung tshabs)
Menopausal disorders

lüsem (lus sems)
Body-mind

lüzung dün (lus zungs bdun)
The seven body constituents

M

ma ning (ma ning)
(Gender) neutral (cf. *tsen nyi ma ning*)

mamin tsawa (ma smin tsha ba)
Unripe fever

marikpa (ma rig pa)
Mental ignorance, the root of all suffering

marutsé (ma ru tse)
One of the two types of uterine *sinbu* (cf. *ngel sin*)

mazhuwa (ma zhu ba)
Indigestion

mé (me)
Fire (element)

médrö (me drod)
Digestive heat, metabolism

mélung gyi lung (me rlung gyi rlung)
Fire-wind wind, corresponds to de-oxygenated air

mélung tsawa (smad rlung tsha ba)
Lower hot wind

menbu (rmen bu)
Glands or lymph nodes

menbu gongön nyi (rmen bu mgo sngon gnyis)
The cervical lymph nodes, lit. "the two blue-headed glands"

menbu karpo nyi (rmen bu dkar po gnyis)
The thigh lymph nodes, lit. "the two white glands"

menmar (sman mar)
Medicinal butter

menmo (sman mo)
Class of feminine (lake) spirits who dwell in the countryside

menpa (sman pa)
Sowa Rigpa practitioner, lit. "healer" or "medicine person," title given to practitioners (syn.: *amchi*)

menpa (sman pha)
"Medicine father", title given to physicians who protect their patients like their own children

menpa jangchup sempa (sman pa byang chub sems dpa')
Bodhisattva doctor

menpé gyu druk (sman pa'i rgyu drug)
The six good qualities required of physicians

menyön chenpo (sman yon chen po)
"Great healing qualities," a subtle wind branching from *soklung a* during week 27 of fetal development

menzhap (sman zhabs)
Nurse, the assistant of physicians

métok düpa (me tog sdud pa)
"Collecting flowers," a subtle wind branching from *soklung a* during weeks 31 to 35 of fetal development

métok dzinpa (me tog 'dzin pa)
"Holding flowers," a subtle wind branching from *soklung a* during week 28 of fetal development

métok trengwa (me tog phreng ba)
"Flower garland," a subtle wind branching from *soklung a* during week 29 of fetal development

métsa (me btsa)
Moxibustion

méwel (me dbal)
Shingles (herpes zoster) and cold sores (herpes simplex), lit. "flame tongue"

mik (mig)
Eye(s)

mik gi tawa (mig gi lta ba)
Visual diagnosis

mik shé (mig shes)
Eye consciousness

ming zuk (ming gzugs)
Name and form (cf. *tendrel yenlak chunyi*)

mo (mo)
Female, feminine

mo né (mo nad)
Gynecology, one of the eight branches of medicine

motsi (mo rtsi)
Female essence or hormone

muchu (dmu chu)
Final stage of edema

münpa (mun pa)
Natural psychic energy carrying wind in embryonic form (cf. *sem kyi rangzhin gyi nüpa sum*)

N

na (sna)
Nose

namkha (rnam kha)
Space (element), ether, sky

namkhé dül (rnam kha'i rdul)
Space element particle

nampar jépa (rnam par byed pa)
"Differentiating" wind, branch of *soklung a* during week 9 of fetal development

nampar shépa (rnam par shes pa)
Consciousness (cf. *tendrel yenlak chunyi*)

namshé tsok druk (rnam shes tshogs drug)
The six aggregates of consciousness, the six sense cognitions

nang gi buga (nang gi bu ga)
Internal nutritional passage(s)

nang gi drongkhyer (nang gi grong khyer)
Inner city or citadel, tantric term for *khorlo*

nangrik (gnang rigs)
A type of physician, descendant from a royally permitted family lineage

nangtsa (nang rtsa)
Internal nerves, lit. "inner channels"

nawa (rna ba)
Ear(s)

nawé chinang jönshing zhi (rna ba'i phyi nang ljon shing bzhi)
The ears' four external and internal blood vessel trees (cf. *nyen gyi rétak zhi*)

né (gnas)
Location, one of the nine branches of the unhealthy humors tree

néyok (nad g.yog)
Assistant or helper of patients (cf. *menzhap*)

nga (nga)
(Sense of) I, me

ngak gi driwa (ngag gis dri ba)
Diagnosis by verbal questioning, anamnesis

ngel dzinpa (mngal 'dzin pa)
Conception

ngel dzinpé tak (mngal 'dzin pa'i rtags)
Signs of conception

ngel peltsül (mngal 'phel tshul)
Fetal development

ngel sin (mngal srin)
Uterine *sinbu* or microorganism (cf. *marutse, aso*)

ngelchak rikpa (mngal chags rig pa)
Embryology (syn.: *chaktsul rikpa*)

ngüldön (rngul 'don)
Sweating, an external therapy indicated for bile imbalance

niruha (ni ru ha)
Strong enema

nö druk (snod drug)
The six hollow or vessel organs, lit. "the six containers"

nö kyi zangpo druk (snod kyi bzang po drug)
The six superlative medicines for the hollow organs

nöjin (snod sbyin)
Harmful spirit

nor gyi bangdzö (nor gyi bang mdzod)
Reproductive fluids, lit. "storehouse of treasures" (syn.: *khuwa*)

norlhagyel lung (nor lha rgyal rlung)
"King of wealth" minor wind (syn.: *zhulégyel gyi lung*)

nötri (snod mkhris)
Gallbladder, one of the *nö druk*

nowa (rno ba)
Sharp, *tripa* characteristic

nü jor (nus sbyor)
Compounding medicine according to the power of the ingredients of a formula

numpa (snum pa)
Oily, *tripa* and *béken* characteristic

nüpa (nus pa)
Potency, power

nya dang ship dra (nya ldang gshibs 'dra)
Occiput and neck muscles "like hanging fishes"

nyamyig (nyams yig)
Body of written texts of practitioners' collected experiential knowledge

nyé gyu (nye rgyu)
Immediate causes, one of the nine branches of the unhealthy humors tree

nyéma (gnye ma)
Rectum (syn.: *tsilshup karnak*)

nyen (gnyan)
Wild sheep, evil spirit

nyen gyi rétak zhi (gnyan gyi re thag bzhi)
The "four head binding cords," the main blood vessels of the head (cf. *nawé chinang jönshing zhi*)

nyen né (gnyan nad)
Aggressive infectious (viral) disease

nyengyü (snyan brgyud)
Secret hearing transmission, whispering lineage

nyenrim (gnyan rims)
Infectious (viral) disease

nyépa sum (nyes pa gsum)
The three humors

nyépé tünmong gi lé (nyes pa'i thun mong gi las)
The collective functioning of the humors

nyi nang (gnyis snang)
Dualistic appearance, duality

nyikma (snyigs ma)
Waste product, residue, impurity

nying (snying)
Heart

nying a chö kyi khorlo (snying a chos kyi 'khor lo)
Heart chakra of phenomena

nyingtop (snying stobs)
Natural psychic energy carrying earth and water in embryonic form (cf. *sem kyi rangzhin gyi nüpa sum*)

nyingtsé (rnying tshad)
Chronic fever or inflammation

nyojé (smyo byed)
Madness

nyoktsé (snyogs tshad)
Turbid fever

nyönmongpé lung (nyon mong pa'i rlung)
Mental affliction wind

nyönmongpé yi (nyon mong pa'i yid)
Mental affliction mind, the deluded mind

O

ö sel ('od gsal)
Clear light, the fundamental nature of the mind (cf. *sem*)

o so ('o so)
Milk teeth

or ('or)
Anemic fluid retention, second stage edema

P

parpata (parpa ta)
An agressive type of *sinbu* that causes *nyenrim* diseases

partsa ('phar rtsa)
Pulsing (dark blood) channels, referring to the arterial system

pawo (dpa' bo)
Hero, warrior; title that designates a Sowa Rigpa practitioner who treats without fear

péma (pad ma)
Lotus; lotus wind, branch of *soklung a* during week 15 of fetal development

po (pho)
Male, masculine

ponya (pho nya)
Messenger (cf. *jikté*)

powa (pho ba)
Stomach, one of the *nö druk*; collective term for the major digestive organs

powé pu (pho ba'i spu)
Gastro-intestinal villi, lit. "stomach hair" (syn.: *gyumé pu*)

potsi (pho rtsi)
Male sex hormone (testosterone), lit. "male essence"

pungpé menbu gongön nyi (dpung pa'i rmen bu mgo sngon gnyis)
The auxillary lymph nodes, lit. "the two upper arm blue-headed glands"

R

rak lüpa (rag lus pa)
To depend on

rangzhin dün (rang bzhin bdun)
The seven body constitutions

ratna (ratna)
Jewel (wind) nerve channel group

rekpa (reg pa)
Contact, touch (cf. *tendrel yenlak chunyi*)

rikpa (rig pa)
Awareness, the knower (cf. *sem*)

rilbu (ril bu)
Pill(s)

rimtsé (rims tshad)
Infectious fever, (viral) infection

rinchen rilbu (rin chen ril bu)
Precious pill(s)

ring gyu (ring rgyu)
Distant causes of disease, one of the nine branches of the unhealthy humors tree

ro druk (ro drug)
The six tastes

ro jor (ro sbyor)
Compounding medicine according to taste of the ingredients in a formula

rotra (ro bkra)
Anatomy

rotsa (ro btsa)
Vital energy, reproductive fluid and sex hormone function

rotsawa (ro btsa ba)
Aphrodisiac(s), one of the eight branches of medicine

rübel gyi lung (rus sbal gyi rlung)
Turtle minor wind

rüpa (rus pa)
Bone, one of the *lüzung dün*

S

sa (sa)
Earth (element)

sa chü lung (sa chu'i rlung)
Earth-water wind, corresponds to oxygenated air

sadül (sa rdul)
Earth element particle

samséu (bsam se'u)
Seminal vesicle, also refers to ovaries and testicles

samten (bsam gtan)
Meditative concentration, one of the six perfections

sang ngak (gsang sngags)
Secret mantra, tantra

sangné dékyong gi khorlo (gsang gnas bde skyong gi 'khor lo)
The bliss-guarding chakra of the secret place (syn.: *sangwé khorlo*)

sangwé khorlo (gsang ba'i 'khor lo)
Secret chakra, often referring to the reproductive organs (syn.: *sangné dékyong gi khorlo*)

sangyé (sangs rgyas)
Buddha, fully awakened being

sangyé kyi chö kyi chökü rangzhin (sangs rgyas kyi chos skyi chos sku'i rang bzhin)
"Buddha-Dharma dharmakaya nature," the primordial Buddha-nature

sawa (sra ba)
Hard, *lung* characteristic

sawar jépa (sra bar byed pa)
Hardening wind, branch of *soklung a* during week 10 of fetal development

sélong chi longwar gyi zhungtsa (sre long phyi long bar gyi gzhung rtsa)
Inferior extensor retinaculum nerve channels

sem (sems)
Mind or consciousness

sem kyi né sum (sems kyi gnas gsum)
The three seats or abodes of mind

sem kyi ranzhin gyi nüpa sum (sems kyi rang bzhin gyi nus pa gsum)
The three natural psychic energies

sem rakpa (sems rags pa)
Gross mind

sem trawa (sems phra ba)
Subtle mind

semtsor (sems tshor)
Mental sensation or feeling

sépa (sred pa)
Craving, desire (cf. *tendrel yenlak chunyi*)

sha (sha)
Flesh, muscle tissue, meat, one of the *lüzung dün*

sha né (sha gnad)
Vital muscle

sham (gsham)
The lower middle mother lungs

shama (bsha' ma)
Placenta

shangwa (bshang ba)
Feces (syn.: *drichen*)

shel (bshal)
Purgation

shépa (shes pa)
Consciousness, cognition (cf. *sem*)

shérap (shes rab)
Wisdom, one of the six perfections

sherchu (gsher chu)
Liquid glandular secretion

sherchü gyulam (gsher chu'i rgyu lam)
Lymph vessels, lit. "waterish liquid pathways"

shermen (gsher rmen)
Endocrine glands

shermen chutsa (gsher rmen chu rtsa)
Endocrine channels

sherwa (gsher ba)
Wet, *tripa* characteristic

shintu tenpa (shin tu brtan pa)
"Very stable" wind, branch of *soklung a* during week 20 of fetal development

shintu trawa (shin tu phra ba)
"Extremely subtle" wind, branch of *soklung a* during week 19 of fetal development

shintu trawé sem (shin tu phra ba'i sems)
Very subtle mind

silwa (bsil ba)
Cool, *béken* characteristic

sin né (srin nad)
Sin diseases, related to parasites and microbes

sinbu (srin bu)
Microbe, bacteria, parasite, lit. "worm"

sipa (srid pa)
Existence (cf. *tendrel yenlak chunyi*)

sipé tsachen zhi (srid pa'i rtsa chen bzhi)
The four great channels of existence

so (so)
Tooth, teeth

so nyil (so rnyil)
Gums

sok (srog)
Life energy, life force

sok gi lung (srog gi rlung)
Lifespan wind, life fuel wind; life-sustaining wind disorder, potential cause of serious psychiatric problems

sok chenpö tsa (srog chen po'i rtsa)
The great life-holding channel (syn.: *tsa uma*)

sok gi yukpa (srog gi dbyug pa)
The "life rod," the central wind channel (syn.: *tsa uma*)

soklung a (srog rlung a)
Fundamental life-wind

soktsa (srog rtsa)
Principal life(-holding) channel(s) (cf. *tsa chen sum*); the aorta

soktsa karpo (srog rtsa dkar po)
White life-holding channel (cf. *tsa kyangma*); used in this book specifically for nerves, but may also refer to lymph vessels

soktsa marpo (srog rtsa dmar po)
Red (blood) life channel (cf. *tsa roma*)

soktsa nakpo (srog rtsa nag po)
Dark (blood) life channels, veins

sönam (bsod nams)
(Good) fortune (cf. *bépé tsé yi kawa sum*)

sormö rekpa (sor mos reg pa)
Diagnosis by touch, mostly refers to pulse diagnosis

sotsa déjé (so rtsa ldad byed)
Jawbone and teeth channels

surya (sur ya)
A severe skin disease

T

ta gom chö sum (lta sgom spyod gsum)
Right view, meditation, and conduct

ta mel né me (tha mal nad med)
Health, obtained through balance

ta zhi so chung (mtha' bzhi'i so chung)
Wisdom teeth, lit. "four junior peripheral teeth"

tak go (stag mgo)
Right and left tips of the mother lungs, lit. "tiger head"

takpé dügo (ltag pa'i sdud sgo)
Occipital bone

takzur pukhyil (ltag zur spu 'khyil)
Occipital bone edge point, corresponds to acupoint GB20 in Chinese medicine

tang (thang)
Decoction

tangka (thang ka)
Tibetan scroll painting

tapshé (thabs shes)
Skillful means and wisdom, method and knowledge

tarka (gtar ka)
Bloodletting

té mik (rte mig)
One of the four son lungs

tébong pukyé chutsa (the bong spu skyes chu rtsa)
Foot extensor nerve channels, lit. "thumb hair-growth water channel"

tendrel yenlak chunyi (rten 'brel yan lag bcu gnyis)
The 12 links of interdependent origination, as taught by the Buddha

tengchok (theng chog)
Panacea, instant cure-all (syn.: *daryaken*)

tenpa (brtan pa)
Stable, *béken* characteristic

terma (gter ma)
Hidden treasure; a Tibetan Buddhist literary genre

tertön (gter ston)
Treasure revealer of ancient hidden texts (cf. *terma*)

tétak (lte thag)
Umbilical cord, lit. "navel thread" (syn.: *butak*)

téwa trülpé khorlo (lte ba sprul pa'i 'khor lo)
Navel emanation chakra

tiklé (thig le)
Essential drop, sometimes also refers to reproductive fluids

tiksak (thig bsags)
Necrosis

timuk (gti mug)
Closed-mindedness, confusion, distant cause of the phlegm humor

tingpé chutsa (rting pa'i chu rtsa)
Achilles tendon, lit. "heel water channel"

tokpé kyen (thogs pa'i rkyen)
"Obstructing condition," a subtle wind branching from *soklung a* during week 38 of fetal development

töl (rtol)
Animal born from a she-yak crossed with an ox, a yak-cow hybrid

tölung silwa (stod rlung bsil ba)
Upper cold wind

tongpa zhi (stong pa bzhi)
The four great stages of emptiness that are part of subtle mind dissolution when dying

tongtsé (stong tshad)
Empty fever

trak (khrag)
Blood, one of the *lüzung dün*

trak rik dün (khrag rigs bdun)
Seven blood types

trak tarwa (khrag gtar ba)
Bloodletting (syn.: *tarka*)

traksin (khrag srin)
Blood microorganism or "parasite," may refer to red blood corpuscles

traktsa (khrag rtsa)
Blood vessels or channels

traktsa marpo (khrag rtsa dmar po)
Red blood channels, arteries

traktsa nakpo (khrag rtsa nag po)
Black blood channels, veins

traktsap (khrag tshabs)
Premenopausal stage disorders

trasin (phra srin)
Microorganism (cf. *sinbu*)

trawa (phra ba)
Subtle, *lung* characteristic

trawé jungwa nga (phra ba'i 'byung ba lnga)
Five subtle elements

trawé lung (phra ba'i rlung)
Subtle wind

trawé lung gi dültren (phra ba'i rlung gi rdul phran)
Minute subtle wind particle

tren (skran)
Lump, swelling, benign tumor (cf. *dré*)

trényel ('phred nyal)
One of the three main skull bone channel groups, lit. "lying on one's side"(cf. *bönpo tö*)

trésam (tres sam)
Medicinal calcinated ash (powder)

tri né ('khri nad)
"Attachment disease," pregnancy symptoms

trikhu (mkhris khu)
Bile juice, waste product of bile

trikmé chutsa (mkhrig ma'i chu rtsa)
Wrist channels

tripa (mkhris pa)
Bile

tripa chi (tripa spyi)
General bile

tripa dangyur (mkhris pa mdang 'gyur)
Color-transforming bile, one of the five bile branches

tripa doksel (mkhris pa mdog gsal)
Complexion-clearing bile, one of the five bile branches

tripa drupjé (mkhris pa sgrub byed)
Accomplishing bile, one of the five bile branches

tripa jujé (mkhris pa 'ju byed)
Digestive bile, one of the five bile branches

tripa tongjé (mkhris pa mthong byed)
Seeing bile, one of the five bile branches

tripé rangzhin (mkhris pa'i rang bzhin)
Bile constitution

tripé tsenyi dün (mkhris pa'i mtshan nyid bdun)
Bile's seven characteristics

trisin (mkhris srin)
Bile microorganisms and parasites (especially pinworms), mainly originating from the small intestine

tritsa (mkhris rtsa)
Bile channel

tru né (khru nad)
Diarrheal disorders

trujam (bkru 'jam)
A type of enema suitable for wind-bile disorder

truktsé ('khrugs tshad)
Disturbed fever

trumalen (bkru ma slen)
A type of enema suitable for wind-phlegm disorder

truwa ('khru ba)
Purgative, *tripa* characteristic; diarrhea

tsa (rtsa)
Channel(s), root

tsa chen sum (rtsa chen gsum)
The three principal channels

tsa duk (tsha dugs)
Salt fomentation

tsa kar (rtsa dkar)
White (life-holding) channels, vague term mostly referring to nerves (cf. *soktsa karpo*)

tsa kyangma (rtsa rkyang ma)
The left lateral, lunar channel (cf. *chutsa*)

tsa roma (rtsa ro ma)
The right lateral, solar channel

tsa uma (rtsa dbu ma)
Central (wind) channel

tsadrip (rtsa 'grib)
Channel contamination or obscuration

tsagak (rtsa 'gags)
Constipation

tsajong (rtsa sbyong)
Blood channel purification

tsakhor (rtsa 'khor)
Chakra, lit. "channel wheel" (cf. *khorlo*)

tsalung (rtsa rlung)
A yogic transformative, (self-)healing practice; lit. "channels and winds"

tsangpé lung (rtsang pa'i rlung)
Nose minor wind

tsap né (tshabs nad)
Gynecological disease

tsawa (tsha ba)
Hot disorder, fever; hot, *tripa* characteristic

tsawa ritang tsam (tsha ba ri thang mtshams)
"Hill meets plain" fever

tsawé béken nga (rtsa ba'i bad kan lnga)
The five principal phlegm branches

tsawé lung nga (rtsa ba'i rlung lnga)
The five principal wind branches

tsawé tripa nga (rtsa ba'i mkhris pa lnga)
The five principal bile branches

tsé (tshe)
Lifespan (cf. *bépé tsé yi kawa sum*)

tsé guk (tshe 'gugs)
Long-life gathering ritual (cf. *laguk*)

tsé yi lung (tshe yi rlung)
Life energy wind

tsé yi tsa (tshe yi rtsa)
Life energy channel

tsen nyi ma ning (mtshan gnyis ma ning)
Intersex, hermaphrodite (cf. *ma ning*)

tsenbar dölwa (mtshan bar rdol ba)
Anal fistula

tsétru (tshad 'khru)
Dysentery

tsil (tshil)
Fat, one of the *lüzung dün*

tsilshup karnak (tshil shub dkar nag)
Rectum (syn.: *nyéma*)

tsip (tshibs)
The upper middle mother lungs

tso lung ('tsho rlung)
Life-nurturing wind or air, oxygenated air

tsojé dartsa (tsho byed dar rtsa)
(the network of) skalp blood channels

tsojé menpa ('tsho byed sman pa)
Healer-physician, a title for a qualified Tibetan medical doctor

tsön (mtshon)
Wounds, traumatology, one of the eight branches of medicine

tsöndrü (rtson sgrus)
Effort, one of the six perfections

tsorwa (tshor ba)
Feeling, sensation, emotion (cf. *tendrel yenlak chunyi*)

tsultrim (tshul khrims)
Moral discipline, one of the six perfections

tsupa (rtsub pa)
Coarse, rough, *lung* characteristic

tuk khap (thugs khab)
Heart-protecting son lungs, lit. "heart castle"

tülwa (brtul ba)
Blunt, *béken* characteristic

tumo (gtum mo)
(Yogic practice of) inner heat

turché (thur dpyad)
Surgery

turma (thur ma)
Surgical spoon or lancet

U

uk (dbugs)
Breath, respiration, breathing wind

uk mi déwa (dbugs mi bde ba)
Breathing disorder

W

wangpo go nga (dbang po sgo lnga)
The five sense organs

wangpo yül la charwé tsa (dbang po yul la 'char ba'i rtsa)
Sensory perception channels

Y

yangdakpar düpa (yang dag par sdud pa)
"Fully collected," subtle wind branch of *soklung a* during week 5

yangdakpar kyöpa (yang dag par bskyod pa)
"Thoroughly agitated" wind, branch of *soklung a* during week 21 of fetal development

yangwa (yang ba)
Light, *lung* and *tripa* characteristic

yenlak gi lung nga (yan lag gi rlung lnga)
The five minor wind branches

yenlak nga (yan lag lnga)
The five extremities (arms, legs, and head)

yéshé kyi lung (ye shes kyi rlung)
Transcendental wisdom wind (cf. *lung gi dangma*)

yi (yid)
Conceptual mind, the intellectual faculty

yi zangma (yid bzang ma)
"noble lady" heart channel

yidak (yi dags)
Preta being, hungry ghost

yidam (yi dam)
Chosen (meditation) deity, tutelary deity

yiga chüpa (yi ga chus pa)
Anorexia

yongsu dakpar dzinpa (yong su dag par 'dzin pa)
"Completely held," Subtle wind branching from *soklung a* during week 23 of fetal development

yönpö go (yon po'i sgo)
Crooked gate wind, branch of *soklung a* during week 12 of fetal development

yowa (g.yo ba)
Mobile, *lung* characteristic

Z

za (gza')
Planet, mainly refers to Rāhula, which induces epilepsy

zak na (zags sna)
One of the five mother lungs, lit. "dripping/dropping edge"

zangpo druk (bzang po drug)
The six superlative medicines

zangtsak lugu go (zang tshags lu gu mgo)
Duodenum (syn.: *gyusor chunyi*)

zé drülwé sinbu (zas 'brul ba'i srin 'bu)
Intestinal flora, gut microorganisms

zé jutsül (zas 'ju tshul)
The digestive system or process

zé juwa (zas 'ju ba)
Food digestion

zertsa (gzer rtsa)
One of the three main skull bone channels, lit. "pain-making channels" (cf. *dungtsuk*)

zhakgor khyil dra (zhag sgor 'khyil 'dra)
The crown head muscle, which is coiled like fat

zhangdrum (gzhang 'brum)
Hemorrhoids

zhédang (zhe sdang)
Anger and hatred, the distant cause of the bile humor

zhu shül tang dra (gzhu bshul btang 'dra)
Fontanel muscle "like a slackened bow"

zhulégyel gyi lung (gzhu las rgyal gyi rlung)
"Victory over asura" wind (syn.: *norlhagyel lung*)

zöpa (bzod pa)
Patience or tolerance, one of the six perfections

zung (zungs)
Constituent, *dangma* passage (cf. *buga*)

REFERENCES

Arya pa sangs yon tan. *Bod kyi gso ba rig pa'i lo rgyus kyi bang mdzod g.yu thog bla ma dran glu.* Neuchâtel: Bedurya Publications, 2021.

Bi ci. *Bi ci'i pu ti kha ser.* Lha sa: Bod ljongs mi dmangs dpe skrun khang, 2005.

Blo bzang rgya mtsho [Rgyal dbang lnga pa chen po]. *Gang can yul gyi sa la spyod pa'i mtho ris kyi rgyal blon gtso bor brjod pa'i deb ther rdzogs ldan gzhon nu'i dga' ston dpyid kyi rgyal mo'i glu dbyangs.* Ldi li: Bod gzhung shes rig par khang, 1981.

Brang ti dpal ldan rgyal mtshan. *Brang ti lha rje'i rim brgyud kyi man ngag gser bre chen mo.* Lha sa: Bod ljongs mi dmangs dpe skrun khang, 2005.

Brang ti dpal ldan 'tsho byed. *Bdud rtsi snying po yan lag brgyad pa gsang ba man ngag gi rgyud kyi spyi don shes bya rab gsal.* Delhi: Tashigang, T. Y., 2005.

'Brong rtse lha sras rgya mtsho. *Rje 'brong rtse lha sras rgya mtsho'i mdzad pa'i be'u bum dkar po,* n.d.

'Brug chen bzhi pa padma dkar po. *Jo bo nA ro pa'i khyad chos bsre 'pho'i gzhung 'grel rdo rje 'chang gi dgongs pa gsal bar byed pa.* Delhi: Tibet House, 1983..

Bsam gtan. *Gso rig snying bsdus skya rengs gsar pa.* Bod ljongs mi dmangs dpe skrun khang, 1997.

Bstan 'dzin rnam dag. *Sangs rgyas kyi bstan rtsis ngo mtshar nor bu'i phreng ba.* Ka ling sbug, 1961.

Byams pa 'phrin las. *Gangs ljongs gso rig bstan pa'i nyin byed rim byon gyi rnam thar phyogs bsgrigs.* Pe cin: Mi rigs dpe skrun khang, 1990.

Dar mo sman rams pa blo bzang chos grags. *G.yu thog gsar rnying gi rnam thar.* Smanrtsis Shesrig Spendzod. Leh (Ladakh): Tashigang, D. W., 1984.

———. *Rgyud bzhi'i 'grel chen mes po'i zhal lung.* Krung go'i bod kyi shes rig dpe skrun khang, 1991.

Dbang 'dus. *Gso ba rig pa'i tshig mdzod g.yu thog dgongs rgyan.* Pe cin: Mi rigs dpe skrun khang, 1983.

De'u dmar bstan 'dzin phun tshogs. *Dpyad mchog gtar ga'i gdams pa nyes 'khrugs snyogs drung 'byin byed kar ke ta,* undated.

Dge 'dun chos 'phel. *Deb ther dkar po.* Pe cin: Mi rigs dpe skrun khang, 2004.

———. *'Dod pa'i bstan bcos.* Ldi li: Gdong thog bstan pa'i rgyal mtshan, 1967.

Dpal 'byor don grub. "Mdo sngags thams cad kyi rgyal po rgyud sde bzhi'i rtsa ba ma rgyud thams cad kyi snying po bskyed rim lhan cig skyes ma rdzogs rim rlung sems gnyis med gsal bar ston pa dpal na ro pa chen po'i chos drug nyams len gsal ba'i sgron me." In *Rtsa rlung 'phrul 'khor,* edited by Thub bstan phun tshogs, 61–484. Si khron: Si khron mi rigs dpe skrun khang, 1995.

Geshe Rabten. *The Mind and Its Functions.* Translated by Stephen Batchelor. Le Mont-Pèlerin: Rabten Choeling, 1992.

'Gos lo tsa ba gzhon nu dpal. *Deb ther sngon po.* Sarnath, Varanasi: Vajra Vidya Library, 2002.

Grags pa rgyal mtshan. *Gso dpyad rgyal po'i dkor mdzod.* Rda ram sa la: Shes rig dpar khang, undated blockprint.

G.yu thog yon tan mgon po. *Bdud rtsi snying po yan lag brgyad pa gsang ba man ngag gi rgyud.* Bod ljongs mi dmangs dpe skrun khang, 1993.

———. *G.yu thog snying thig gi chos skor.* New Delhi: Bkra shis g.yang 'phal, undated blockprint.

Hassnain, F. M., and Tokan D. Sumi. *Bhaiṣajyaguru Sūtra.* New Delhi: Reliance Publishing House, 1995.

'Ju mi pham pa. "Bdud rtsi snying po'i rgyud kyi 'grel pa drang srong zhal lung las dum bu bzhi pa phyi ma rgyud kyi rtsa mdo chu mdo'i ti ka." In *Gso rig skor gyi rgyun mkho gal che ba bdam bsgrigs*, 255–303. Pe cin: Mi rigs dpe skrun khang, 1988.

Karma gling pa. *Zab chos zhi khro dgongs pa rang grol las bar do thos grol gyi skor*. Dharamsala: Tibetan Cultural Printing Press, 1995.

Karma ngag dbang yon tan rgya mtsho. "Ring 'tsho'i cho ga sgrub pa'i rnam gzhag tshe dbang dga' 'khyil thig le." In *Gsang chen thabs lam nyer mkho rnal 'byor snying nor*, edited by Dor zhi gdong drug snyems blo, 204–58. Pe cin: Mi rigs dpe skrun khang, 1991.

Karma 'phrin las. *Lus khams nyi ma'i gnyen po*. Bod ljongs mi dmangs dpe skrun khang, 1993.

Lati Rinbochay, and Jeffrey Hopkins. *Death, Intermediate State, and Rebirth in Tibetan Buddhism*. Boulder, CO: Snow Lion Publications, 1985.

Lati Rinbochay, and Elizabeth Napper. *Mind in Tibetan Buddhism*. Boulder, CO: Snow Lion Publications, 2013.

Lo chen dharma shri. "'Byung rtsis man ngag zla ba'i 'od zer." In *Dbyangs 'char dang nag rtsis kyi skor*, edited by Byams pa 'phrin las, 3: 486–516. Bod kyi rtsis rig kun 'dus chen mo. Si khron: Si khron mi rigs dpe skrun khang, 1998.

Mar pa lo tsa ba. "Bde mchog snyan rgyud kyi gtum mo dang thabs lam gyi 'phrul 'khor." In *Rtsa rlung 'phrul 'khor*, edited by Thub bstan phun tshogs, 1–20. Si khron: Si khron mi rigs dpe skrun khang, 1995.

Mkhas btsun bzang po. *Bod du sgrub brgyud shing rta chen po mched brgyad las snga 'gyur gsang chen rnying ma'i bla ma brgyud pa rjes 'brangs dang bcas pa'i rnam thar ngo mtshar rgya mtsho'i stod cha*. Rda ram sa la: Bod kyi dpe mdzod khang, 1973.

Mkhyen rab nor bu. "Dpal ldan rtsa ba'i rgyud kyi sdong 'grems gso rig rga mtsho'i snying po" In *Bla sman mkhyen rabs* [sic] *nor bus mdzad pa'i lha ldan sman rtsis khang gi chos spyod*, 83–111. Rda ram sa la: Bod gzhung sman rtsis khang, 1984 (1924).

Pasang Yonten Arya. *Dictionary of Tibetan Materia Medica*. Translated by Yonten Gyatso. Delhi: Motilal Banarsidass Publishers, 1998.

Pha khol [Slob dpon rta byangs]. "Yan lag brgyad pa'i snying po bsdus pa" In *Gso rig pa'i rtsa 'grel bdam bsgrigs*, edited by Rdo rje rgyal po, 112–756. Bstan 'gyur nang gi gso ba rig pa'i skor gyi dpe tshogs. Pe cin: Mi rigs dpe skrun khang, 1989.

Phyag sman rin rgyal. *'Bum khu tshur*. Pe cin: Mi rigs dpe skrun khang, 2004.

Rechung Rinpoche Jampal Kunzang. *Tibetan Medicine: Illustrated in Original Texts*. London: Wellcome Institute of the History of Medicine, 1973.

Sa skya pa rgyal mtshan dpal bzang. "Rdo rje lus kyi sbas bshad." In *Gsang chen thabs lam nyer mkho rnal 'byor snying nor*, edited by Dor zhi gdong drug snyems blo, 1–108. Pe cin: Mi rigs dpe skrun khang, 1991.

Sde dge'i drung yig gu ru 'phel. "Srid gsum gtsug rgan si tu chos kyi 'byung gnas kyi zhal lung dngul chu btso chen dang rin chen ril bu'i sbyor sde zla ba bdud rtsi'i thig le ces bya ba bi dza ha ram." In *Rin chen dngul chu sbyor sde phyogs bsdebs*, 303–92. Dharamsala: Library of Tibetan Works and Archives, 1986.

Sde srid sangs rgyas rgya mtsho. *Dpal ldan gso ba rig pa'i khog 'bugs legs bshad vaidurya'i me long drang srong dgyes pa'i dga' ston*. Kan su'i mi rigs dpe skrun khang, 1982.

———. *Gso ba rig pa'i bstan bcos sman lla'i dgongs rgyan rgyud bzhi'i gsal byed vaidur sngon po'i mali ka*. Rda ram sa la: Bod gzhung sman rtsis khang, 1994.

———. *Man ngag lhan thabs*. Mtsho sngon mi rigs dpe skrun khang, 1992.

Shan ting gharba. "Gso dpyad rin po che'i 'khrungs dpe bstan pa zhe bya ba'i rgyud." In *Gso rig sman gyi ro nus ngos 'dzin gsal ston phyogs sgrig rin chen sgron me*, edited by Dpal brtsegs bod yig dpe rnying zhib 'jug khang nas bsgrigs, 73–208. Pe cin: Skrung go'i bod rig pa dpe skrun khang, 2007.

Sman dpyad zla ba'i rgyal po. Pe cin: Mi rigs dpe skrun khang, 1985.

Stag lo shes rab rin chen. "Sman bla'i rnam gzhag cho ga nyams len bde 'jug." In *Sman bla'i mdo dang mdo chog phyogs sgrig rin chen sgron me*, edited by Dpal brtsegs bod yig dpe rnying zhib 'jug khang nas bsgrigs, 229–53. Pe cin: Krung go'i bod rig pa dpe skrun khang, 2007.

Sum ston ye shes gzung. "'Grel ba 'bum chung gsal sgron nor bu'i 'phreng mdzes." In *Cha lag bco brgyad*, 158–312. Kan su'u mi rigs dpe skrun khang, 1999a.

———. "Brgyud pa'i rnam mthar med thabs med pa." In *Cha lag bco brgyad*, 690–96. Kan su'u mi rigs dpe skrun khang, 1999b.

Tshul khrims gyal mtshan. "Sa dpyad kyi rtsis rig ji ltar dar ba'i lo rgyus rten 'brel me long." In *Skar nag rtsis kyi lo rgyus skor*, edited by Byams pa 'phrin las, 1: 500–524. Bod kyi rtsis rig kun 'dus chen mo. Sichuan: People's Publishing House, 1998.

Zur mkhar blo gros rgyal po. *Rgyud bzhi'i 'grel pa mes po'i zhal lung.* Mtsho sngon mi rigs par khang, 1991.

———. *Sman pa rnams kyis mi shes su mi rung ba'i shes bya spyi'i khog dbubs.* Bod kyi gso rig dpe rnying phyogs sgrig gang ri dkar po'i phreng ba. Si khron mi rigs dpe skrun khang, 2001.

ILLUSTRATION CREDITS

Figure 1.1 (Medical Thangka 1), Figure 1.2 (Medical Thangka 77), Figure 3.1 (Medical Thangka 1), Figure 3.3 (Medical Thangka 2), Figure 5.6 (Medical Thangka 5), Figure 5.7 (Medical Thangka 19), Figures 9.2–9.10 (Medical Thangka 47), Figure 11.1 (Medical Thangka 2), Figure 13.4 (Medical Thangka 6), Figure 14.1 (Medical Thangka 50), Figure 14.5 (Medical Thangka 49), Figure 16.1 (Medical Thangka 47), Figure 21.1 (Medical Thangka 2), Figure 21.3 (Medical Thangka 3), Figure 21.5 (Medical Thangka 4), Figure 21.7 (Medical Thangka 2): © Dharmapala Thangka Centre, Kathmandu, Nepal (www.thangka.de)

Figure 1.3: © Himalayan Art Resources / Private collection (item no. 58141)

Figure 2.2: Personal collection of the author

Figure 2.3: © Bundesarchiv (image 135-S-15-46-24)

Figure 4.1: © Royal Ontario Museum (object no. 994.40.1)

Figure 4.2, Figure 4.4, Figure 5.1, Figure 6.2, Figure 9.5, Figure 13.3, Figure 14.5, Figure 17.7, Figures 18.3–18.4, Figure 20.2, Figure 20.4, Figure 20.6, Figure 20.8, Figures A.1–A.2: © Sylvie Béguin

Figure 2.1, Figure 4.3, Figures 5.2–5.5, Figure 6.1, Figures 6.3–6.4, Figures 7.1–7.2, Figures 8.1–8.2, Figure 10.1, Figures 11.2–11.4, Figures 13.1–13.2, Figures 14.1–14.4, Figures 14.6–14.8, Figures 15.1–15.7, Figure 16.1, Figures 17.1–17.6, Figures 17.7–17.11, Figures 18.1–18.2: © Tiana Morici

ABOUT THE AUTHOR

Prof. Arya Pasang Yonten was born in 1955 in Dölpo (Dol po), a small village in Kyirong (Skyid grong), Tibet. He fled with his parents to Nepal in the wake of the Chinese invasion and was later admitted to Syabru Bensi refugee school. Through the guidance and advice of his teacher, Gowo Lopzang Tendzin, Pasang Yonten joined Men-Tsee-khang (the Tibetan Medical and Astro-science Institute) in 1973, in Dharamsala, India. There, he was instructed in Tibetan medicine, astrology, and Buddhist philosophy by eminent masters such as Prof. Barshee, Dr. Jamyang Tashi of Tsona, and Dr. Lobsang Dolma Khangkar, graduating first of his class in 1977. Consequently, he was offered the rare opportunity for further specialization in pharmacy. In 1982, he participated in the alchemical practice of mercury purification under Dr. Tenzin Choedrak, completing his studies. He was then appointed as a teacher at the Tibetan medical college, also acting as the secretary of the scholars' committee. In 1984, he became professor and college principal, a post he held until 1989. Under his mentorship, many physicians graduated who later took up important roles as professionals both in India and abroad. During these years, Prof. Pasang Yonten received many sutra and tantra teachings from H. H. the Dalai Lama and other gurus, including the *Yutok Nyingtik* (*G.yu thog snying thig*) empowerment from Dilgo Khyentse Rinpoché. He moved to Ladakh in 1989, working as the main lecturer in the newly founded Amchi Medicine section of the Central Institute for Buddhist Studies. He received further teachings there, particularly on *Nāropā's Six Dharmas* (*Na ro'i chos drug*) and related yogic techniques.

Under challenging circumstances, Pasang Yonten authored three works in Tibetan based on his personal textual-historical study and clinical practice. These were among the first research publications on Sowa Rigpa to come out in exile: an award-winning account of Tibetan medical history (Jammu-Kashmir Best Book award, 1989), a highly practical clinical manual for inexperienced physicians (1990, 1995), and an extensive dictionary of medical ingredient names (1991). The latter was translated to English as *Dictionary of Tibetan Materia Medica* (1998), and appeared in an expanded German edition in 2001.

In 1990, Pasang Yonten was invited to give a seminar series in Montreal (Canada), where he came into contact for the first time with geriatric diseases such as Alzheimer. In the same year, Dr. Pasang also traveled to Russia and Mongolia, as the only layperson in the goodwill delegation funded by the Tibetan exile government's Council for Religious Affairs in the context of the International Symposium on Buddhist Culture and Traditions (Asian Peace Conference, Ulaanbaatar). After several short visits to Europe, he settled in Italy in 1994. Through the support of Dr. Walburg Marić-Oehler and later under the umbrella of the Institut für Ost-West Medizin founded by her daughter Sonja Marić, he acted as guest professor in Tibetan medicine for DÄGfA (the German Medical Association for Acupuncture) for more than two decades. Over time, he gradually refined his insight into the body-mind by teaching and learning from medical doctors and complementary medicine specialists. Motivated by enthusiastic students, he then founded the New Yuthok Institute (NYI) in 1999 in Milan, where he taught a four-year weekend course on Sowa Rigpa until recently, in addition to related subjects such as advanced pathologies, astrology, psychology, and yoga. Together with a group of dedicated practitioners, a 10-day Medicine Buddha retreat was held for 15 years under the auspices of the Buddha Bedurya Center. Through his efforts, Tibetan medicine was added to the national list of complementary medicines in Italy in 2003 after a meeting with member of parliament Francesco Paolo Lucchese. In the same year, he was also invited to the European Parliament in Brussels for a lecture by Nuala Ahern (then-president of the Intergroup on Complementary and Natural Medicine).

Dr. Pasang furthermore shared his expertise on medicinal plants and pharmacy with scientists working in the laboratory of PADMA (2001–2008), a Swiss pharmaceutical company that exclusively produces registered medicines and supplements based on Tibetan formulas. This collaboration contributed to the formulation of several PADMA products which are still available across Europe. In 2005, he and one of his senior students, Sylvie Béguin, founded the nonprofit organization TME - Tibetan Medicine Education Center in Switzerland. Since then, hundreds of students have had the opportunity to participate in three-year, advanced, and short medical courses by means of online seminars, tailored texts and audiovisual materials, as well as on-site intensive practical workshops in Neuchâtel.

Arya Pasang Yonten is now one of the most senior and respected Tibetan medical teachers in the West. Currently, he is the director of NYI and president of TME. He is in the process of carrying out historical research on the Arya family tree while writing down his autobiography on his personal Tibetan-language website. Through Bedurya Publications, which has already republished his pioneering early works after being out of print for decades, he aims to produce several more volumes of medical teachings based on his lifelong experience. In the past few years, his focus also shifted to introducing *tsalung* as a practical healing therapy that complements Sowa Rigpa's more material approach to treating the body-mind complex, resulting in a rare teaching cycle being offered for the first time as an innovative yet systematic training course.